Introduction to
MEDICAL SCIENCE

Introduction to
MEDICAL SCIENCE

CLARA GENE YOUNG

Retired Technical Editor and Writer (Medical),
U.S. Civil Service; formerly Instructor, Medical
Terminology, Good Samaritan Hospital,
Phoenix, Arizona

JAMES D. BARGER, M.D., F.C.A.P.

Pathologist, Sunrise Hospital Medical Center,
Las Vegas, Nevada

with 104 illustrations

THIRD EDITION

THE C. V. MOSBY COMPANY

Saint Louis 1977

THIRD EDITION

Copyright © 1977 by The C. V. Mosby Company

Previous editions copyrighted 1969, 1973

Printed in the United States of America

Distributed in Great Britain by Henry Kimpton, London

Library of Congress Cataloging in Publication Data

Young, Clara Gene.
    Introduction to medical science.

    Bibliography: p.
    Includes index.
    1. Medicine.   I.   Barger, James D., joint author.
II.   Title.
R130.Y68 1977   616   76-26713
ISBN 0-8016-5657-5

CB/CB/B 9 8 7 6 5 4 3 2 1

PREFACE

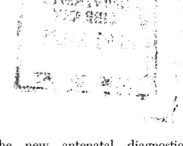

In this third edition the basic content and organization of the book have not been changed. The emphasis here is on the incorporation of the latest information on the diseases, with the addition of some diseases not included in previous editions. This has been done in an attempt to keep abreast of new medical findings and in view of recognition of a more widespread prevalence of certain diseases. For example, Reye syndrome, while still relatively rare, is now being recognized more often. This is also true of Prinzmetal's variant angina pectoris, which is now considered to be a distinct entity of angina.

Some revision of diseases has been necessitated by a change in nomenclature; for example, the term "coal worker's pneumoconiosis" (CWP) is now used instead of "black lung disease." All dust inhalation diseases have been grouped together in the new nomenclature under the term "pneumoconioses," which includes such diseases as silicosis, siderosis, and anthracosis. Hepatitis is no longer described as either infectious or serum but is now designated A or B, and the latest information on its mode of transfer has been included.

In the field of congenital and inherited diseases, there is new information on sickle cell anemia, chromosomal aberrations and their association with congenital abnormalities, and Down's syndrome or mongolism, including the factors that represent risks for transmission of defects to off-spring. The new antenatal diagnostic methods or techniques for detecting abnormalities or chromosomal aberrations are given.

The chapter on drug and chemical injury has been extensively revised in order to give current information on effects of drug abuse. Drugs that have received particular attention in this revision are alcohol and narcotics. Since heroin is now the chief drug in illicit drug traffic in the United States, the health hazards involved in its use are discussed at length. The popularity of glue sniffing among youngsters necessitated including the latest findings on this practice. Amphetamines and cocaine have been added to the discussions on harmful drugs.

There are many new scientific breakthroughs in the field of neoplasia, but most of these are in therapy or new drugs, which are not subjects for discussion in this book. The new diagnostic techniques, however, are of interest, and these have been added where applicable. Reports of some additional tumors have been added to the selection of neoplasia.

The chapter on allergies has been updated to include the latest information on food and drug allergies and some of the recently discovered mechanisms for causing asthma and other allergies. The chapter on infectious diseases has also been revised, with the table now including the new nomenclature and findings. Some diseases, such as herpes zoster, have been added.

v

The discussion of venereal diseases, which are becoming epidemic in the United States, has been revised to include recent findings on mode of transfer.

The chapter on symptomatology has been rather extensively revised to reflect the latest information on a number of diseases. Myasthenia gravis has been added to the list of diseases under muscular weakness, and corneal transplants and retinitis pigmentosa are additional discussions under loss of vision. The inclusion of some of these diseases has been prompted by an upsurge in national interest and establishment of foundations to study causes and effects and to search for possible cures or new ways of treatment. Some of the diseases that received particular attention in updating are multiple sclerosis, parkinsonism, cerebral palsy, and chronic obstructive pulmonary disease (emphysema).

Many new references have been added to reflect recent literary contributions from various medical journals. Some references in this book might seem to the reader to be outdated because they are not recent, but in medical science the causes of many diseases have been known for years, so there is nothing new to add to this particular aspect of the disease. However, new information on diagnostic techniques and new discoveries of effects of a disease have been added to discussion and references given as to source. Through extensive literary research, every attempt has been made to bring this book up to date on knowledge of the most commonly encountered diseases. It is hoped that the reader will find this a welcome and useful addition to the storehouse of knowledge of diseases.

Clara Gene Young
James D. Barger

CONTENTS

Introduction

Medical science as we know it today embraces both the art of medicine, which lays down the foundation for the quest for solution of a clinical problem, and the use of scientific advances or methods for diagnosis and treatment of illnesses. For many centuries medicine was solely an empirical art, since basic sciences were unknown and almost nothing was known about anatomy.

In the fifth century B.C., physicians relied mainly on their senses of taste, smell, inspection, and palpation for the diagnosis of diseases. Hippocrates, the Father of Medicine, was the first to lift medicine out of its mystic existence and establish the rational basis for the study of diseases. But even his knowledge was confined to the art of medical practice in recognizing symptoms and treating patients accordingly. With his rational concept that a train of symptoms would produce a certain disease, the quest began for the cause and the ultimate effect. Thus throughout the centuries since Hippocrates' time the quest has continued until the number of basic scientific disciplines and departments with which modern medicine collaborates has increased tremendously.

With this growth of medical science the rapport of the physician-patient relationship has been invaded by a third party or parties—the paramedical personnel, who are the by-products of modern medicine. The care of patients has now become an increasingly complex division of labor and of specialized activity. Modern medicine, regardless of where it is practiced—the hospital, the clinic, the laboratory, the doctor's office, or the public health and governmental medical agencies—requires teamwork of doctors and paramedical or ancillary personnel. Each is dependent on the other for either diagnostic tests or therapeutic measures that will aid in the restoration of the patient to a state of health or well-being. Such paramedical personnel as secretaries, statisticians, clerks, medical social workers, and record librarians are also a part of this teamwork, regardless of the fact that their work may not necessitate close contact with the patient.

Although the doctor's superior knowledge of disease and therapy is unquestioned, almost daily those who assist the doctor are confronted with areas of uncertainty, imperfect knowledge, or confusion about disease. This lack of knowledge of disease stems mainly from the fact that their didactic training or education was acquired mainly in a narrow field devoted to the services they were to perform. At one time this might have been acceptable, but with the expanding field of medicine and the social pressures for improved medical care, knowledge of disease has become a part of the responsibility of those who care for the sick and injured, directly or indirectly, in a paramedical capacity. No longer is it deemed sufficient just to be able to carry out or mechanically perform a service or diagnostic procedure. Today the person performing the service has the obligation to carry out the assignment with knowledge as well as efficiency. Thus the expanding field of education, with paramedical specialization, demands that all those assisting the doctor in any capacity be motivated by the desire to acquire and augment knowledge of disease as it relates to the services they perform.

Knowledge of disease cannot be attained solely through the mechanics of performing a service. To understand disease it is necessary to be aware of the dynamic processes involved in the chain of events leading to a specific impairment of function or structure, or both, of the bodily organs and systems. Knowledge of anatomy and physiology, of course, is a prerequisite to understanding disease. If you are lacking in knowledge of normal anatomy and physiology, you cannot understand the departures from this norm that result in disease.

As a result of the shortage of doctors and the necessity for extending adequate medical care to small communities and remote rural areas, a movement has begun to solve the problem by making better use of the skills of paramedical personnel. To a more limited extent, this might be true of crowded urban medical facilities. The paramedical personnel who assist the physician, supervise a clinic, or even in some remote areas assume more responsibility in caring for patients, are referred to as physicians' assistants. These assistants require training beyond that of those who are employed in well-staffed hospitals and clinics where there is no shortage of doctors. First and possibly foremost, the physician's assistant must have a good background in knowledge of diseases and the signs and symptoms they might provoke. Although not a diagnostician in any sense of the word, he should be able to differentiate between patients who require only minor or routine treatment and those whose illness requires immediate attention of a physician. Using as a guide the profile of major symptoms given in Chapter 18, the assistant can save the physician valuable time in interrogation of patients to ascertain their past and present complaints before they are presented to the doctor for physical examination and further interview. The profile of symptoms is not complete but represents the major complaints in most diseases. To this profile can be added other complaints such as vomiting, loss of weight and appetite, pain, edema, rash, and passing of blood in urine, feces, vomitus, and sputum. A careful interview of the patient, or members of his family if the patient is a child or mental retardee, will usually establish a profile of his illness on which the doctor can elaborate in the examination.

Some states in cooperation with state medical societies have begun to establish guidelines for the duties that can be performed by paramedics without jeopardizing the life or health of patients or giving to them medical authority that can only be exercised by doctors. The services that a paramedic will perform in assisting a doctor must, of course, always be subject to the limitations imposed by the doctor and be under his control and supervision.

Many fire departments, particularly in the larger cities, have added paramedical employees to the force. These employees are specially trained in administering first aid and in other life saving techniques. They respond to emergency calls in ambulances or vehicles that have been called "emergency rooms on wheels." In most instances the paramedic units maintain two-way communication with the doctors in an emergency room of a hospital. In this way vital information on the condition of a patient is transmitted and in turn emergency treatment is prescribed by a doctor.

HOW TO USE THIS BOOK

This book is probably different from anything you have ever studied before. It combines a text type of material with a modified version of programmed instruction. Programmed instruction is a new educational tool for teaching, which has been widely adopted in industry, medicine, and various types of training and educational fields. In the standard type of programmed instruction, however, no text material is presented as such; all the information is incorporated in a series of steps requiring a response from the student. To increase the usefulness of this book for classroom instruction or a self-directed type of learning and to provide a ready reference, the information is presented in both text form and in a series of statements called steps designed for self-instruction.

Beginning with Chapter 1 on basic principles of pathogenesis and in each succeeding chapter some phase vital to your understanding of disease is introduced. These concepts range from how and why disease occurs, to which organs are injured and which are capable of regeneration or repair, to a discussion of the etiologic factors involved. Representative diseases in each etiologic category are included in the discussions. In Chapters 1 through 17 there is a series of steps containing statements and questions requiring answers on the most important points you should know concerning disease. Thus the reader actively participates in this type of instruction. The correct responses are given before the references at the end of the chapter. However, to learn most effectively, you should write out the answer before looking ahead. The correct responses will be found in the statements preceding the questions or in the text, or you may be referred to a table or illustration.

The step exercises in all etiologic categories have been designed to stress the important concepts of disease production from its very beginning in cells. This information will be useful to you in studying the last section of the book on clinical manifestations of disease (symptomatology).

When studying the illustrations in the section on symptomatology, you can increase your knowledge of anatomy by pinpointing the location of diseases in organs.

Some illustrations show how a disease process develops (pathogenesis), and others show the ultimate effects on an organ. As paramedical personnel you do not possess the highly developed skill of such medical specialists as the radiologist, the pathologist, or the surgeon, who can through various procedures discover areas of deficiencies in function and structure and ascertain the reasons for their existence. You often have to rely on a mental image of destructive elements operating inside the body, information you have gained from your basic knowledge of disease. By careful study of the illustrations, however, you will be able to visualize how diseases affect organs.

QUESTIONS TO ASK YOURSELF ABOUT DISEASES

When confronted with an unfamiliar disease, you should ask yourself the following questions:

1. What is the disease? Is it an infection, inflammation, allergy, trauma, tumor, congenital defect, mechanical obstruction, circulatory disturbance, metabolic defect, or nutritional disorders? Most diseases will fall somewhere within this standard etiologic classification. A medical dictionary or other medical reference will define the disease in terms of these factors, when known. There will, of course, be some instances when the etiology is unknown but is suspected.

2. How does the disease affect the patient? The answer to this question refers to the signs and symptoms of illness. These may be present initially, or they may develop during the course of the disease. Among the more common signs and symptoms are fever, headache, generalized or localized pain, anorexia, malaise, vomiting, diarrhea, persistent cough, rash, edema, oliguria, anuria, dyspnea, choking, wheezing, vertigo, diplopia, paralysis, hypertension or hypotension, leukocytosis, leukopenia, anemia, mental confusion or disorientation, delirium, and coma. Not all these, of course, will or could be present

in all diseases, but some of them are present in most every type of illness.

3. Which organ or bodily system is involved? The answer to this question gives you the possible or probable seat of the trouble. Through the interrelationship of organs or systems an illness may provoke a whole chain of events involving one or more organs or systems. The primary injury may be in one organ and secondarily affect the function of another. This is the famous law of the dominoes—"if one falls, others fall."

4. How does the disease affect the organ, organs, or bodily systems? The answer to this question relates to whether the organ structure or the function or both have been injured by the disease. You will not know the answer to this question, of course, unless you know how a particular disease affects an organ or system to which it belongs, whether it is a temporary malfunction, or whether the cellular damage has destroyed vital tissue.

5. Can the injured organ or organs be repaired? Repair in this instance relates mostly to tissue damage from disease. In any illness or injury the body's inbuilt defense mechanisms are called into play, and they attempt to repair the damage. In the case of a simple wound or slight illness all that may be necessary for repair lies in the ability of the body's inherent defense mechanisms to overcome injury. However, in more complicated illnesses exogenous measures (therapy) may be instituted to aid the body in its own defense. These measures may be surgical procedures or administration of drugs as antibiotics in infections. You will not know whether an organ can recover completely with residual damage, but through a study of repair or regeneration of tissues as given in a later chapter you will know which organs or tissues are capable of repairing damage in most instances. For example, you will know that a fracture of a bone can be repaired by the growth of new bone to fill the defect. Only the doctor is qualified to make the prognosis, that is, to say whether the patient will recover completely, or whether the damage is so extensive that there will be permanent injury. But from a knowledge of diseases you will learn which are likely to be fatal or irreversible and which can be reversed. For example, you know that cancer if extensive is ultimately fatal in most instances. In this disease it is usually found that the organ or organs have been severely impaired and that complete repair of the damage cannot be expected. This does not mean that the affected tissue cannot be removed or that the cancerous growth cannot be arrested, but it does mean that no new normal tissue or organ can ever replace the defect. On the other hand, you know that a common cold or simple infection, without complications, can reasonably be expected to subside with complete restoration of the affected organs to normalcy. Each disease carries with it, therefore, the implication that its course may or may not be reversed either by the body's defense mechanisms or exogenous influences or a combination of both.

PATHOGENESIS

CHAPTER 1

Basic principles of pathogenesis

Pathogenesis is the development of a morbid process or disease. All diseases of the body are produced either by an alteration in structure or an alteration in function, or both, of an organ, organs, or system. The function of an organ may be impaired and its structural elements unchanged. Functional disorders are seen in many diseases triggered by psychic or psychophysiologic factors, such as occur in many mental disturbances in which there is no lesion in the brain tissue itself. Conversely, the normal structure of an organ may be altered but the function is not impaired. For example, the heart of an athlete may be enlarged beyond that of the normal limits as a result of physical exertion, but the function will not be affected. In pregnancy the uterus and the breasts undergo physiologic enlargement, but we would not speak of this as a disease or a symptom of a disease just because the usual structure was altered. For a disease to be considered as caused by structural derangement, the organ or organs involved must be altered in such a way that they represent a pathologic entity. For a disease to be considered caused by functional and structural derangements, the normal function of the organ must be impaired by a structural defect in such a way that the organ is hampered in carrying out its duties.[3]

DIAGNOSIS

The recognition of a disease from its signs and symptoms or from scientific determinations is called diagnosis. The diagnosis of a disease is based on a number of factors. The clinical manifestations alone may point toward a specific diagnosis. The patient's past illnesses, any heritable diseases in his family, or a familial tendency toward a disease are contributing factors in the diagnosis. However, other tests may be necessary for establishment or confirmation of a diagnosis.

The vital organs, the brain and heart, are often studied by means of the electroencephalogram (EEG) and electrocardiogram (ECG), respectively, as a means of diagnosing functional disturbances. Particularly in the case of the heart, functional disorders may have their basis in structural derangements. This is also true of many functional disorders of the brain, which might be diagnosed by encephalographic means. Of course, the basis of the trouble may also be a structural defect such as a tumor.

One form of disease more or less elusive to diagnosis is disease produced by psychogenic disturbances. The clinical symptoms presented may fall within the pattern of a number of diseases, functional and organic, but no basis in fact may be found for the cause of the disturbance. It is known that psychologic factors may be either entirely responsible for a patient's complaints or may adversely affect somatic ailments. Organic illness in these cases is usually ruled out by appropriate tests and examinations. The list and causes of these types of illness are too broad for exploration here, but a great many of the minor psychogenic disorders are attributable to environmental factors.[2]

Some widely used diagnostic procedures are described in the following discussions.

Pathology specimens of tissue[5]

All specimens of tissue removed in the operating arena (surgical specimens) are examined grossly (for structure) and, if warranted, microscopically (cellular study). A *biopsy* is a small piece of tissue removed for pathologic examination. It is widely used for detection of malignant cells. Pathologic examinations, gross and microscopic, are the methods of assessing tissue and organ damage at autopsy and of establishing the cause or contributing causes of death. Most diseases are dynamic processes that in the course of their evolution sooner or later produce lesions or abnormal tissue alterations, which can be studied by gross or microscopic means. Yet there are a number of diseases that present only functional disorders, biochemical or metabolic derangements, that are not observable in tissue examinations.[3] Psychiatric disorders cannot be diagnosed by the pathologic examination of tissue because their manifestations are abnormal behavioral patterns, which are not detectable as tissue changes. However, if the abnormal behavior were the result of structural damage to the nervous system, the disease would be considered a result of primary damage of tissues and not a true psychiatric disease.

Exfoliative cytologic studies[5]

Exfoliative cytology is the study of cells in exfoliated, abraded, and aspirated material. Exfoliated and abraded material contains cells found on the surfaces of mucous membranes, glands, and skin, as well as in secretions from these sources. The cells are exfoliated in sputum, urine, transudates, and exudates. Aspirated cells are cells obtained by needle puncture of any organ or tumor or other diseased area, as well as cells obtained by gastric or colonic lavage, proctoscopy, proctosigmoidoscopy, bronchoscopy, and duodenal drainage. The technique most often used in exfoliative cytology is the Papanicolaou technique, which is often shortened to "Pap smear."

Radiography[6]

Since x rays pass through an object that is normally opaque, they are used to view the internal functions and structure of the body to pinpoint disease or an anomaly. In addition to routine x-ray examinations, for example, chest films and the skeletal views, there are many special diagnostic procedures that reveal more specific information about the function of an organ or organs. For these types of x-ray examination a contrast medium (liquid, powder, gas, or pill), keyed to examination of a particular organ or organs of the body, is injected or given orally or by enema. The contrast medium opacifies the organ or organs under study. Thus function of an organ or organs can be studied by x-ray films, fluoroscopy, or cineradiography (motion pictures). Each of these special procedures has a specific name. The first part of the term usually designates the organ under study, and the second part the procedure; for example, cholecystography (gallbladder); pyelography (kidneys); angiocardiography (great vessels and heart); arteriography (arteries); bronchography (bronchial tree); myelography (spinal subarachnoid spaces); cerebral ventriculography (ventricular system of the brain); cystography (urinary bladder); cystourethrography (urinary bladder and urethra during voiding); and lymphangiography (lymphatic channels). The exceptions to this general rule are the administration of a barium meal for examination of the esophagus, stomach, duodenum, and small intestines, and the barium enema for examination of the colon.

Clinical laboratory procedures[5]

Blood and lymph flow through every organ of the body and are in contact with all the tissue cells. Each tissue contributes chemical substances and cells. By examining the blood and noting chemical and physical properties and cytologic patterns and comparing these with normal constituents of blood, much valuable diagnostic information is obtained. Other body fluids and materials or contents are also examined. These include the cerebrospinal fluid, sputum, saliva, transudates, exudates, gastric contents, body wastes (feces and urine), and bone marrow.

Because of the wide range of clinical laboratory studies the laboratory is usually divided into branches that perform specific examinations. Broadly speaking, these branches and the tests or studies performed in each are hematology (morphology of blood and blood-forming organs), urinalyses (urinary constituents and kidney function), blood banking (typing and cross matching, blood group systems, transfusion reactions), chemistry (blood constituents such as enzymes, electrolytes, hormones, nitrogen, carbohydrates, and blood lipids), toxicology (identification of poisons), immunology (immunity studies), bacteriology (bacteria), parasitology (protozoal and helminthic organisms), mycology (fungi), and virology and rickettsia (isolation and identification of viruses and rickettsiae).

Radioisotopes[6]

The diagnosis of diseases by means of radiopharmaceuticals is based on the principle that radioactive isotopes can be traced through the body by sensitive instruments (Geiger counter or scintillation counter) that count the rays given off by radioactive atoms moving through the body or congregating at various points. The procedure of systematically mapping the distribution of a radioactive substance in the human body is known as scanning, and the map produced is called a scintigram. An example of a radioisotope widely used in both diagnosis and therapy is radioactive iodine or radioiodine, which is used in studies of function of the thyroid gland or therapy of thyroid lesions. It can also be incorporated into human serum albumin to determine the plasma volume of patients, and it is used to label dyes such as rose bengal in order to study the function of the liver. Another example is radiogold, which is used in studying the functional integrity of the liver and also in bone marrow function studies. The use of radiopharmaceuticals is much too broad a subject to be discussed in this book. However, one should know that radioisotopes have been found to be valuable adjuncts in confirming and amplifying the results of some existing diagnostic techniques (for example, x-ray, laboratory), and in many instances have supplanted others.

• • •

In all the diagnostic procedures previously mentioned, it can be readily seen that modern medicine offers many methods for arriving at a true diagnosis of a disease. The functional and structural alterations of organs and tissues in disease can be studied in various ways in pathogenesis. In the selected diseases covered in the following chapters the major diagnostic procedures are given to increase your knowledge of the disease under discussion.

CLASSIFICATION OF DISEASES

The cause or etiology of disease is usually classified into a specific category. Most of the diseases will fall somewhere within a broad classification of etiologic categories as follows:

1. Congenital abnormalities or anomalies (existing at or before birth)
2. Hereditary and familial predisposition
3. Inflammations and infections
4. Intoxications—allergies, poisons
5. Trauma and physical agents
6. Circulatory disturbances
7. Disturbances of innervation or psychic control
8. Static mechanical abnormalities (obstructions, calculi, ectopic organs or

tissue, twisting or volvulus of an organ)
9. Neoplasms
10. Metabolism, growth, or nutrition
11. Mental deficiencies (psychogenic disturbances and true psychoses)

In recording the diagnosis of any disease caused by one of these etiologic factors the name of the organ or system is supplied if it is pertinent to the understanding of the disease process. For example, if paralysis is a factor, the part of the body affected will be given. In duplicate organs, such as the kidneys and lungs, if only one is involved, the side (right or left) is a part of the diagnosis; if both are involved, the term "bilateral" is added. If a disease is peculiar to a specific organ or if the term itself applies only to one organ or tissue, it is not necessary to give the name of the organ with the diagnosis. For example, you do not need the term "liver" when the diagnosis is hepatitis (*hepa* refers to liver); nor do you need the term "eyes" when the diagnosis is total blindness.

STEP-BY-STEP EXERCISES

Step 1. Any definite morbid process usually having characteristic symptoms and at times physical signs is defined as a disease.

Complete the blanks in the following statement.

A disease is a morbid process usually

having _____ symptoms and

at times _____ signs.

Step 2. A disease may primarily affect one organ or multiple organs and their parts. It may have a target organ or part and secondarily affect other organs. Its etiology, pathology, and prognosis may or may not be known (as shown below).

Step 3. The structural elements of an organ may be altered, but the essential functions remain unchanged. For example, the heart may be enlarged, and it will continue to carry on its labor of pumping blood to the body. Conversely, the function may be impaired and the structure remain unchanged. For example, the structural elements of the brain may remain normal when there is mental illness. In some diseases both the function and the structure may be impaired. For example, in emphysema both the structure and the function (respiration) may be impaired.

Mark the following statements *T* for true or *F* for false.
1. The function of an organ may be impaired without its having structural defects. ___
2. The structure of an organ and its function are always impaired in disease. ___
3. Structural elements and functional impairment never occur simultaneously. ___

Step 4. Read the discussion on diagnosis (p. 7) and then complete the blanks in the following statements.
1. A diagnosis is sometimes made from

Indicate the comment that best applies to the following statements.

	Always	Sometimes	Never
1. A disease affects only one organ.	—	—	—
2. A disease affects multiple organs.	—	—	—
3. There may be a target organ but other organs may be secondarily affected.	—	—	—
4. The etiology is known.	—	—	—
5. A disease is diagnosed by gross microscopic examination.	—	—	—
6. The prognosis is known.	—	—	—

_____ and _____,
which are clinical manifestations.

2. A diagnosis sometimes requires

_____ determinations.

3. Surgical specimens of tissue are examined _____ for structure, and _____ for cellular pathology.

4. A small piece of tissue taken from an organ or tissue, usually for microscopic study, is called a _____.

5. Exfoliated, abraded, and aspirated cell and materials are subjects of

_____ _____

studies.

6. The most commonly used technique in exfoliative cytology is the _____ _____.

7. The diagnostic procedure used to view the internal functions and structures of the body is called _____.

8. The tests performed on blood and its constituents, urine, cerebrospinal fluid, feces, sputum, gastric contents, and so on are called _____ _____ procedures.

9. A relatively new diagnostic procedure is that of tracing _____ through the body by sensitive instruments, such as the Geiger counter.

10. An electrocardiographic examination is performed for diagnostic purposes in _____ diseases.

11. Functional disturbances of the brain are studied by means of the _____ in certain diseases.

NOTE: The following steps present important information about diseases not included in the text. Read each statement carefully before you attempt to make a response.

Step 5. For the body to remain healthy the functions of elimination, secretion, absorption, movement, support, circulation, respiration, and manufacture of hormones must be normal.

In the spaces provided indicate which of the following might be signs or symptoms of disease.

1. Diarrhea __
Regular bowel movement __
2. Loss of sensation of pain __
Awareness of applied painful stimuli __
3. Paralysis __
Free and uninhibited movement __
4. Malnutrition __
Well nourished appearance __
5. Arrhythmia (irregular heart beat) __
Regular cardiac rhythm __
6. Dyspnea (shortness of breath or difficult respiration) __
Regular respiratory movements __
7. Hemoptysis (spitting of blood) __
No hemorrhagic tendencies __
8. Goiter __
No enlargement of thyroid __

Step 6. The primary requirement for survival of the human organism is the maintenance and safeguarding of physiologic equilibrium for the individual cells that make up the sum of the body and its parts.[1] All living organisms are never at rest but are in a constant state of dynamic internal change in order to maintain an internal equilibrium despite the pressures of environment. This dynamic state is called homeostasis (from *homeo* referring to same or similarity; *stasis* meaning standing or stability).[1]

Would you assume from this statement that the maintenance of internal equilibrium is the basis of health?

Yes __ No __

Step 7. There are many disturbing elements that have the manifest tendency to destroy the existing order within the organs and to bring about their total destruction, alter their structure, or handicap their function.[4] These disturbing elements may be exogenous (developing or originating outside the body) or endogenous (developing or originating within the body). (*Exo* means outside; *endo* means inside.)

Complete the blanks in the following statement.

Disturbing elements that destroy tissue coming from outside the body are called _____; those that originate or develop within the body are called _____.

Step 8. The disturbing elements referred to in step 7 may exert an unremitting influence on an organ or group of organs, which are then forced to take counteraction against these elements to survive and to maintain physiologically acceptable conditions.[4] A person is healthy if his organs have at their disposal mechanisms sufficiently powerful to neutralize the effects of pathologic disturbances without therapeutic measures. If the function of the organ is impaired and the body's inbuilt mechanisms of defense are unable to repair the damage or if the pathogen onslaught is overwhelming, the end result is disease.

Mark the following statements *T* for true or *F* for false.

1. The body has inbuilt defense mechanisms to counteract or aid in counteracting disease. ___
2. The body's defense mechanisms can often neutralize pathogens before they can do harm. ___
3. The body is defenseless against the attack of disease-producing biologic agents. ___

Step 9. The vital physiologic values in the body that must be kept at constant level if you are to survive in good health include among others average blood pressure, normal body temperature, normal osmotic pressure of body fluids, and normal blood sugar levels.[4] Nature invariably operates in such a manner as to govern and adjust appropriate physiologic values compatible with good health. If any one of these vital physiologic values in the body is grossly de-

ranged, disease results. (It is assumed that you have studied physiology.)

Indicate which conditions are indicative of deranged vital physiologic values.

1. Hypertension ___; hypotension ___; average blood pressure ___
2. Fever ___; 98.8° body temperature ___
3. Edema (swelling of tissues) ___
4. Diabetes mellitus ___; normal glucose tolerance test ___

Step 10. Nature cannot always overcome or repair damaged organs or tissues. There is, however, a normal physiologic breakdown of organs with age because of wear and tear. These include such changes as graying of the hair, wrinkling of the skin, and atrophy of some organs, such as the uterus. We are said to start to die, the minute we are born, for the human body is not indestructible and death of the organism is inevitable. However, in the aged there may be a breakdown of vital organs, such as the heart and blood vessels, with degenerative conditions. These constitute disease. Arteriosclerosis (hardening of the arteries) and osteoarthritis (degenerative joint disease) to some extent are usually present in the aged who come to autopsy, but in the lifetime of the individual they may have been asymptomatic (without symptoms).

1. Would normal physiologic aging evidenced by graying of hair and atrophy of the uterus in a woman of 70 years be considered a disease?

Yes ___ No ___
2. Would loss of skin elasticity in the aged be a sign of disease?

Yes ___ No ___
3. In a man of 75 years would arteriosclerosis and osteoarthritis accompanied by characteristic symptoms be a disease?

Yes ___ No ___

Step 11. The functions of some vital organs are interrelated in that normal function of one often depends on normal function of the other. This is true of the lungs, the heart, and the kidneys. When one of these organs is damaged in certain diseases, you might expect the damage to be reflected in all or some of them. For example, hypertension may involve the kidneys and the heart. Emphysema (a lung disease) may affect the heart eventually, causing it to become enlarged. If the kidneys fail in their functions with subsequent uremia, the heart may be affected.

Complete the following blanks with the name of the organ that might be involved *secondarily* by primary disease in the systems given.

1. _____
   Circulatory system—hypertension

2. _____
   Respiratory system—emphysema

3. _____
   Urinary system—uremia

Step 12. Diseases are usually referred to as reversible or irreversible. When a disease is irreversible, it means that despite therapeutic measures the damage is such that it cannot be repaired or returned to a state of normalcy. Complete recovery structurally or functionally is not possible. Reversible diseases are those that respond to therapy and in which complete recovery can be expected.[3]

Complete the blanks in the following statements.

1. Diseases that maim structures and functions of an organ or system beyond repair would be called _____ conditions.

2. Diseases that respond to treatment with restoration to a normal or near normal state are called _____ conditions.

Step 13. Diseases are also described according to stages, such as acute, subacute, or chronic. Acute diseases have a short and relatively severe course. Subacute is an intermediary term used to describe the course of a disease somewhere between the acute and chronic phase. It is more or less a term

of choice, and not all doctors use it. The chronic phase is one in which there is persistence of the injurious agent for weeks or even years. An acute phase may regress inta a subacute or chronic form. Not all subacute or chronic diseases, however, have their origin in an acute focus. In many instances the stimulus is low grade or the organisms are of low toxicity, and the full-blown acute stage is never reached.[3]

Complete the blanks in the following statements.

1. A disease with a short and relatively severe course is called _____.

2. A disease that persists for weeks or years is called _____.

3. The intermediary phase between acute and chronic is called _____.

Responses

Step 1: characteristic; physical

Step 2: 1 through 6. sometimes

Step 3: 1. T; 2. F; 3. F

Step 4: signs; symptoms; 2. scientific; 3. grossly; microscopically; 4. biopsy; 5. clinical cytologic; 6. Papanicolaou technique; 7. radiography or radiographic; 8. clinical laboratory; 9. radioisotopes or radioactive substances; 10. heart; 11. encephalogram

Step 5: 1. diarrhea; 2. loss of sensation of pain; 3. paralysis; 4. malnutrition; 5. arrhythmia; 6. dyspnea; 7. hemoptysis; 8. goiter

Step 6: Yes

Step 7: exogenous; endogenous

Step 8: 1. T; 2. T; 3. F

Step 9: 1. hypertension; hypotension; 2. fever; 3. edema; 4. diabetes mellitus

Step 10: 1. No; 2. No; 3. Yes

Step 11: 1. kidneys; 2. heart; 3. heart

Step 12: 1. irreversible; 2. reversible

Step 13: 1. acute; 2. chronic; 3. subacute

REFERENCES

1. Cannon, W. B.: The wisdom of the body, ed. 2, New York, 1963, W. W. Norton & Co., Inc.
2. Lief, H. I., Lief, V. F., and Lief, N. R., editors: The psychological basis of medical practice, New York, 1963, Hoeber Medical Division, Harper & Row, Publshers.
3. Robbins, S. L.: Pathology, ed. 3, Philadelphia, 1967, W. B. Saunders Co.

4. Wagner, R.: Triangle (Sandoz Journal of Medical Science) 5:322, Oct., 1962 (the principle of biological regulation).

5. Young, C. G., and Barger, J. D.: Medical specialty terminology, vol. 1, Pathology, clinical cytology, and clinical pathology, St. Louis, 1971, The C. V. Mosby Co.

6. Young, C. G., and Likos, J. J.: Medical specialty terminology, vol. 2, X-ray and nuclear medicine, St. Louis, 1972, The C. V. Mosby Co.

CHAPTER 2

Cellular injury in disease

The cell is the building block from which tissues, organs, and systems are constructed. (*Cyte* is a term for cell.) When the cell is the seat of injury, this is a manifestation of disease. The alterations in cells in disease may be minor or irreversible, depending on whether cell injury is slight or severe. In total destruction of cells, as in myocardial infarction, the damage is irreversible.

A prerequisite to understanding disease should include knowledge of the normal cell and tissue, for all alterations in cell structure and function are merely a greater or lesser degree of departure from a relatively fixed norm. The study of cell structure and function is called cytology. The practical and technical application of this science to the diagnosis and treatment of disease is the subject of numerous medical textbooks and other medical writings. Obviously it would be impossible in a book of this scope to cover these subjects in detail. From your previous studies of physiology it is assumed that you have sufficient knowledge to understand cell structure and functions. However, since cell injury is very important in disease, some of the dynamic manufacturing complexities of cells as well as cellular structure are briefly reviewed.

CELL STRUCTURE AND FUNCTIONS[2, 3]

Cells are the smallest living parts of the body, and the body contains millions of them. They are too small to be seen without a microscope or an electron microscope.

They vary in form and shape, but all have many physical properties in common. All cells are composed of a watery, gelatinous substance called *protoplasm,* a complex chemical material that composes all living things. Its most abundant elements are oxygen, nitrogen, carbon, and hydrogen. Its main components are water, inorganic salts, proteins (including enzymes), carbohydrates, lipid, and nucleic acids. The basic activities of protoplasm are irritability (response to stimulus), conductivity (transmission of impulses), contractility (contraction or movement), and metabolism (utilization of foods to furnish it with energy and the synthesis of various compounds). Protoplasm is also able to reproduce itself. The cell is surrounded by a very thin membrane composed of lipid and protein molecules. The membrane maintains the cell's integrity and its organization and determines which substances are allowed to enter or leave the cell. This two-way traffic consists of molecules of water, foods, gases, wastes, and many kinds of ions. The passage of these particles takes place mainly by diffusion and osmosis.

The protoplasm has two main parts—*cytoplasm* and *nucleus.* The cytoplasm is located between the cell membrane and the nucleus. It is not the homogeneous substance that it was once thought to be, but it contains different kinds of small structures, called *organelles* (little organs). These organelles consist of molecules that perform some function necessary for maintaining the life of the cell or for its reproduction. The membranous organelles are the endoplasmic reticulum, Golgi apparatus, mitochondria, and lysosomes. The endoplasmic reticulum contains the ribosomes (attached to the rough type) that synthesize proteins. The ribosomes are composed mainly of ribonucleic acid (RNA), with a lesser amount of protein molecules. The Golgi apparatus synthesizes large carbohydrate molecules and combines them with proteins, a secretion called glycoprotein. The mitochondria have been called the cell's powerhouse, since they are believed to generate the power for cellular work. The lysosomes contain hydrolytic enzymes capable of dissolving most of the compounds present in the cells. They can digest large molecules and large particles, such as bacteria. They are present in phagocytic cells.

The nucleus is the spherical body located in the center of the cell. It is surrounded by a nuclear membrane, said to contain pores that allow communication with the cytoplasm. Within the nucleus are the chromosomes. The chromosome is composed mainly of deoxyribonucleic acid (DNA) plus protein. The DNA molecules consist of lines of genes, which determine heredity. The nucleus also contains nucleoli, which are small spherical bodies composed mainly of ribonucleic acid (RNA) and some protein. The nucleoli are believed to serve as the sites where ribosomal RNA (referred to above) combines with protein, forming a complex which then migrates out of the nucleus to the cytoplasm where it becomes organized into the ribosomes. (See Fig. 2-1 for cell structure.)

From the foregoing cellular structures

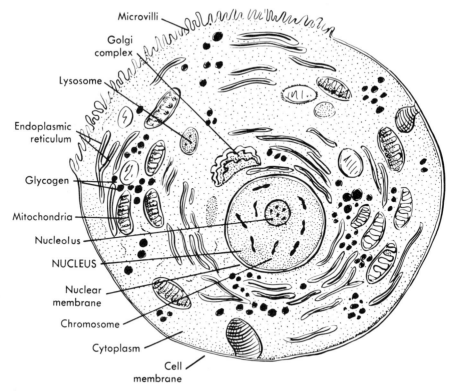

Fig. 2-1. Typical cell with cell structures as might be seen by an electron microscope. (From Young, C. G., and Barger, J. D.: Medical specialty terminology, pathology, clinical cytology, and clinical pathology, St. Louis, 1971, The C. V. Mosby Co.)

it can be seen that the cell is composed of highly specialized parts, constituting a dynamic manufacturing complex, whose functions are secretion, absorption, conduction, and contraction, all of which the well-being of the body depends upon.

To carry out these activities, cells are of different types, each with specialized functions, such as muscle, nerve, blood, epithelial, connective, and reproductive. These cells through a division of labor all contribute something to the structure and function of the body as a whole. The division of labor is orderly, however, since specialized cells join together to form organs and tissues with similar abilities or functions.

The body tissues are of four main types—nervous, muscular, epithelial, and connective. The nervous tissue activates and integrates the body as a whole through its special powers of irritability, conductivity, and integration. The muscular system excels in contractility, which is the power of the body and its parts to move and to relax. The epithelial tissue in different forms (squamous, stratified, columnar, cuboidal, and transitional) provides a protective covering for the body and lines the organs. The connective tissue lends support wherever the body needs it, as in tendons, fascia, ligaments, and bone. Injury to the cells of any one of these tissues may result in total or partial destruction of an organ or tissue with resultant impairment of predestined functions. The injury, however, may be of the type that can be repaired, as discussed in the chapter on repair of tissues.

The role of the cell in disease will become more apparent to you as you proceed in your studies of inflammation repair, and etiologic factors (for example, metabolism, growth, nutrition, trauma, and allergies) in the chapters that follow this basic discussion.

STEP-BY-STEP EXERCISES

Step 1. Cells are the building blocks of organs, and when they become injured, the result is disease. The injury may be permanent or temporary.

Which statement best defines cellular injury?

1. A factor in disease ___
2. In no way influencing disease ___

Step 2. Necrosis, from the Greek word *nekrosis* meaning deadness, refers to the circumscribed cell or tissue death within the living body. Necrobiosis refers to the physiologic death and replacement of certain cells, a constant occurrence, for example, blood cells and epidermis. Somatic death is death of the body as a whole, occurring when respiration and cardiac action cease. Some individual cells and tissues, however, may remain alive for a variable but short period of time after somatic death; for example, mitotic activity in progress at the time of death may proceed to complete division of cells.[1]

Complete the blanks in the following statements.

1. Circumscribed cell or tissue death within the living body is called

   _____.

2. The process of physiologic death and replacement of certain cells is called

   _____.

3. Death of the body as a whole, occurring when respiration and cardiac action cease, is called _____.

Step 3. Cell necrosis may be caused by the following agents[1, 5]: (1) ischemia (loss of blood supply to a tissue) and anoxia (lack of oxygen), (2) physical agents (for example, trauma, extremes of temperature, x rays, radioactive materials, sunlight, and electrical energy), (3) chemical agents (for example, mercury, arsenic, and carbon tetrachloride), (4) biologic agents (bacteria, viruses, rickettsiae, protozoa, and fungi), and (5) hypersensitivity (severe allergies —the simple allergies may not cause necrosis).

Complete the blanks in the following statements.

1. When cell death results from deprivation of oxygen, it is called _____; when it is caused by lack of blood supply, it is called _____.
2. When necrosis results from overexposure to x rays, radioactive materials, or sunlight, this is classified as caused by a _____ agent.
3. When necrosis results from bacteria, viruses, rickettsiae, protozoa, or fungi, the agent involved is called a _____ agent.
4. When a drug or inhalant causes a severe reaction with cell necrosis, this would be the result of _____.
5. When cell death is attributed to arsenic or mercury, the agent would be _____.
6. Exposure to freezing temperature with cell death would be the effect of a _____ agent.
7. Cell necrosis of the lining of the intestinal tract because of protozoa would be caused by a _____ agent.
8. Cell death resulting from contact with a high tension electric wire would be caused by a _____ agent.

Step 4. All the above agents capable of causing cell death act first by impairing the metabolic and biochemical activities of the cell. The extent of the cell necrosis and tissue damage depends upon the following factors of the specific noxious agent: virulence, duration of exposure, susceptibility of individual cells to a particular agent, and mode of invasion or entrance.

Mark the following statements T for true or F for false.
1. The virulence of an agent is not a factor in cell necrosis. ___
2. There is less chance of cell death if the duration of exposure is short. ___
3. The specific noxious agent is not a factor in individual cell damage. ___
4. The metabolic and biochemical activities of the cell are not disturbed in cell injury. ___
5. The mode of invasion or entrance influences cell necrosis. ___

Step 5. Anoxia destroys brain tissue more readily than other body tissues. (The brain requires a large amount of oxygen to function.) Chemicals are more destructive to the kidneys and liver than to the brain. Poisons, such as corrosives introduced orally, are particularly damaging to the esophagus, since in this instance it is the passage through which the poison gains entrance to the stomach. Radiant energy from sunlight produces erythema (redness) of the skin. Thus there is a difference in the way organs react to injury from specific noxious agents.[5]

Mark the following statements T for true or F for false.
1. The brain is more subject to chemical agents than are the kidney and the liver. ___
2. Anoxia produces its greatest destruction in the kidneys. ___
3. Corrosive agents taken orally damage the esophagus. ___
4. The cells of the skin are susceptible to injury from overexposure to the sun's rays. ___

Step 6. Cells react to injury causing necrosis in different ways, depending upon the initiating physical agent. In physical trauma, cell membranes rupture, disrupting the normal relationships of the cell elements. Some chemical solutions cause local destruction of cells and tissues by derangement of the osmotic equilibrium in cells, whereas others cause their damage by immediately destroying the tissue at the point of entrance, where the concentration is higher. Some chemical agents are damaging after systemic absorption and transport by the blood to organs like the liver, and they later cause necrosis of cells when excreted by the kidneys and colon. Bacteria cause necrosis by elaboration of toxic products.[4, 5]

Read the previous statement carefully and then by analytical application see if you can identify the mode of destruction in cells in the following statements.

1. A volatile liquid damaging to the liver is inhaled and carried by the blood to this organ. Would this be an example of systemic absorption?

Yes ___ No ___

2. Mercury has been taken orally and absorbed through the stomach, causing initial damage, but later causes further cell necrosis in the colon and kidneys. Would this be an example of injury produced by both absorption and excretion?

Yes ___ No ___

3. Suppose you have an infection caused by bacteria and there is necrosis of cells. Would this be the result of elaboration of toxic products?

Yes ___ No ___

4. Suppose you have suffered a gunshot wound. Would the impact of the bullet cause disruption of the cell membranes?

Yes ___ No ___

Step 7. Bacteria cause necrosis of cells by elaboration of toxic substances. If these toxins are constituents of the bacterial cells, they are called *endotoxins* (*endo* meaning within).[4] If the toxins formed by the bacteria are found outside the cell, they are known as *exotoxins* (*exo* meaning outside).

The viruses and parasites (protozoa and rickettsiae) cause cell necrosis by the production of destructive enzymes or toxic fractions.

Complete the blanks in the following statements.

1. Toxins that are constituents of the bacterial cell are called _____.

2. Toxic substances formed by bacteria and found outside the cells are known as _____.

3. Cell necrosis resulting from invasion of viruses or parasites is caused by production of destructive _____

or _____ _____.

NOTE: For the reader or student who would like to have more specific knowledge of the types of necrosis, as reported in tissue examinations (pathology reports), the following is included. No response is indicated.

If you were to study cell death in tissues, you would discover that necrosis is a dynamic process and that the morphologic changes have occurred over a period of time in sequences of changes. These changes have been labeled coagulation necrosis, liquefaction necrosis, caseous necrosis, and gangrenous necrosis. In coagulation necrosis there is a persistence of the cellular outline for a long period of time. It is seen when the arterial supply to a tissue is cut off and the tissue becomes ischemic. It is also seen in cell death by bacterial toxins, as in typhoid fever and streptococcal infections, and in chemical intoxications, such a mercurial poisoning of the kidneys. Liquefaction necrosis is a fairly rapid total enzymatic dissolution of cells with complete destruction of the entire cell. This type is encountered in brain cells damaged by anoxia or ischemia. It is also found in all tissues in bacterial infections where there is pus formation.

Caseous necrosis is produced by the tubercle bacillus (in tuberculosis), in which the destroyed cells lose their cell detail and are converted into granular, friable masses of amorphous fat and protein. These resemble soft friable pieces of cheese.

Gangrenous necrosis is a combination of cell necrosis by ischemia and superimposed bacterial infection. The initial event may have been bacterial infection followed by ischemia, or the infarction (ischemia) may have come first followed by invasion of bacteria. This type is seen in acute gangrenous appendicitis and in gangrene of the extremities.[1,5]

Responses

Step 1: 1. X

Step 2: 1. necrosis; 2. necrobiosis; 3. somatic

Step 3: 1. anoxia; ischemia; 2. physical; 3. biologic; 4. hypersensitivity; 5. chemical; 6. physical; 7. biologic; 8. physical

Step 4: 1. F; 2. T; 3. F; 4. F; 5. T

Step 5: 1. F; 2. F; 3. T; 4. T

Step 6: 1. Yes; 2. Yes; 3. Yes; 4. Yes

Step 7: 1. endotoxins; 2. exotoxins; 3. enzymes; toxic fractions (or equivalent response)

REFERENCES

1. Anderson, W. A. D.: In Anderson, W. A. D., editor: Pathology, ed. 6, St. Louis, 1971, The C. V. Mosby Co. (degenerative changes and disturbances of metabolism).
2. Anthony, C. P., and Kolthoff, N. J.: Textbook of anatomy and physiology, ed. 9, St. Louis, 1975, The C. V. Mosby Co.
3. Finerty, J. C., and Cowdry, E. V.: In Anderson, W. A. D., editor: Pathology, ed. 6, St. Louis, 1971, The C. V. Mosby Co. (cells and their behavior).
4. Hopps, H. C.: In Anderson, W. A. D., editor: Pathology, ed. 6, St. Louis, 1971, The C. V. Mosby Co. (bacterial diseases).
5. Robbins, S. L.: Pathology, ed. 3, Philadelphia, 1967, W. B. Saunders Co.

CHAPTER 3

Inflammation

Whenever cells are injured or destroyed as in necrosis, an immediate protective response occurs in the surrounding tissues at the site of injury. This is called inflammation. Usually we think of an inflammation as being caused by bacteria, such as we see in an infected cut on the skin with formation of pus; this is an infection. Or we may think of it as being redness of the throat tissue when we have a cold that results from a virus. Both these concepts are correct, for both represent inflammatory response. Actually all the agents capable of causing necrosis of cells, which were discussed in the previous chapter, act as harmful or destructive influences and evoke inflammatory reactions in injured tissues under attack or exposure. In addition to the initial response provided by the noxious agent itself many of the agents are sufficiently violent to cause death of cells, releasing noxious substances from these cells which also serve as injurious agents and add to the inflammatory response.[4]

Not all inflammations are characterized by necrosis of cells; some are simple, in which there is no pus or other inflammatory product. This type heals in a short time, and no permanent damage to tissues results in the process. In necrotic inflammatory responses there may be permanent tissue damage, for although the body acts to repair any damage to tissue, it is not always able to reconstitute cells or tissues, and the result will be scarring or distortion of tissue. This is further discussed in Chapter 4.

Basically the immediate inflammatory response to tissue injury is almost always the same, regardless of the nature of the inciting injurious agent—its virulence and toxicity. This response is the same for simple inflammation as it is for more profound injuries. The immediate response consists of a complicated sequence of physiologic and structural adjustments to injury and includes the blood vessels, the fluid (exudate) and cellular components of the blood, and the surrounding connective tissue. Although all these physiologic and structural changes follow a fairly regular pattern and occur in sequence, the final outcome depends upon the extent and severity of the tissue changes and other factors relating to the host as well as the invading agent. For example, a simple burn on the finger produces a blister that will heal without damage to the cells or tissue within a reasonably short time. But if bacteria invade the wound, there may follow more extensive tissue damage.[3, 4]

The state of health and the age of the host are important factors to be considered in inflammatory response to injury. Younger healthy people have a greater capacity than the aged to resist disease and recover more quickly partly because of better nutrition and a more adequate blood supply. In many older people who suffer from inadequate nutrition or who have preexisting diseases of the blood vessels such as arteriosclerosis, vascular adjustment to injury may be impaired. Adequate circulation and tissue drainage are essential, as is nutrition, since the healing processes of injuries exert a great demand on body stores of all nutrients.[6] In short, any disorder that impairs the general physical condition also becomes an important predisposing factor to infection. Human beings are constantly exposed to a number of harmful invaders, bacteria in particular, which need only a suitable host and a portal of entry. Their success in surviving after gaining entrance to the body is dependent to a great extent on the ability of the body's protective and defensive measures to react to injury in the inflammatory process. The inflammatory response serves a protective and defensive purpose, since it attempts to neutralize and destroy noxious agents at the site of injury and prevent their dissemination to other organs. This it does through its blood supply and through the cellular components active in the defense of the body that dilute, phagocytize (*phago* is a term meaning to eat), or wall off the invading noxious agents as well as the tissue cells that may have been injured.[7, 8]

STEP-BY-STEP EXERCISES

In the following steps you will learn how the inflammatory response is organized and how it is an expression of the body's inherent defense system to protect itself from injury.

Step 1. Tissue response to injury is called inflammation. It is a protective response occurring in the tissues surrounding an injured membrane or at the site of injury. It is characterized usually but not always by four cardinal symptoms: heat, redness, pain, and swelling.[8] An additional symptom may be loss of function; this depends upon the site and extent of injury and is not considered a cardinal symptom, since its occurrence is variable.

Complete the blanks in the following statements.

1. _____ is a condition into which tissues enter as a response to injury.
2. The cardinal signs of tissue injury, if acute, are _____, _____, _____, and _____. An additional sign may be _____.

Step 2. Both heat and redness of an inflammation are caused by increased vascularity in areas of injury. When cells or tissues are injured, there is vasodilatation (dilatation of blood vessels) and increased permeability of capillary walls (walls are altered, which allows escape of plasma). With vasodilatation an increased supply of blood is delivered to the injured area; this results in congestion. We recognize congestion as heat and redness from the abnormal accumulation of blood in the injured part. The increase in blood supply to an injured area is the first step in inflammatory response. It occurs within minutes after an injury.

Indicate the statements that give characteristics of vascular changes in injury, producing heat and redness.

1. There is an increased blood supply. ___
   There is no vasodilatation. ___
2. Plasma escapes because capillary walls are more permeable. ___
   The increased permeability of capillary walls has nothing to do with plasma escape. ___
3. The abnormal accumulation of blood in an injured part results in congestion. ___
   Blood does not accumulate in an injured part. ___

Step 3. The vasodilatation of vessels (arterioles, venules, and capillaries) is believed to be initiated by release of histamine-like substances.[7] This vasodilatation permits circulating cells (white blood cells for phagocytosis), antibodies (immune substances), oxygen, and nutrients to be carried to the site of injury. These are all measures of the inflammatory response to protect the body against injury.

Mark the following statements *T* for true or *F* for false.

1. White cells or phagocytic cells are carried by the blood to the site of injury to aid in destroying the enemy invader. ___
2. Antibodies, although carried by the bloodstream to the site of injury, have

nothing to do with protective measures. ___

3. Nutrients carried by the bloodstream to the site of injury aid in the protective mechanisms. ___

Step 4. In the inflammatory response to injury the nutrients serve to support the metabolic activities of the cells under attack as well as supporting the defensive cells.[7] Plasma fluid is increased for exudation, which serves a protective purpose.

From the information given in this step and the one immediately preceding it, which of the following are protective measures initiated by the increased blood supply?

1. Increase of white blood cells ___
2. Oxygen ___
3. Destruction of antibodies ___
4. Exudation ___
5. Prevention of phagocytosis ___
6. Nutrients ___

Step 5. When the blood supply is increased to an inflamed area, not only does it bring in protective cellular elements as discussed in the previous steps, but also it is able to carry off more toxic products, thus preventing them from accumulating and adding to the injury. Fibrin may be precipitated in both the blood vessels and the surrounding lymphatics to block dissemination of bacteria. Fibrin in the focus of inflammation forms a meshwork that aids in localizing and trapping bacteria and hindering their spread. The migratory white cells remove bacteria and foreign matter from the injured area.[7]

Indicate the correct response by placing a check in the space provided.

1. An increased blood supply aids by carrying away toxic products ___ or localizing toxic substances at the site of injury. ___
2. The precipitation of fibrin with formation of a clot aids by blocking dissemination of bacteria ___ or permitting bacteria to escape from the inflamed focus through the fibrin meshwork. ___

Step 6. Pain at the site of inflammation is believed to be the result of either injury to the nerve fibers within the inflammatory focus or irritation caused by the release of chemical substances in the tissues. The intensity of pain varies with the extent of the injury, the physical pressure of swelling, or the introduction of pyogenic agents. Thus, while an inflammatory response is provoked in any injury, a small inflamed cut will not produce the same amount of pain as a large wound. Pain may be immediate or delayed, but it is a cardinal symptom of inflammation. Mark the following statements *T* for true or *F* for false.

1. Pain is more intense when there is pyogenic infection. ___
2. The physical pressure of swelling at the site of injury has an effect on pain. ___
3. The extent of injury has a direct bearing on the intensity of pain. ___

Step 7. Edema generally refers to increased volume of extracellular (outside of cells), intravascular (inside of vessels) fluid.[8] This excess localized or generalized accumulation of fluid is within tissue spaces and serous cavities. Swelling or edema is likely to occur in inflammation. It is more marked in soft or spongy tissues, for example, subcutaneous tissues. (See Chapter 9 for further details.)

Mark the following statements *T* for true or *F* for false.

1. Excess localized or generalized accumulation of fluid within tissue spaces and serous cavities is known as edema. ___
2. Edema is not so marked in soft or spongy tissues as it might be, for example, in compact tissues. ___

Step 8. As a review of the signs and symptoms of inflammation, complete the blank with the sign or symptom that corresponds with the description given.

1. Increased blood supply and capillary

   permeability _____
2. Accumulation of fluid in extracellular

   or interstitial spaces _____

3. Sensitization of nerve endings _____
4. Increased temperature of skin around

a wound _____

Step 9. In acute inflammations there is often a purulent or suppurative exudate, called pus. This is made up of a thick fluid of viable and dead white cells and necrotic debris. Another type of exudate, called catarrh, is composed of mucinous secretions and can be found only in organs possessing a mucus-secreting membrane, for example, nose, pharynx, lungs, intestinal tract. In the nose you are familiar with it as the running nose. When coughed from the lungs, it is called sputum.[7]

Complete the blanks in the following statements.

1. If the nasal mucous lining is inflamed,

the discharge is called_____.
2. The mucinous secretions from the

lungs are called _____, which is a catarrhal type of exudate.

Step 10. A severe localized collection of pus caused by suppuration in a tissue, an organ, or a confined space is called an abscess. It is often produced by pyogenic bacteria. It may be deep seated but can burrow to the surface and discharge its contents by rupture.[7, 8]

Complete the blank in the following statement.

A severe localized collection of pus caused by pyogenic bacteria would be

called an _____.

Step 11. An ulcer is a focal defect or excavation of the surface of an organ or tissue. It is produced by sloughing or shedding of inflammatory necrotic tissue. Ulcers are commonly found in focal inflammatory necrosis of the mucous membrane of the mouth, stomach, and intestines and in the subcutaneous inflammations of the lower extremities of elderly people who have circulatory disturbances that predispose to extensive necrosis.[7, 8]

Complete the blanks in the following statements.

1. The sloughing or shedding of inflammatory necrotic tissue in an inflammatory focus of the stomach might

produce an _____.
2. Elderly people with inflamed subcutaneous tissues of the lower extremities and circulatory disturbances predisposing to extensive necrosis are

prone to develop an _____ in these tissues.

Step 12. Both systemic and local white cell response occurs in inflammation, since the leukocyte is the body's first line of defense against unwelcome intruders that might provoke injury. Although the exact mechanism is not known, when an organ or tissue is under attack by injurious influences, white cells mobilize from all over the body and rush to the site of injury. These scavenger cells are called phagocytes because their function is to destroy the harmful inciting agents. The process is called phagocytosis.

Complete the blanks in the following statements.

1. Scavenger cells that attempt to destroy toxins entering the body from

injury are called _____.
2. The process of destruction of the

toxins is called _____.

Step 13. The cells that mobilize for defense against invasion of harmful agents are the leukocytes. A temporary or symptomatic increase of total circulating leukocytes is called leukocytosis.[8] (There is also an increase in circulating leukocytes in leukemia, but the increase is permanent and progressive.) The normal value for both sexes (adult) varies between 5,000 and 10,000 per cubic millimeter.[1] A significant rise above this number occurs in most diseases of an infectious nature. A physiologic increase in the leukocyte count occurs in the first few days of life, during and immediately following strenuous exercise, in anxiety states, and during emotional stress.[5] An increase is also observed at the time of menstruation, in the later months of pregnancy, and during or after labor.[5] These increases, although leukocytosis, are not pathologic. A decrease in the number of leukocytes is called leukopenia.

Complete the blanks in the following statements.

1. The temporary or symptomatic increase of total circulating leukocytes is called _____.
2. A decrease in the number of white cells is called _____.

Step 14. The basic types of white cells that take part in an inflammatory reaction fall into three categories: (1) granulocytic leukocytes (neutrophils, eosinophils, and basophils); (2) lymphocytes; and (3) monocytes (including the large mononuclear phagocytes known as macrophages). The granulocytic leukocytes are called polymorphonuclear leukocytes, deriving their name from the appearance of their nucleus. The procedure for determining the different types of white blood cells and their percentage of the total white count is called the differential count. The key to the type of infection is often reflected in the relative frequency of a particular white cell in the differential count. Usually the increase is in only one type of cell. The name of the principal type of cell so involved is used to indicate the cellular increase, for example, neutrophilic leukocytosis, eosinophilia or eosinophilic leukocytosis, and lymphocytosis. An absolute increase is one in which the total number of any cell per cubic millimeter of blood is increased; a relative increase is one in which only the percentage is increased, because the other types of cells are decreased.[21]

Complete the blanks in the following statements.

1. The three categories of white cells taking part in an inflammatory reaction or response are _____ _____, _____, and _____.

2. The white cells deriving their name from the appearance of their nuclei are called _____ _____; they include three types of white cells as follows: _____, _____, and _____.

3. The procedure for determining the different types of white blood cells and their percentage of the total white count is called _____ _____.

4. The increase in the total number of any cell per cubic millimeter of blood is called _____; when only the percentage is increased because of decrease of other types, it is called _____.

Step 15. Of all the polymorphonuclear leukocytes, the neutrophils are the most important in defense against infection, particularly of the pyogenic type (staphylococcic, streptococcic, pneumococcic, gonococcic, and meningococcic). Neutrophils are the first to arrive at the scene in response to inflammation, and they are the most numerous types found in acute reactions. They comprise about 65% to 75% of circulating leukocytes in normal circulating blood.[1] A significant increase (relative) about 80% is called neutrophilic leukocytosis.[5] The neutrophil is an actively phagocytic cell that can engulf foreign material of a size equal to its cell body. On its death and dissolution valuable enzymes that cause proteolytic digestion of necrotic cells and bacteria are released in the inflammatory focus. This is an important mechanism for the removal of bacteria and other useless refuse.[7] In addition to their role of defense against pyogenic agents, the neutrophils are also increased for lesions that produce tissue injury and necrosis (for example, burns, crush injuries, strangulated hernias, torsion of viscera, and thrombosis of blood vessels with infarct formation). They are also increased following hemorrhage into tissues or serous cavities, and in malignancies when there is necrosis, hemorrhage, and secondary infection.

Neutropenia is a decrease in the number of neutrophils below normal biologic levels for healthy individuals. An absolute decrease would be below 2,000 per cubic millimeter.[5] They may be decreased because of defective formation and delivery or because of a rate of loss or destruction greater than the rate of formation and delivery. Neutrophils are suppressed in certain infectious diseases such as typhoid fever, brucellosis, measles, mumps, hepatitis, poliomyelitis, and malaria. There is neutropenia in some blood diseases such as pernicious anemia, aplastic anemia, lupus erythematosus, and acute leukemia.

Indicate which statements best describe neutrophils.

1. Neutrophils are important in defense against pyogenic infections. ___
2. On their death neutrophils release valuable enzymes that cause proteolytic digestion of necrotic cells and bacteria. ___
3. Lesions that produce necrosis and tissue injury are associated with neutrophilic leukocytosis. ___
4. Neutropenia is a significant decrease ___ or increase ___ in neutrophils.
5. Neutropenia may be a feature in pyogenic infections ___, malaria ___, typhoid fever. ___

Step 16. The eosinophils are normally 1% to 4% of the total white cell count,[1] or from 45 to 400 eosinophils per cubic millimeter of blood. Eosinophilia is said to exist if there is an increase of eosinophils in the peripheral blood greater than 500 per cubic millimeter.[5] Eosinophilic leukocytosis or eosinophilia occurs in a number of diseases, notably in allergies such as asthma, hay fever, urticaria, eczema, angioneurotic edema, and reactions to foreign proteins. An increase may also be indicative of a parasitic infestation, such as trichinosis.

A decrease in eosinophils is called eosinopenia. It occurs in situations of stress (shock, severe burns, blood loss, and severe infections).

Indicate which statements best describe eosinophils.

1. Eosinophils are decreased in bronchial asthma. ___
2. Eosinophils are increased in parasitic infestation. ___
3. Eosinophils are increased in hay fever. ___
4. Eosinophils are decreased in situations of stress. ___

Step 17. The exact role of basophils in the control of inflammation is not clear. Normally they comprise about 1% of the circulating white blood cells.[2] On disintegration they liberate histamine and heparin. They are decreased in situations following stress and after corticosteroid administration.[5] They are increased in chronic granulocytic leukemia, polycythemia vera, and in chronic hemolytic anemias.[2]

Indicate which statements best describe basophils.

1. Basophils are increased ___ or decreased ___ following stress.
2. Basophils are increased in chronic granulocytic leukemia. ___

Step 18. Lymphocytes (large and small) comprise about 20% to 25% of all circulating white cells.[1] They do not appear as a rule until late in an inflammatory process, and they are characteristic of chronic inflammation. An increase of lymphocytes is called lymphocytosis, which may be either physiologic or pathologic. Physiologic lymphocytosis occurs in newborns and small children.[2] Pathologic lymphocytosis occurs in overwhelming infections, in viral diseases, and in nonpyogenic infections such as tuberculosis, typhoid fever, and malaria.[2, 5] Relative lymphocytosis occurs in those diseases in which there is neutropenia. Both absolute and relative lymphocytosis occurs in lymphocytic leukemia, infectious mononucleosis, mumps, whooping cough, and syphilis. In the chronic inflammatory reactions the lymphocytes are the predominant cells.

Lymphopenia is a decrease in lymphocytes. Lymphopenia is likely to occur in conditions marked by neutrophilic leukocytosis, such as acute pyogenic infections. Both relative and absolute decrease in lymphocytes occurs in active tuberculosis and in Hodgkin's disease.[5]

Indicate which conditions best describe the role of lymphocytes in inflammation.

1. Lymphocytes do not appear as a rule until late in an inflammatory process. ___

2. Lymphocytes are increased in chronic inflammation. ___

3. Pathologic lymphocytosis occurs in typhoid fever ___, malaria ___, infectious mononucleosis ___, syphilis ___, newborns. ___

4. Lymphocytes are decreased relatively and absolutely in active tuberculosis. ___

Step 19. Monocytes comprise 3% to 8% of the circulating white blood cells.[1] Monocytosis is an increase in monocytes in the peripheral blood greater than 10%.[5] The neutrophilic leukocytes constitute the initial response to injury but they are followed by the monocytes, or the mononuclear phagocytes (monocytes and macrophages), and lymphocytes. It has been postulated that the monocytes emigrate concurrently with the neutrophils to the site of injury but that they persist after the latter have disappeared and that they later become transformed into tissue macrophages.[8] For this reason the mononuclear phagocytes have been called the body's second line of defense against acute inflammation. Some consider the macrophages found in peripheral blood to be large forms of monocytes.[8] The life history of the monocytes to date has not been fully established.

Monocytosis is a frequent finding in tuberculosis, and in active cases the range may be from 15% to 30%.[5] An increase in monocytes also occurs in various mycotic diseases, rickettsial diseases, virus infections, and disease caused by protozoa. Monocytes are also increased during the recovery and convalescent stages of pyogenic infections.[5]

Indicate the conditions that best describe the behavior of monocytes.

1. Monocytes are phagocytic cells. ___

2. Monocytes are increased in active tuberculosis ___, mycotic diseases ___, rickettsial diseases ___, and diseases caused by protozoa. ___

3. Mononuclear phagocytes are the body's first ___ or second ___ line of defense against infection.

4. Monocytosis occurs during the recovery of convalescent stages of pyogenic infections. ___

Responses

Step 1: 1. inflammation; 2. heat; redness; pain; swelling (list in any order); loss of function (additional symptom)

Step 2: 1. there is an increased blood supply; 2. plasma escapes because capillary walls are more permeable; 3. the abnormal accumulation of blood in an injured part results in congestion

Step 3: 1. T; 2. F; 3. T; NOTE: In 1. macrophages are present in some tissues, but for the most part this is "true."

Step 4: 1. X; 2. X; 4. X; 6. X

Step 5: 1. carrying away toxic products; 2. blocking dissemination of bacteria

Step 6: 1. T; 2. T; 3. T

Step 7: 1. T; 2. F

Step 8: 1. heat and redness; 2. edema; 3. pain; 4. heat

Step 9: 1. catarrhal; 2. sputum

Step 10: abscess

Step 11: 1. ulcer; 2. ulcer

Step 12: 1. phagocytes; 2. phagocytosis

Step 13: 1. leukocytosis; 2. leukopenia

Step 14: 1. granulocytic leukocytes, lymphocytes, monocytes (including macrophages); 2. polymorphonuclear leukocytes; neutrophils; eosinophils; basophils; 3. differential count; 4. absolute; relative

Step 15: 1. X; 2. X; 3. X; 4. decrease; 5. malaria; typhoid fever

Step 16: 2. X; 3. X; 4. X

Step 17: 1. decreased; 2. X

Step 18: 1. X; 2. X; 3. typhoid, malaria, infectious mononucleosis, syphilis; 4. X

Step 19: 1. X; 2. X, X, X, X; 3. second line; 4. X

REFERENCES

1. Anthony, C. P., and Kolthoff, N. J.: Textbook of anatomy and physiology, ed. 9, St. Louis, 1975, The C. V. Mosby Co.
2. Bauer, J. D.: In Frankel, S., Reitman, S., and Sonnenwirth, A. C., editors: Gradwohl's clinical laboratory methods and diagnosis, ed. 7, St. Louis, 1970, The C. V. Mosby Co. (white blood cell pathology).
3. Bostwick, W. L.: Oral Surg. 2:425, 1949 (vascular-cellular dynamics of inflammation).
4. Dible, J. H.: Ann. R. Coll. Surg. Engl. 6:120, 1950 (inflammation and repair).
5. Diggs, L. W.: In Miller, S. E., editor: A textbook of clincal pathology, ed. 7, Baltimore, 1966, The Williams & Wilkins Co. (diseases primarily affecting leukocytes).
6. Haley, H. B., and Williamson, M. B.: Surg. Clin. North Am. 42:15, 1962 (wound healing).
7. Robbins, S. W.: Pathology, ed. 3, Philadelphia, 1967, W. B. Saunders Co. (inflammation).
8. Wilhelm, D. L.: In Anderson, W. A. D., editor: Pathology, ed. 6, St. Louis, 1971, The C. V. Mosby Co. (inflammation and healing).

CHAPTER 4

Repair and regeneration

The terms *repair* and *regeneration* are not synonymous, but both refer to healing. Repair is the replacement of damaged tissue by connective tissue; regeneration is the replacement of a single type of cell by proliferation of its type or kind.[7]

When a tissue or organ is injured, nature makes a valiant effort to heal the defect. This effort is not always successful, but nevertheless a number of protective measures are initiated when there is even a small threat of danger to any of the body parts through injury.

In modern medicine we are prone to think of recovery from a disease or surgery as coming only from the beneficial influences and measures instituted by humans through therapy. This is certainly true to a great extent, since therapeutic measures are helpful in almost all diseases to bring about complete recovery or to prolong life. We forget, however, to give credit to the body's own inherent ability to overcome disease or injury or at least to put up a fight for its own existence. A surgeon may remove an organ or part whose existence is a threat to life, but he cannot heal the wound that results; this is the exclusive property of the tissue cells. Otherwise, all that would remain of the surgeon's efforts would be a gaping hole or incisional wound that would not heal and would remain a real threat to life. Manmade machines or devices can function efficiently only so long as breakdowns can be repaired by able mechanics. The body has its own repair shops, which diligently attempt to correct all disorders that handicap its efficient functioning. The physician treating any disease relies upon this factor, so the success of restoration to health becomes a teamwork between the doctor and the body's inherent ability to fight for its own survival.

In the preceding chapter you have learned about nature's first and second lines of defense, the neutrophils, monocytes, and macrophages. You have also learned about the role of the lymphatic supply and blood supply in draining and resorbing the inflammatory exudate or blocking the dissemination of harmful materials to structures beyond the site of injury. The mere removal of these harmful invaders, however, cannot restore the tissues to normalcy, particularly if the cells have been damaged in the attack. Nature then must have some other method to restore the preexistent status quo of tissues that are injured and also to restore the cells that are worn out through normal usage. Replacement is accomplished by the ability of the tissues through proliferation of their cellular components to replace the dead or damaged cells with healthy cells. Specifically it guarantees the continuity of life through the replacement of cells dead or damaged by normal wear and tear.

The reconstructive phase for tissues damaged through disease or injury is closely bound to the inflammatory response, since it begins during the active phase of inflammation. It can only be completed after all injurious influences have been neutralized or removed from the seat of injury. The new healthy cells are derived from either the parenchyma or from the connective tissue stroma of an organ. The parenchyma comprises the essential or functional elements of an organ, for example, the organ cells. The stroma forms the ground substance or framework of an organ, for example, the connective and fibrous tissue supporting the functioning cells. Whether an organ or tissue will be reconstituted to its former normal structure with functions unimpaired depends upon which type of cells (parenchymal or stromal) were active in the process. If the healing of a damaged organ or tissue is accomplished solely by the proliferation of the parenchymal elements, a perfect or near perfect reconstitution of the original structure may result. On the other hand, if the connective tissue stromal elements of an organ are called upon to repair a defect, the result will be fibrosis or scarring. Replacement of an organ or part by fibrosis is usually undesirable, since the scarring is permanent and function may be impaired. It is therefore obvious that the most important factor in the repair or reconstitution of an injury lies in the inherent capacity of the parenchymal cells of a tissue to regenerate and thus to replace the old worn-out or damaged cells with healthy new ones.[6, 7]

Not all the cells of the body have the same capacity for regeneration. The functioning cells in the brain, for example, are incapable of proliferation and therefore cannot restore damaged parenchymal cells. When a neuron or nerve cell is lost in the central nervous system, it is gone forever. Wounds of either the brain or the spinal cord are repaired by proliferation of the cells of their stroma (the glial-supporting tissue),[1] but usually the result is fibrosis as in other tissues, particularly muscles. The peripheral nerve tissues cannot regenerate unless the neurilemma is present.

There are many parenchymal cells in the body that under normal physiologic circumstances continue to multiply throughout life replacing worn-out or destroyed cells.

The examples of this are the epithelial surfaces throughout the body—skin, oral cavity, vagina, cervix, uterus, respiratory tract, excretory ducts, and urinary tract. In these organs the surface cells exfoliate or drop off continually throughout life, but the integrity of the epithelium is not lost, since there is a constant replacement of discarded cells with new healthy ones. This same capacity to replace cells with new ones is evident in the healing of injury. Consequently, when epithelial cells are lost through injury, perfect restoration may occur by regeneration of the marginal preserved functional or parenchymal cells. A good example of the capacity of epithelial cells to regenerate and to replace desquamated (shed) cells is the shedding of the endometrial lining of the uterus during menstruation. There is a prerequisite for the growth of newly replaced parenchymal cells, and this is the persistence of the underlying supporting tissue (stroma). An underlying framework or supporting stroma for the parenchymal cells must be present to permit healing.[3] When there is a deep ulcer or abscess, the new cells from the marginal epithelium cannot grow across the defect until there is a suitable supporting surface. This is accomplished by the filling in of the defect with a granulation tissue to form a support for the cells.[4, 5]

The cells of lymphoid and hematopoietic systems (blood-forming organs) are also capable of regeneration. For example, the life of a red blood cell is about 120 days, and it is replaced by a new cell in healthy individuals at the end of its life-span. Bone marrow cells are a good example of active proliferation throughout life.[6, 7]

Many glands of the body are made up of cells capable of regeneration but that do not ordinarily multiply vigorously throughout life, although retaining a latent capacity to do so if spurred to proliferate under appropriate stimulation. These include the cells of the liver, pancreas, salivary glands, endocrine glands, and kidney tubules as well as the sweat and sebaceous glands of the skin. The skin glands and hair shaft follicles, however, are usually totally destroyed in deep skin wounds and extensive burns. The epithelium may be reconstituted, but the loss of hair and secretions of the glands is permanent.

Also included among the cells capable of regeneration but that do not multiply repeatedly throughout life for physiologic reasons are the fibroblasts (fibrous tissue cells), osteoblasts (bone), and chrondroblasts (cartilage). The process of bone reconstitution is sometimes referred to as knitting, which is the physiologic process of healing a fracture.[6]

However, if a major gland such as the liver is completely destroyed, this is usually incompatible with life, and there would be no possibility of regeneration.[6, 7]

PROCESS OF HEALING

As stated previously, reconstructive activities begin soon after the initiation of an inflammatory response. First, there is removal of the inflammatory exudate by drainage or resorption followed by regeneration of parenchymal elements when possible.[1, 3] In some instances this may be all that is necessary to complete the repair of damage. However, if the damage to cells or tissues is severe or extensive, the stromal elements may be called upon to make a contribution concomitant with that of the parenchymal elements. This form of healing occurs in connective tissue by the proliferation of fibroblasts and capillaries. This proliferation of fibroblasts and capillaries creates an actively growing, highly vascularized connective tissue known as granulation tissue.[4, 6] Granulation tissue fills the gap of a wound or surgical incision and provides the necessary supporting framework or stroma for the advancement of epithelial elements from the margins of the wound to fill the gap.[2] The granulation tissue may be the sole reparative effort, or it may be parallel with the regeneration of parenchymal elements when possible. When tissue damage is extensive involving both the parenchymal and stromal elements, a scar or fibrosis will form that is permanent.[3] Fibrosis or scarring always occurs when permanent cells are destroyed, as in deep skin wounds. The steps of healing in a wound are amply illustrated and explained in Fig. 4-1.

CONDITIONS MODIFYING HEALING

The adequacy of healing is governed by the conditions under which it occurred. In general these are the same factors that modify inflammatory response, such as the physiologic condition of the host—his age and state of health. Nutrition is extremely important in healing of damaged tissue, since a great demand on body stores of nutrients is exerted. These nutritional factors are a diet adequate in carbohydrates, proteins, and vitamins. Vitamin B complex is necessary for maintaining cellular integrity and enzymatic functions. Vitamin A is important in maintaining epithelial structures, and vitamin K is necessary for clot formation.[4, 5]

The importance of the blood supply in tissue healing cannot be overestimated, for it is the blood that brings in oxygen, nutrients, immune substances (antibodies), and defensive cells. In addition, tissue fluid and deoxygenated venous blood may accumulate in tissue because of the inability of the circulation to carry away these substances. This is a deterrent to the healing processes. Adequate circulation and drainage are also important for carrying away bacteria, foreign bodies, and tissue necrotic debris. Persistence of infection and inflammatory exudate slow or block the healing process.[2, 4]

The immobilization of wound margins, as in fractures and soft tissue wounds and surgical incisions, speeds up healing. This lessens the gap between the margins of the wound or fracture and provides a firm base for the repair processes.[6]

The extent of injury and the type of tissue involved are also important factors in healing. Perfect restoration cannot take

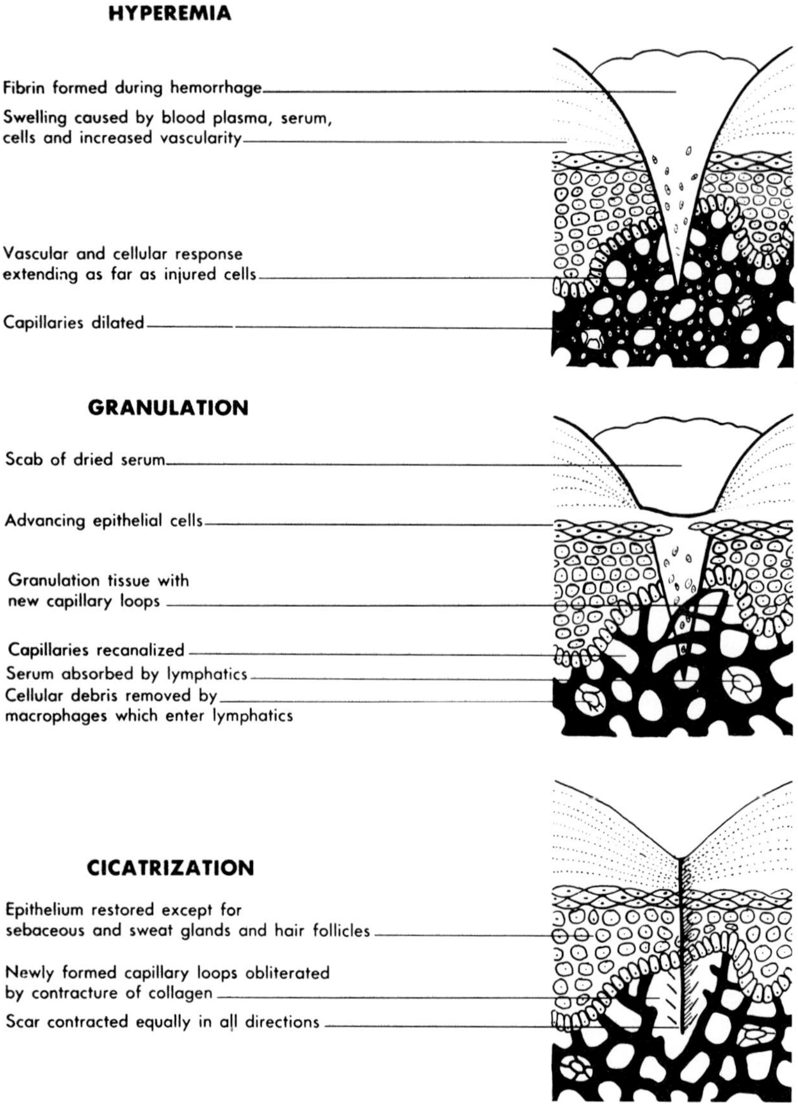

HYPEREMIA

Fibrin formed during hemorrhage

Swelling caused by blood plasma, serum, cells and increased vascularity

Vascular and cellular response extending as far as injured cells

Capillaries dilated

GRANULATION

Scab of dried serum

Advancing epithelial cells

Granulation tissue with new capillary loops

Capillaries recanalized

Serum absorbed by lymphatics

Cellular debris removed by macrophages which enter lymphatics

CICATRIZATION

Epithelium restored except for sebaceous and sweat glands and hair follicles

Newly formed capillary loops obliterated by contracture of collagen

Scar contracted equally in all directions

Fig. 4-1. The stages in wound healing are overlapping. By the fourth day, however, fibroplasia has begun, and by the end of two weeks healing usually is completed. Bleeding occurs immediately after the wound has been made. Clotting in the wound and capillaries is caused by fibrin. **HYPEREMIA,** This vascular and cellular response may be caused by a chemical substance and by local axonal reflex. Tissues react by increasing the blood supply to the involved part and by attracting phagocytic cells. **GRANULATION,** Capillaries have been recanalized and have grown across into granulation tissue. Plasma and serum are absorbed by the lymphatics. Epithelium is advancing across granulation tissue under the protection of the scab. The epithelium is at first one cell layer thick. Stratified squamous epithelium develops from these epithelial cells. **CICATRIZATION,** Contraction occurs in length, width, and depth. (After Berman, J. K.: Principles and practices of surgery, St. Louis, 1950, The C. V. Mosby Co.; from Therap. Notes **71:**71, March, 1964, Parke, Davis & Co.)

place when permanent cells have been destroyed. However, regeneration of parenchymal cells cannot always reconstruct a perfect replacement of large areas of damaged tissue, and the result is scarring or fibrosis.[1, 6]

The important concepts to remember in the outcome of an inflammatory and reparative response are as follows: (1) Not all injuries will result in permanent damage. Some will resolve or be followed by regeneration with a relatively perfect replacement of damaged tissue. (2) The usual residual of tissue damage is fibrosis or scarring, which is most often the ultimate outcome of the reparative process.[1, 6]

This has been a rather lengthy discussion of repair and regeneration, but it is important to your understanding of the end result of many injuries or diseases. If you understand something of the principles of the repair and regeneration of tissue, it is easier to understand temporary or permanent impairment of the organs in disease or injury.

STEP-BY-STEP EXERCISES

Step 1. Restoration of destroyed tissue is by the replacement of dead or damaged tissue cells by new healthy cells derived from either the parenchymal or stromal connective tissue elements of the tissue involved. Parenchyma means the essential or functional elements of the organ, for example, the organ's functioning cells. Stroma means the framework or supporting elements.

On the lines to the left write *parenchyma* or *stroma*, whichever matches the description that follows.

1. _____ functional or essential elements of a tissue

2. _____ framework or supporting elements of a tissue

Step 2. Healing of an injury with stromal connective tissue elements and healing with parenchymal tissue elements differ in their effects on the reconstitution of the damaged tissue. If healing is by parenchymal elements, a perfect or near perfect reconstitution of the organ's functions will result. If, on the other hand, the major part of the healing process is contributed by the stromal elements through fibroblastic proliferation, the result will be scarring or fibrosis, with loss forever of the parenchymal reserve cells. Function will be impaired and the tissue permanently damaged in that it will not be an exact replica of the preexisting tissue before damage.

Mark the following statements *T* for true or *F* for false.

1. Reconstruction of the organ will be perfect or near perfect if healing is by parenchymal elements. ___

2. Reconstruction of the organ will be perfect or near perfect if healing is by stromal elements. ___

3. Fibroblastic repair of damaged tissue will result in permanent scarring or fibrosis. ___

4. Fibrosis is a temporary repair that will later be replaced by new healthy tissue. ___

Step 3. Mitosis or division of cells is necessary for reproduction. Not all the cells of the body are capable of reproduction or regeneration. These include the nerve cells (neurons) of the central nervous system and the muscle cells. Epithelial cells of the skin and those lining the digestive, respiratory, reproductive, and urinary tracts continue to regenerate through life.

Mark the following statements *T* for true or *F* for false.

1. Epithelial tissue cannot regenerate. ___

2. Nerve cells can regenerate. ___

Step 4. Cells of glandular organs, such as the liver and pancreas, and those of the endocrine system are less capable of regeneration than are epithelial cells. The lymphoid tissues, as well as the hematopoietic organs or tissues, are also capable or regeneration; for example, bone marrow cells are in active proliferation throughout life.

Indicate the appropriate verb in the following statements.

1. Bone marrow cells can ___ cannot ___ be replaced by regeneration in the healthy individual.
2. Cells of glands—liver, pancreas, or endocrine organs—are ___ are not ___ capable of regeneration.

Step 5. You may refer to the text or to Steps 3 and 4 to answer the following questions. Your answer will depend upon your knowledge of which tissues are capable of regeneration to the extent that no permanent impairment of function or structure, or both, is involved in injury or disease. In the following conditions the cells of the organs or tissues have been destroyed or damaged.

Mark *No* if the tissue cannot be restored to its former normal state before disease or injury. Mark *Yes* if the cells will regenerate and no permanent injury or impairment will result.

	No	*Yes*	
1.	___	___	Severance of the spinal cord by trauma
2.	___	___	Deep penetrating wound of the abdomen
3.	___	___	Extensive skin burn involving sweat and sebaceous glands
4.	___	___	Minor sunburn of the skin
5.	___	___	Shedding of the endometrial lining of the uterus during menstruation
6.	___	___	Cancer of the lung
7.	___	___	Nasal mucosa following a cold
8.	___	___	Extensive destruction of brain cells by gunshot wound

Step 6. At the site of a deep cut a blood clot normally forms that is both a protective device to stop hemorrhage and an aid to formation of a framework for migration of cellular components from the margins of the wound to fill the gap and to speed repair.

Indicate the factors conducive to repair.

1. Clot formation ___

2. Uncontrolled hemorrhage ___
3. Advance of cells from the marginal parenchyma to fill the gap of the wound ___

Step 7. A surgical incision causes the death of cells in the initial path of the cutting scalpel as well as death of underlying connective tissue elements. The incision is closed by sutures to bring the margins in apposition. The narrow space between the apposed tissues is filled later with a blood clot that seals the defect. This is called healing by first intention or union by intention.[6]

Complete the blank in the following statement.

The blood clot that seals the gap between sutured apposing margins in a surgical incision brings about healing by _____ _____.

Step 8. In a surgical procedure where the loss of cells is extensive because of a large tissue defect and the marginal edges of the defect cannot be apposed (such as occurs in deep abscesses, inflammatory ulcerations, or infected surgical incisions), the parenchymal cells cannot regenerate or are inadequate to fill the gap. Vascularized connective tissue (granulation tissue) grows in from the margins to fill the gap. This is called secondary healing or union or healing by second intention.[6]

Complete the blanks in the following statements.

1. The vascularized connective tissue that grows in to fill a gap when parenchymal cells from the margin cannot bridge the defect is called _____ tissue.
2. In a deep abscess in which the marginal edges of the defect are not apposed the type of healing that takes place is known as _____ _____.

Step 9. Study the information given in Steps 7 and 8 and then complete the following by indicating the appropriate adjective.

1. You have had an appendectomy that

was simple and uncomplicated. The edges of the incision have been apposed. Would the incision be healed by primary ___ or secondary ___ intention?

2. Suppose in another abdominal operation there is a complication of extensive peritonitis and a drain tube has been left in the incision for removal of necrotic material. Would the healing of the incision be likely to occur as primary ___ or secondary ___ union of apposing margins of the wound?

Step 10. The adequacy of blood supply to an injured tissue is important not only for initial protective measures in the inflammatory response but also to speed healing by removal of foreign debris.

In which of the following disorders would you expect healing to be slower than normal or not to occur at all?

1. Gangrene of the feet in an older diabetic person ___
2. The uninfected wound of a young healthy individual ___
3. A wound in an older person in which foreign debris has accumulated and venous circulation is inadequate to carry it away ___

Responses

Step 1: 1. parenchyma; 2. stroma
Step 2: 1. T; 2. F; 3. T; 4. F
Step 3: 1. F; 2. F
Step 4: 1. can; 2. are
Step 5: 1. No; 2. No; 3. No; 4. Yes; 5. Yes; 6. No; 7. Yes; 8. No
Step 6: 1. X; 3. X
Step 7: first intention or union by intention
Step 8: 1. granulation; 2. secondary healing or healing by second intention
Step 9: 1. primary; 2. secondary
Step 10: 1. X; 3. X

REFERENCES

1. Altemeier, W. A., and Stevenson, J. M.: In Davis, L., editor: Christopher's textbook of surgery, ed. 7, Philadelphia, 1960, W. B. Saunders Co.
2. Berman, J. K.: Principles and practice of surgery, St. Louis, 1950, The C. V. Mosby Co.
3. Edwards, L. C., and Dunphy, J. E.: N. Engl. J. Med. **259:**224, 1958 (wound healing).
4. Haley, H. B., Jr., and Williamson, M. B.: Surg. Clin. North Am. **42:**15, 1962 (repair of wounds).
5. Hartwell, S. W.: The mechanisms of healing in human wounds, Springfield, Ill., 1955, Charles C Thomas, Publisher.
6. Robbins, S. L.: Pathology, ed. 3, Philadelphia, 1967, W. B. Saunders Co.
7. Wilhelm, D. L.: In Anderson, W. A. D., editor: Pathology, ed. 6, St. Louis, 1971, The C. V. Mosby Co. (inflammation and healing).

CHAPTER 5

Abnormalities in cell structure

Developmental defects or derangements in cell structure, existing before birth or acquired later, may materially affect the function of an organ. The developmental anomalies existing at birth are discussed in Chapter 15.

Cellular derangements may be quantitative or qualitative. The quantitative derangements represent variations from normal in size and number of the cells. This type of abnormality in cell structure affects the size of an organ or tissue. Qualitative derangements represent cellular abnormalities of growth in individual cells. These include the changes in cells observed by microscopic examination of tissues—metaplasia, dysplasia, and anaplasia. They are not diseases in themselves, and their significance in relation to disorders is a matter of interpretation by the pathologist. It is worthy of note, however, that anaplasia is an important morphologic change significant of malignancy. In anaplasia, adult cells regress toward the more primitive cell types.[1, 2]

The quantitative derangements in cells include atrophy, aplasia, hypoplasia, hypertrophy, and hyperplasia. All these terms practically define themselves when you consider that *a* means not; *trophy* means nourish; *plasia* means form; *hypo* means under; and *hyper* means over.[3]

Atrophy is an acquired defect that is regressive and results from a decrease in cell size or a decrease in the total number of cells or both. It may be physiologic, affecting the size of an organ in the normal aging process, such as atrophy of the uterus, or it may be atrophy of the thymus gland at about the time of puberty. When atrophy is pathologic, it refers to the decrease in size of tissue or organs as a result of disease.

Atrophy can result from disuse,[1, 3] as may occur when immobilizing devices (braces, casts) are applied to a structure, or from an interruption of innervation, as occurs in poliomyelitis. In all these cases there is wasting away of the muscles.

In vascular atrophy the blood supply to an organ or tissue has been reduced to such an extent that the cells of the affected organ or tissue have been deprived of nutrition and oxygen. They then undergo progressive loss of substance. Pressure atrophy and vascular atrophy may both be caused by impairment of blood supply.[1, 3] Narrowing of blood vessels is most often caused by arteriosclerosis, but it may result from pressure such as a tumor. Other tissues and organs may be affected by the pressure atrophy that occurs in such conditions as skeletal deformities and aneurysms.

When an endocrine organ, such as the adrenal, pituitary, or thyroid, is overworked for a long period of time, it may first respond with hypertrophy; and later the functional elements diminish and atrophy results.[3] If the pituitary gland, which is the master of all endocrine glands, fails to elaborate specific trophic hormones for these organs, they will atrophy.

Aplasia or agenesis is the congenital absence of an organ. The term is also used when an organ is represented only by a rudimentary structure that bears little resemblance to a normal organ. If there are twin organs, such as the kidneys, the normal one may be able to carry the load in case of a missing or rudimentary organ.[3]

Hypoplasia is the failure of an organ to reach full adult size. It is much less severe than aplasia, since enough of the functioning cells may be present for an organ or tissue to carry out its intended purpose.[3]

Hypertrophy is an increase in volume of tissues or organs by enlargement of their existing cells. It differs from hyperplasia in that no new cells are added. In hyperplasia the organ or tissue enlarges through the addition of new cells. Hypertrophy and hyperplasia may both be present in an organ or tissue. Hypertrophy is most often observed in the tissues or organs of the body in which the cells are incapable of reproduction, as in the muscular tissues. The enlargement of the heart is a good example. Cardiac hypertrophy may occur in any type of disorder that places an added burden upon the heart to pump blood against resistance. This condition occurs in some congenital heart anomalies and in diseases that result in aortic stenosis (narrowing of the aortic valves). Compensatory hypertrophy of the heart is also often observed in hypertension and pulmonary disorders such as emphysema and fibrosis. The individual muscle fibers may also increase markedly in size in the muscles of athletes. This is often seen in professional wrestlers and boxers. When one kidney is missing congenitally or surgically or is only rudimentary and nonfunctioning, the other kidney may increase in size because of the extra workload. The uterus is an exception to the rule that smooth muscles cannot reproduce, for in pregnancy it enlarges through the increase of muscle fibers and the formation of new muscle cells. Many organs, such as the endocrine glands, enlarge in size because of an increase of the size of existing cells (hypertrophy) and the addition of new cells (hyperplasia). An overproduction of hormone can cause an increase in size of the body, as observed in pituitary giantism, and underproduction of growth hormone will cause dwarfism. Enlargement of the breasts in pregnancy is the effect of stimulation by hormones and is considered a normal physiologic reaction.[1, 3]

STEP-BY-STEP EXERCISES

Step 1. Using the text for a reference, match the cellular abnormalities given on the left with the description on the right by placing the letters A, B, C, D, and E in the spaces provided.

1. Aplasia ___
2. Atrophy ___
3. Hyperplasia ___
4. Hypertrophy ___
5. Hypoplasia ___

A. Decrease in size of organ tissue
B. Increase in size of organ or tissue caused by additional cells
C. Increase in size of organ or tissue caused by growth of existing cells
D. Congenital underdevelopment of an organ
E. Congenital absence of an organ

Step 2. From information given in the text, complete the blanks with the proper cellular abnormality of structure.

1. Enlargement of the heart because of overload of work _____
2. Congenital rudimentary nonfunctioning kidney _____
3. Decrease in size of uterus with aging _____
4. Abnormal increase in the number of cells in the endometrial lining of the uterus _____
5. Physiologic involution of thymus gland at puberty _____
6. Absence of one kidney at birth _____

7. Congenital dwarfed but still functioning testis _____

8. Enlargement of an organ because of an increase in size of existing cells _____ plus an increase in number of cells _____

9. Enlargement of one kidney after removal of the other _____

10. Wasting of muscle caused by immobilization _____

11. Wasting of muscle as a result of innervation _____

12. Decrease in size of an endocrine gland because of lack of hormone supply _____

Responses

Step 1: 1. E; 2. A; 3. B; 4. C; 5. D

Step 2: 1. hypertrophy; 2. aplasia; 3. atrophy; 4. hyperplasia; 5. atrophy; 6. aplasia; 7. hypoplasia; 8. hypertrophy; hyperplasia; 9. hypertrophy; 10. atrophy; 11. atrophy; 12. atrophy

REFERENCES

1. Anderson, W. A. D.: In Anderson, W. A. D., editor: Pathology, ed. 6, St. Louis, 1971, The C. V. Mosby Co. (degenerative changes and disturbances of metabolism).
2. Cowdry, E. V.: Arch. Pathol. 30:1245, 1940 (properties of cancer cells).
3. Robbins, S. L.: Pathology, ed. 3, Philadelphia, 1967, W. B. Saunders Co. (cellular abnormalities).

CHAPTER 6

Neoplasms

Neoplasm is a term derived from the Greek words *neos,* meaning new, and *plasma* meaning formation. Although neoplasm is the term generally used in medical circles to indicate a pathologic overgrowth of tissue, you are possibly more familiar with the term *tumor* to designate such a growth. The neoplasms or tumors are divided into two main groups—benign and malignant. Benign growths are usually harmless (except brain tumors), and most are eradicated by surgery or other means. A malignant growth is often called a cancer—a general term to cover all such growths. Cancer in Greek means crab, which is descriptive of the disorderly growth of tumors. The malignant growths are harmful abnormalities and rank second as the cause of death in the United States, heart disease being first. Because of cancer's incidence, prevalence, and mortality rates, which are climbing yearly, its etiology or cause is the subject of widespread research. Although some light has been shed on the cause of some malignancies, such as those produced by radiant energy or certain irritants, by and large the reason why cells suddenly start growing in a bizarre, haphazard way distorting the structure and function of organs or systems remains a mystery. All tumors, whether benign or malignant, represent a wide departure from normal morphology and growth. These cellular changes can occur in almost all the tissues. Anaplasia, as mentioned previously, is a morphologic change seen in malignant tissue growth.[23]

It is impossible to describe each tumor, benign or malignant, that occurs in the body. Complete textbooks have been devoted to the study of tumors. Since neoplasms represent cellular or tissue changes that occur in almost all tissues and since there are noted variations according to tissue of origin and so on, only the general principles that more or less apply to all of them as a group can be covered here. A table has been included for reference to tissue of origin and site of the major tumors, benign and malignant (Table 1). A few specific neoplasms have been selected for further discussion at the end of this chapter. It is hoped that you will be able to apply the general principles to these specific tumors as well as to others that are not discussed.

BENIGN TUMORS[18, 23]

Generally the term *oma,* meaning tumor, is attached as a suffix to the name of the cell of origin in benign tumors. For example, a tumor arising from fibrous tissue elements is called a fibroma; one with glandular tissue origin is called an adenoma; one with osseous origin is called an osteoma; and so on. When it is necessary to use a term that will be more descriptive of a benign tumor, other more specific combining terms become a part of the word. For example, the smooth muscle tumor is called a leiomyoma, with *leio,* meaning smooth, added to *myoma,* meaning muscular tumor. However, a number of benign tumors will not fit conveniently

Table 1. Classification of tumors[*]

Tumors	Benign	Malignant
Connective tissue and derivatives		
Fibrous tissue	Fibroma	Fibrosarcoma
Myxomatous tissue	Myxoma	Myxosarcoma
Fatty tissue	Lipoma	Liposarcoma
Cartilage	Chondroma	Chondrosarcoma
Bone	Osteoma	Osteogenic sarcoma
Notochordal tissue	Chordoma	Chordosarcoma
Endothelial and related tissues		
Blood vessels	Hemangioma	Angisarcoma
Lymph vessels	Lymphangioma	Lymphangiosarcoma
	Lymphangioendothelioma	Lymphangioendotheliosarcoma (Kaposi's sarcoma)
Synovia	Synovioma	Synoviosarcoma
Mesothelium (lining cells of body cavities)	Mesothelioma	Mesothelialsarcoma
Brain coverings	Meningioma	
Blood cells and related cells		
Hematopoietic cells		Granulocytic leukemia
		Monocytic leukemia
Lymphoid tissue		Malignant lymphomas
		Lymphocytic leukemia
		Multiple myeloma (plasmacytoma)
Reticuloendothelial systems		Reticulum cell sarcoma
		Malignant lymphoma, histiocytic type; Hodgkin's disease ?
Muscle	Myoma	
	Leiomyoma	Leiomyosarcoma
	Rhabdomyoma	Rhabdomyosarcoma
Tumors of epithelial origin		
Stratified squamous	Squamous cell papilloma	Squamous cell or epidermoid carcinoma basal cell carcinoma
Skin and adnexa	Nevi	Melanoma
	Sweat gland adenoma	Sweat gland carcinoma
		Sebaceous gland carcinoma
Epithelial linings		
Ducts and glands	Adenoma	Adenocarcinoma
	Papilloma	Papillary carcinoma
	Papillary adenoma	Papillary adenocarcinoma
	Cystadenoma	Cystadenocarcinoma
		Medullary carcinoma
Respiratory epithelium		Bronchogenic carcinoma
Renal epithelium	Renal tubular adenoma	Renal cell carcinoma (hypernephroid)
Liver cells	Liver cell adenoma	Liver cell carcinoma or hepatoma
Bile ducts	Adenoma	Carcinoma (cholangiocarcinoma)
Urinary tract (transitional)	Transitional cell papilloma	Papillary carcinoma
		Transitional cell carcinoma
		Squamous cell carcinoma
Placental	Hydatid mole	Choriocarcinoma
Mixed tumors	Mixed tumor of salivary gland	Malignant mixed tumor of salivary gland
Renal anlage		Wilms' tumor
Compound (more than one neoplastic cell type derived from more than one germ layer)	Teratoma, dermoid	One or more elements malignant, i.e., squamous cell carcinoma arising in teratoma

[*]From Robbins, S. L.: Pathology, ed. 3, Philadelphia, 1967, W. B. Saunders Co., p. 90.

into this classification or description. These are tumors derived from epithelial elements. This tissue is widespread throughout the body, and there is no clear-cut anatomical or other specific designation of tissue that will adequately describe them. Thus this type of tumor is called an epithelioma, and the site is further designated in the description used in diagnosis. Epithelioma, however, is usually a term applied to malignant tumors of the skin or cervix. Some benign tumors have fingerlike projections seen when examined under the microscope. These have been designated papillomas (papilloma meaning projection). When a term is needed to describe a tumor that has both a papillary and cystic appearance, the word papillary becomes part of the description or diagnosis, followed by the name of the tumor. For example, a cystadenoma arising in glandular tissue would be called a papillary cystadenoma if a combination of these patterns were present.

MALIGNANT TUMORS[18, 23, 40]

Malignant tumors usually follow the same method of designation of origin as the benign tumors but with some notable exceptions to further describe their characteristics of origin. Malignant tumors of mesenchymal tissue origin or from its derivatives, such as muscles, bone, tendons, cartilage, fat, vessels, lymphoid and connective tissue, are called sarcoma (from the Greek word *sarkos*, meaning flesh). When it is necessary to further clarify their origin, other more specific terms are added. For example, a sarcoma of bone would be called an osteogenic (osseous origin) sarcoma; one arising from lymph nodes, spleen, or bone marrow, whose cells are in close contact with the reticulum (network) of the tumor, would be called a reticulum cell sarcoma; one arising from fibrous tissue would be called a fibrosarcoma. And thus through a number of combinations the right term is found to describe a specific tumor.

The malignant tumors of epithelial origin are called carcinoma, and this designation should be used only where such tissue exists.[23] This term, however, is sometimes used erroneously to apply to all malignant tumors. When a further description is needed to specify the particular type of epithelium involved, such as that lining glands that have secreting elements, the word adenocarcinoma is used. The term adenocarcinoma for a tumor can further be expanded by adding the type of cell involved, such as renal cell adenocarcinoma (kidney tumor), or the involved organ can be named, such as adenocarcinoma of the stomach.

In some malignancies more than one type of cell may be involved. These are so-called mixed tumors, or they may be referred to as being pleomorphic (from the Greek words *pleon*, meaning more, and *morph*, meaning form).

By studying Table 1 you can further identify the origin of many malignant tumors.

CHARACTERISTICS OF TUMOR GROWTH[18, 23]

The rate of growth of benign and malignant tumors differs widely. As a rule the benign tumor grows slowly. Malignancies, on the other hand, tend to grow rapidly. Both types, however, are progressive in that they will continue to grow throughout life. Some of them have periods of remission following specific therapy or from other obscure reasons and tend to remain stationary. However, unless a tumor is completely eradicated, the old pattern will persist and growth will be reinstituted after remissions. Benign tumors tend to remain localized, whereas malignancies tend to spread throughout an organ. Benign tumors are usually enclosed in a capsule, which accounts for their tendency to be stationary and also for the fact that they are movable on palpation. Exceptions to this rule, however, are the leiomyomas, which are demarcated but not encapsulated. The nevi, which are pigmented tumors in the skin, and the angiomas, which are tumors of blood vessel origin, are other examples of unencapsulated growths. A capsule, on the other hand, is almost never found enclosing a malignant growth. Malignant tumors are invasive, both eroding and infiltrating the tissues around the original focus as they spread to involve an entire organ and adjacent structures.

Metastasis (from the Greek words *meta,* meaning beyond, and *stasis,* meaning stand) is the ability of tumors to spread beyond the original site or to transfer cells from one organ to another. The secondary growths or nodules at some distance from the original or primary site of the tumor are called metastases. An example of a malignant tumor that usually or almost always remains in one location is the benign basal cell carcinoma of the skin. The nodules produced by metastasis closely resemble those of the cell or tissue of origin (the primary focus). It is not always possible, however, to locate the primary site. For example, adenocarcinomas of the stomach, colon, pancreas, or similar tissues all have glandular elements; therefore a secondary spread from this original site will not pinpoint which of the organs was primarily involved. If, however, the metastatic nodules are from a malignant tumor noted for its particular cellular elements, such as a renal cell carcinoma of the kidney or a thyroid carcinoma that has acini and colloid present, the origin can be more readily identified through these elements.[23]

The usual pathways for dissemination of tumor cells are through the venous, arterial, and lymphatic channels as emboli (broken-off fragments of the primary tumor), through serous cavities, through hollow structures such as the ureters and bronchi, and, rarely, through contact with an apposing structure.[18, 23]

The most common route of dissemination is through the lymphatic vessels. Generally the carcinomas metastasize this way, but the sarcomas favor the venous route. Once tumor cells have gained entrance to lymphatic vessels, the emboli may be carried to a regional lymph node or nodes or they may form a continuous growth within the vessel. In the lymph nodes the cells multiply and eventually invade the pulp of the node and the stroma and then gradually replace the node with a tumor growth. When the primary site of a malignancy is known, the sites for metastases can at times be predicted or surmised. For example, a breast cancer often metastasizes to the axillary nodes. The regional lymph nodes are often the site of metastases in cancer of the prostate, cervix, stomach, rectum, sigmoid, and colon.[18, 23]

As mentioned previously, sarcomas favor spread through the blood channels, but carcinomas may also metastasize in this manner, and this is particularly true of carcinomas of the lung, breast, kidney, prostate, and thyroid gland. The cancer cells from a primary site invade blood vessels as detached tumor emboli or as single cells or at times as cellular aggregates of various sizes. The liver is often the site of metastasis from transport of tumor cells through vascular channels of organs that empty into the portal veins. Metastasis in the lungs often occurs from transport of tumor cells or emboli from primary sites of tumors in organs whose vascular channels empty into the systemic veins. Arterial metastatic spread is hampered by the resistance of the thick walls of arteries to penetrance of tumor emboli. The transport of tumor emboli in either the lymphatic vessels or blood channels may be hampered by obstruction in either of these routes. When the route of the tumor emboli is altered, metastasis may occur in a distant or unusual site.[18, 23]

Transplantation of malignant growth can occur in the body cavities, such as the peritoneum, where the cells break away from one site and transplant in another. A malignant tumor may also be accidentally transplanted to other exposed tissue during surgery by mechanical transference of cells adhering to instruments.

Table 2. Tumor characteristics*

Characteristics	Benign tumor	Malignant tumor
1. Structure and differentiation	Structure often typical of tissue of origin	Structure often atypical, i.e., differentiation imperfect
2. Mode of growth	Usually purely expansive and a capsule formed	Growth infiltrative as well as expansive so that strict encapsulation is absent
3. Rate of growth	Growth usually slow; mitotic figures scanty, and those present are normal	Rapid with many abnormal mitotic figures
4. Progression of growth	Progressive, slow growth may come to a standstill or retrogress	Growth rarely ceases; often rapid and usually progressive to a fatal termination
5. Metastases	Absent	Frequently present

*From Robbins, S. L.: Pathology, ed. 3, Philadelphia, 1967, W. B. Saunders Co., p. 103.

A table of tumor characteristics is included for your reference (Table 2). A careful study of this table will give you valuable criteria in distinguishing between benign and malignant growths.

ETIOLOGY AND PATHOGENESIS[18, 23, 39]

The development of tumors has no one cause. There are a number of initiating or contributing factors, some of which are known. Heredity is believed to play a role in development of some tumors. For example, retinoblastoma of the eye is believed to result from inheritance of a defective gene. Certain tumors of endocrine organs, called multiple endocrine adenoma syndrome, have a tendency to develop on a familial basis. Familial states or conditions that predispose to the development of cancer are multiple polyposis of the large intestine, xeroderma pigmentosum (inherited hypersensitivity to ultraviolet light), and neurofibromatosis (multiple pedunculated soft tumors distributed over the entire body).

Physical agents that lead to the production of cancer include ionizing radiation, which may cause cancer on the hands and other exposed areas of workers in radiation. The malignancy usually results from disregard of safety regulations governing radiation exposure or from accidental overexposure. Overexposure to ultraviolet rays is a factor in the development of skin cancers, particularly among farmers and other workers who spend long hours in sunlight.

Chemists have synthesized several hundred pure chemicals that produce cancer in animals. These chemical carcinogens include many types of compounds that act in different ways. Whereas some produce cancers at the site of contact, others cause cancer at distant sites. Some are weak and require other chemicals, called promoting agents or cocarcinogens, to induce tumors.[39]

Few people are exposed to the high concentrations of chemicals used in laboratories, but there are environmental hazards that are gaining widespread attention and investigation as causes or possible causes of cancer. There are potential hazards in combinations of chemicals and crude products to which people are exposed in large numbers. These combinations include food additives, cosmetics, insecticides, and drugs, as well as smoke and residue of all kinds encountered in industrial and consumer air pollutions. Among human cancers that are conceded to be caused by industrial exposure are: cancers of the bladder in aniline dye workers who handle beta-naphthylamine; bone cancer from swallowing radium; lung cancers resulting from inhalation of chromium compounds, radioactive ores, asbestos, iron, and arsenic; cancer of nasal sinuses and the lung in nickel mine workers; and skin cancers caused by handling some products of coal, oil shale, petroleum, and lignite. These hazards to which industrial groups may be exposed have some implications for the general population. The air may contain impurities, and if these are laden with cancer-producing substances, prolonged exposure to them can lead to cancer. Smoking of cigarettes has been implicated in causing lung cancer; however, the health hazards of smoking are not limited to cancer but also include bronchitis, emphysema, and heart disease. Cancers of the oral cavity are associated with cigar smoking and lip cancers with pipe smoking.[39]

The virus as a possible cause of cancer is under extensive investigation, but the results are still inconclusive for production of cancer in humans. Chronic irritation has been blamed for production of cancers, notably those in the buccal mucosa in relation to a jagged tooth or ill-fitting dentures.[18]

It is not known whether tumors arise from a single cell undergoing mutation or whether they arise from a community of cells that develop an abnormal growth pattern.[18] The exact method by which the multiple and complex factors bring about the irreversible changes in cellular metabolism that result in tumor are still unknown.[18]

SYMPTOMS[18, 23]

The symptoms of cancer can mimic those of many diseases. Pain may not occur until after the tumor has become quite large and invasive and there is impingement on nerves.[18] Loss of weight and cachexia or wasting of musculature and malnutrition are not contsant features, and they may occur in other diseases, notably tuberculosis and Addison's disease. Cachexia in cancer has a number of causes, such as hemorrhage, ulceration, infection, and necrosis in a tumor, as well as the anxiety state of the patient.

Some tumors of endocrine organs, both benign and malignant, produce specific effects in hormone production that are recognizable in certain endocrine diseases and clinical syndromes. These alterations in hormone production may point to the existence of a tumor in an endocrine organ. There are some inconstant effects produced by tumors in the alteration of certain enzymes, serum proteins, and coagulability of the blood, but these are not specific enough to be reliable.[18]

Abnormal bleeding or passage of blood is a danger signal that may indicate cancer, but again there are a number of diseases in which this occurs. An extensive investigation should be made to rule out a malignancy. The blood may be passed in vaginal discharges, urine, vomitus, sputum, and feces.

The appearance of a lump or lumps in the breast may be caused by cancer. Other indications of cancer might be a sore that will not heal, a persistent cough, dyspnea, indigestion or difficulty in swallowing, and a change in bowel or bladder habits.

All these signs and symptoms should be investigated immediately, for if a cancer is discovered before local invasion and spread, there may be a chance for cure or at least prolongation of the patient's life. The signs and symptoms of cancer are further discussed in the section of this chapter devoted to specific neoplasms.

DIAGNOSIS OF TUMORS

Biopsy is a widely used procedure for detection of malignant cells in tissues. It is a reliable source of identification of malignant cells and is often used prior to more definitive surgery. A biopsy is a small piece of tissue or other material removed for microscopic examination.

Sometimes when the patient is undergoing surgery, a piece of tissue is removed by the surgeon and submitted to the pathologist for study. The tissue is first frozen and then cut by a microtome into thin slices that are stained. This is called a frozen section. It is a speedy type of examination, since the report on whether the tissue is malignant can be given to the surgeon within a short time. This type of examination is often performed in surgery of breast lesions that are suspected to be malignant and when there is a question as to whether the surgeon should perform a radical mastectomy (removal of breast and axillary lymph nodes).

Another procedure widely used, especially for detection of malignant cells in vaginal secretions, is the cytologic examination or smear. This is often referred to as the Papanicolaou examination,[21] after its discoverer. It is also used for examination of secretions from other areas of the body such as respiratory, intestinal, and urinary tracts. The findings are usually classified on a graded basis from class I through class V. Classes I and II are considered benign; class II is suspicious but not diagnostic and warrants repetition of the test for further identification; class IV is highly suspicious of malignancy; class V is considered to be malignancy.[21]

The x ray is an invaluable diagnostic tool for detection of tumors.[41] Special radiographic procedures using contrast media to opacify organs are used to pinpoint obstructive lesions in the gastrointestinal, respiratory, and urinary tracts.[41] These obstructions may prove to be tumors. Diagnosis of bone tumors is often made on x-ray examination, which ranks second to the actual biopsy of these tumors as the most important single means of identification of lesions. These are several special radiographic procedures for locating intracranial lesions and discovering the extent of compression or distortion of parts of the brain. Often the findings of a routine chest x-ray examination will reveal lesions that warrant further study on the basis of suspected malignancy.

The use of radioisotopes (radiopharmaceuticals) in the diagnosis of diseases is a new modality in modern medicine.[41] It is based on the principle that radioisotopes can be traced through the body by sensitive instruments such as the Geiger counter or scintillation counter, which counts the number of telltale rays given off by the radioactive atoms moving through the body or congregating at various points. Radioisotopes are used to detect the existence of a tumor (for example, in the brain, liver, kidney, or thyroid) or to give information about its size and location.

Ultrasonic scanning or ultrasonography has proved successful in diagnosis of space-occupying lesions in intraperitoneal or retroperitoneal locations.[27] The ultrasonic beam is sensitive to the difference between acoustics and interference. An ultrasonic beam passing from one type of tissue into another will usually produce an echo. This allows for mapping of the boundaries of a pathologic lesion. Solid tumors because of their internal heterogenicity produced by blood vessels, ducts, or connective tissue stroma, usually give rise to echoes. On the other hand, fluid-containing hematomas or cysts are much more homogeneous and do not give rise to internal echoes. It is therefore possible to distinguish between a solid mass and a collection of fluid.[27]

NOTE: As a preliminary to the study of tumors and as an aid in identifying their site and origin, as well as other characteristics, the following list of combining forms relating to tissues, fluids, cells and other body substances is given. Not only will this information prove invaluable in the study of tumors, but also some terms can be applied to infections and many other disorders that will be discussed later.

Adeno—gland
Angio—vessel
Astro—star-shaped nerve cell
Blast—germ cell
Chondro—cartilage
Cyst—sac
Cyte—cell
Fibro—fibrous
Hem, hemato—blood
Leiomyo—smooth muscle
Lipo—fat

Lympho—lymph
Melano—black pigment
Meningo—meninges
Myo—muscle
Myxo—mucus; slime
Neuro—nerve
Osteo—bone
Retino—retina
Sarco—flesh

STEP-BY-STEP EXERCISES

Step 1. Neoplasm means a new growth. In this sense it means a growth that is not normally a part of the body structure. Neoplasms, therefore, are overgrowths of the existing tissues of the body, which may have a disorderly and sometimes bizarre arrangement of cells, resulting from wild proliferation of the existing cells. Tumors or neoplasms will always fall into two types —malignant (harmful) and benign (usually not harmful except in the brain).

Complete the blanks in the following statements:

1. An overgrowth of tissue independent of its surrounding structures with no physiologic value called _____.

2. The two types of tumors are _____ and _____.

3. The harmful type of tumor is _____; the type that is usually not harmful is _____.

Step 2. Tumors involve the structure and function of organs. The cellular changes found in tumors may occur in almost all tissues with notable variations according to the tissue of origin. The term *oma* means tumor, and its use in medical terminology will be in this connection.

Complete the blank in the following statement.

The suffix attached to other medical combining forms to designate a tumor is

_____.

Step 3. Refer to the preceding list of combining medical terms and using the suffix *oma*, give the names of the benign tumors that match the following definitions.

1. _____ Tumor of the bone

2. _____ Tumor of the muscle

3. _____ Nerve tumor

4. _____ Fibrous tissue tumor

5. _____ Tumor with fatty elements

6. _____ Blood vessel tumor

7. _____ Tumor of lymph tissue

Step 4. Refer to the list of combining medical terms or to Table 1. In this response it will be necessary to combine more than one of the terms with the suffix *oma* to identify the tumors described below, for example, neuroblastoma (neuro meaning nerve + blast meaning germ + oma)—a nerve tumor derived from primitive germ cells.

1. _____ Tumors with fibrous and sarcomatous elements

2. _____ Smooth muscle tumor

3. _____ Tumor with both cartilaginous and sarcomatous elements

4. _____ Tumor with osseous and cartilaginous elements

5. _____ Tumor with osseous and sarcomatous elements

6. _____ Tumor arising in lymphatics with sarcomatous elements

7. _____ Carcinoma of glandular origin

8. _____ Osseous tumor deriving from primitive germ cells

9. _____ Tumor arising from retinal germ cells

10. _____ Tumor consisting of melanoblasts
11. _____ Angioma containing fibrous tissue
12. _____ Cystic and adenomatous tumor

Step 5. The rate of growth, mode of growth, destruction of tissue, and vessel invasion differ widely in benign and malignant tumors. Refer to Table 2 and complete the following blanks with _benign_ or _malignant_.

1. Rapid growth _____

2. Slow growth _____

3. Little tissue destruction _____

4. Infiltrative _____

5. Encapsulated _____

6. Unencapsulated _____

7. Invasion of blood vessels _____

8. No invasion of blood vessels _____

Step 6. Metastasis is the ability of tumors to spread beyond the original site or to transfer cells from one organ to another. The secondary nodules or growths, which may be at some distance from the original or primary focus, are called metastases. Benign tumors do not metastasize, although metastases are frequently present in malignancy.

Complete the blanks in the following statements.

1. The process by which the spread of tumor cells is possible is called

   _____.

2. Secondary nodules or growth of tumor cells are referred to as _____.

3. Tumors that do not metastasize are called _____.

4. Secondary tumor nodules found at some distance from a primary tumor site are from a _____ tumor.

Step 7. The characteristic pathways for metastatic dissemination are venous, arterial, and lymphatic channels, or direct transplantation. Carcinomas tend to metastasize through the lymphatics. Sarcomas are more prone to favor the venous route. It is easier for tumor cells to invade the venules and veins than the arteries because of the thick walls of the latter. The usual method of transport through vessels is by tumor emboli, which are detached tumor cells.

Complete the blanks in the following statements.

1. Metastases from a sarcoma are more likely to spread through _____ channels.

2. Carcinoma of the breast is more likely to spread through _____ channels.

3. Detached tumor cells carried in vessels are called _____.

Step 8. A small piece of tissue or other material removed for microscopic examination to determine malignancy is called a biopsy. Cytologic examination of smears of body fluids, such as sputum, vaginal, breast, and prostate secretions, and gastric washings, is called a Papanicolaou smear, after its discoverer. During a surgical procedure for removal of organs a piece of tissue is often removed and sent to the pathology laboratory or department for immediate examination when there is a question of malignancy. This is called a biopsy for frozen section.

Complete the blanks in the following statements by indicating the type of examination performed.

1. A routine vaginal smear is called a

   _____ _____.

2. A single lump in a breast is to be removed for carcinoma, and tissue from an axillary lymph node is submitted for _____ _____ while the patient is still under anesthesia in the operating room.

3. A patient is believed to have a malig-

nant tumor or metastasis of the liver; a piece of tissue is removed for examination and this is called a _____.

4. A smear of vaginal secretions was class IV, and a piece of tissue was later removed from the cervix for examination. The vaginal smear was a _____ _____; the piece of tissue was a _____.

5. A man was suspected of having a malignancy of the prostate gland, and fluid was removed for a _____ _____.

Step 9. Mark the verb in the following statements that best typifies present knowledge of the pathogenesis or etiology of tumors.

1. All cancers are __ or are not __ caused by viruses.
2. Cancers can __ or cannot __ be familial.
3. Chronic irritation has __ or has not __ been implicated in cancers of the mouth from ill-fitting dentures.
4. Overexposure to ionizing radiation can __ or cannot __ cause cancer.
5. Overexposure to ultraviolet rays can __ or cannot __ be the cause of skin cancers.

Step 10. Indicate the conditions that might be indicative of cancer.

1. Abnormal bleeding from an organ __
2. Passage of blood in urine, sputum, vomitus, or feces __
3. Coughing from minor upper respiratory infection __
4. Skin lesions that heal without subsequent breakdown and bleeding __
5. A palpable lump in the breast __

Step 11. Complete the blanks in the following statements.

1. Organs are opacified with a _____ _____ to pinpoint an obstruction that might be a tumor.
2. _____ can be traced through

the body by sensitive instruments to detect tumors or give information as to their size and location.

REPRESENTATIVE NEOPLASMS FROM VARIOUS ORGANS
Uterine and cervical neoplasms[11, 29]

The neoplasms considered here are divided into those that occur in the neck of the uterus, in the cervix, and in the body of the uterus proper.

Carcinoma in situ literally defines itself as cancer confined to one location. It occurs most often in younger patients. This tumor develops in the squamous epithelium along the surface of the cervix without stromal invasion. It is usually discovered by random biopsy, by endocervical curettage, or from a suspicious cytologic vaginal smear. Since it is a local tumor, it is responsive to treatment, usually by surgical intervention.

Squamous cell carcinoma of the cervix is the most common form of genital cancer in women. (See Figs. 18-3 and 18-28, *C*.) It occurs more frequently in women between the ages of 40 and 60 years who have borne children.[11] It usually develops at the junction of the squamous and columnar epithelium and is an infiltrative tumor. It may extend into the pelvic wall, vagina, bladder, rectum, and above the pelvic brim and may spread by the lymphatics. The mortality rate is high in untreated patients, within the first 3 years after discovery, since regional lymph node involvement may have occurred before the time of clinical recognition.[29]

Adenocarcinoma of the cervix originates in the endocervical glands and mucosa anywhere from the internal os to the external os. (See Figs. 18-3 and 18-28, *C*.) It occurs more frequently in unmarried patients than does the squamous cell type. This tumor is first confined to the cervix and then invades the adjacent portions of the uterus. It next involves the adnexa uteri and infiltrates the parametrial tissue, including the rectum or the bladder or both. The

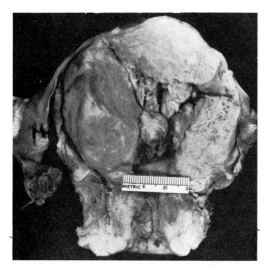

Fig. 6-1. Carcinoma of endometrium. (From Hertig, A. T., and Gore, H.: In Anderson, W. A. D., editor: Pathology, ed. 6, St. Louis, 1971, The C. V. Mosby Co.)

average age of patients is 50 years, but the range is from 17 to 80 years.[11]

Endometrial carcinomas, those arising from the endometrium (Fig. 6-1) of the uterus, are usually glandular and are only about one third as common as cervical carcinomas, with an age range from the third to the ninth decade, the peak being the sixth decade.[11, 29] They occur more commonly in unmarried persons and married nulliparous persons or those with few children. The spread of endometrial carcinoma is slower than that of cervical cancer. It tends to invade the uterine wall and later to involve the parametrial structures. It may metastasize to the ovaries and elsewhere in the peritoneal cavity. Distant sites of metastases are the lungs and liver.

Bleeding is the most common symptom of uterine cancer, occurring between menstrual periods of patients in this age group and after the menopause in the older group. This is not invariable, however, since some cancers that have been detected did not present this symptom. Enlargement of the uterus is a late symptom, as are pain and fixation.

Metastases from distant sites may involve the uterus. These are usually from pelvic viscera, with the most common metastatic endometrial tumor being from a primary focus in the ovary. Metastatic tumors of the uterus from extrapelvic sites are most commonly from the breast and stomach, but in this connection it must be remembered that these latter organs have a high incidence of cancer.

Fibroids or *leiomyomas* (smooth muscle tumors) are the most common benign neoplasmas of the uterus. (See Fig. 18-3.) Their incidence is greater in the black than in the white race.[11] They may occur anywhere within the uterus, being subserosal, intramural, or submucosal. They may be pedunculated and may lose their attachment to the uterine wall and become parasitic on a neighboring organ through adhesions. Twisting on their pedicles causes strangulation and pain. Degenerating fibroids or leiomyomas may become necrotic and are prone to become inflamed. Leiomyomas are multiple as a rule and are well demarcated from the surrounding muscle. The symptoms are pressure or bleeding, enlargement of the uterus, and anemia if bleeding has been profuse or prolonged.

Cervical polyps arising from the endocervical mucosa are common (Figs. 18-3 and 18-28, *C*). They may be multiple or single and are pedunculated. They are more common in women between 40 and 50 years of age who have borne children. They have a low potential for malignancy. Bleeding may be severe. In the younger group they may cause sterility by blocking the cervical canal.[29]

Breast neoplasms[9, 16, 23]

Cancer of the breast may occur in both sexes and may affect either breast or accessory breast tissue. The incidence is far greater in women than in men. Carcinoma of the breast has an incidence nearly twice that of malignancy at any other site in women. The lesion occurs most commonly near, during, or shortly after menopause. In older patients, past the menopause, a

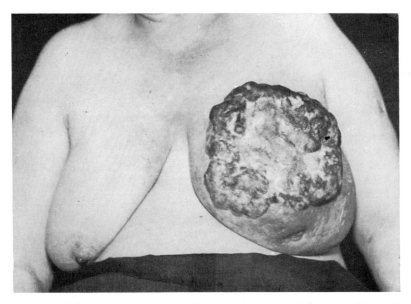

Fig. 6-2. Advanced fungating carcinoma of breast of 6 months' duration. (From Meissner, W. A., and Warren, S.: In Anderson, W. A. D., editor: Pathology, ed. 6, St. Louis, 1971, The C. V. Mosby Co.)

single lump in the breast is in all probability a cancer. It is more common in single women, nonparous women, or those who have married late in life; this suggests that the role of unopposed estrogen activity during a long reproductive period is an important factor. However, as in most cancers, the etiology is not completely known.

The tumor arises frequently in the upper outer quadrant of the breast from the epithelium of the duct system. Most of the tumors are adenocarcinomas, but other types are comedo, mucinous, acute inflammatory, papillary, medullary carcinomas, and Paget's disease of the nipple. All of them are of the infiltrating type (Fig. 6-2).

The symptoms are variable according to type. Any lump in the breast that is not movable but is fixed to breast structures is suspicious for malignancy. In contrast, benign lesions are usually freely movable. Another presenting symptom is nipple retraction or dimpling of the skin. The axillary lymph nodes may also be palpable. In Paget's carcinoma of the nipple the red, granular, crusted, or eczematous appearance of the nipple is often noted before a definite mass is palpated. Late symptoms are edema, skin infiltration, ulceration, peau d'orange (dimpling of skin caused by lymphatic edema; also called pigskin), and a bloody or watery discharge from the nipple.

Women are being urged to perform a periodic self-examination to determine if there is a lump or lumps in the breast. The early discovery of a lump that proves to be malignant often spells the difference between life and death. This self-examination is of such importance that the National Cancer Institute, Bethesda, Maryland 20014, distributes a free leaflet, Public Health Service Publication No. 48, which through diagrams describes how a woman can examine the breasts for possible lumps. The American Cancer Society has been foremost in the promotion of breast self-examination and has made available not only literature but movies as well.

Thermography is a new method for breast cancer detection, which relies on infrared (IR) sensing techniques. But as

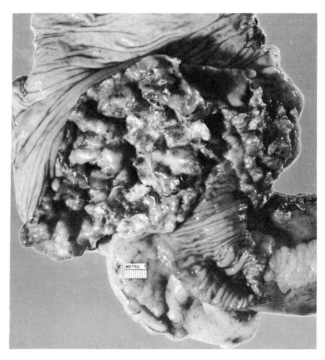

Fig. 6-3. Characteristic bulky, ulcerated carcinoma of right side of colon (in cecum). (From Horn, R. C., Jr.: In Anderson, W. A. D., editor: Pathology, ed. 6, St. Louis, 1971, The C. V. Mosby Co.)

a technique it has been somewhat disappointing. However, x-ray mammography has now been developed into a fairly reliable tool for the discovery and diagnosis of small, early carcinomas of the breast.

The principal route for metastasis is the lymphatic channels, with the axillary lymph nodes showing the greatest involvement, but the lower cervical chain, the supraclavicular and infraclavicular lymph nodes, as well as the intercostal, retrosternal, and mediastinal routes may also be involved. These latter routes are often involved with cancer in the medial and lower quadrants of the breast. Occasionally the opposite breast becomes involved by extension. The multiple nodular skin metastases of the chest wall are known as cancer *en cuirasse,* meaning cancer about the skin of the thorax. Metastases to the viscera occur most commonly in the lungs and pleura (Fig. 6-11), but the liver, bone, brain, adrenals, and spleen may also be involved, in this order of frequency.

Gastrointestinal neoplasms

Cancer of the colon and rectum.[13, 20, 23, 30] Cancer of the large intestine is second only to carcinoma of the lung as the leading cause of death from cancer in the United States. Cancer of the colon (Fig. 6-3) is more frequent in women, whereas cancer of the rectum has a higher incidence in men. The age group is mainly those between 50 and 70 years, but it has been reported in children. (See Fig. 18-1, *F.*)

The cause is unknown. Statistical evidence, however, has indicated a relationship between cancer of the colon and chronic ulcerative colitis and congenital or familial polyposis. (See Figs. 16-2 and 18-11.) If ulcerative colitis has been of long standing (10 years or more), there is a higher incidence of cancer of the colon associated with this lesion. Congenital polyposis intestinalis is hereditary. In this condition, multiple polyps in the colon and rectum have a distinct tendency to become malignant. About three fourths of the cancers of the large intestine occur in the rectum and sigmoid colon. Their occurrence in these locations presents a more favorable prognosis than do those occurring in other sites of the large intestine, since they can be detected by sigmoidoscopy or rectal examination in the early stages.

The symptoms are variable according to location of the tumor and stage of development but are more or less persistent. Often the first symptom is a change in bowel habits, which may be constipation or diarrhea, followed by abdominal discomfort and weight loss. Later there may be blood, mucus, or both in the stools, and pain. When there is occult bleeding, anemia results. Because of the tumor's growing circumferentially around the intestine, the lumen is narrowed, causing dilatation and hypertrophy of the proximal colon, which later progresses to partial or complete obstruction of the bowel.

Colonic carcinomas break through the intestinal wall by local invasive growth and from there are spread by the lymphatics and the venous bloodstream. When there is venous spread, however, there is usually well-established extensive growth of the tumor with lymphatic involvement.

Barium enema is the principal method of detection of colon cancer other than sigmoidoscope and colonoscope, which provide direct observation.[20] Recently, fiber colonoscopy (examination of the entire colon by fiber optics) has proved helpful in detection of colon cancer. If treated early, cancer of the colon is highly curable and about 71% of patients have a 5-year survival rate after surgery of localized disease.[20]

Stomach cancer.[13, 31] For the past several decades the incidence of carcinoma of the stomach (Fig. 6-4) has been decreasing. This is particularly true in the United

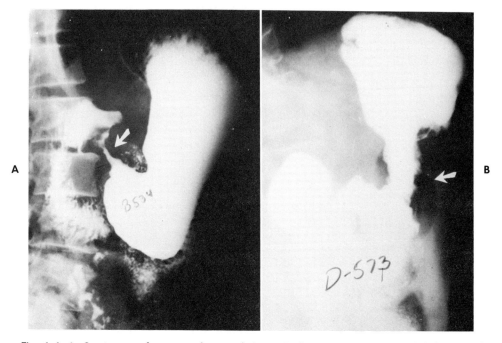

Fig. 6-4. A, Carcinoma of antrum of stomach (arrow), showing narrowing and deformity of the antrum. **B,** Adenocarcinoma of body of stomach (arrow). (From Young, C. G., and Likos, J. J.: Medical specialty terminology, x-ray and nuclear medicine, St. Louis, 1972, The C. V. Mosby Co.)

States. The incidence is higher in men than in women, and in the United States it is higher in nonwhite than in white persons.

The cause is unknown, but there has been much speculation that diet and preparation and preservation of food are contributing factors.

Most cancers of the stomach arise from the muscus-secreting cells. All parts of the stomach may be the seat of cancer, but the antrum or the greater curvature is the most common site (Fig. 6-4, A). The ulcerative types have a predilection for areas near the greater curvature and the pylorus. The less malignant types grow more in the lumen of the stomach, whereas others are more invasive and penetrate the gastric wall. As a rule the fungating type arising in the region of the cardioesophageal junction becomes extensive locally with lymph node involvement before giving any symptoms. A diffuse spreading type is known as linitis plastica, in which the wall of the stomach is thickened more or less uniformly with fibrous tissue production, giving the shrunken stomach a leather bottle appearance.

The symptoms of cancer of the stomach are prone to mimic those of any less serious digestive illness. The first symptoms may be vague digestive discomfort following a meal, later progressing to pain. Other prominent symptoms that develop late are blood in the stool, vomiting of blood, rapid weight loss, generalized weakness, and anemia. At the time most of the symptoms occur, the malignant tumor may have been present for a number of months and already have invaded adjacent lymph nodes and spread to other organs, such as the liver or lungs. Good prognosis depends upon early detection. These include blood counts, analysis of acidity of stomach, and radiographic contrast media studies as well as gastroscopy.

Metastasis to lymph nodes along the curvatures of the stomach is frequent, with extension into other nodes in the region. Metastatic spread to the left supraclavicular lymph nodes by way of the thoracic duct may be one of the first symptoms in some types. When the tumor is located high in the stomach, the spread to the esophagus and mediastinal lymph nodes is a prominent feature. Occasionally the pulmonary lymphatics and bone marrow may be permeated; this is an early manifestation. Metastasis to the liver occurs from invasion of the tributaries of the portal venous system. Peritoneal spread and carcinomatosis may also occur. Carcinoma of the stomach, as well as other gastrointestinal cancers, may metastasize early to ovaries, so that the ovarian tumors, called Krukenberg tumors, dominate the clinical picture.

Diagnosis of cancer of the stomach may be made by roentgenographic studies and fluoroscopy following a barium meal. These studies reveal the tumor as a filling defect and also disclose areas of rigidity, and ulceration and deformity of the mucosa. Gastroscopy (visualization of the lesion with instruments equipped with optical means and gastrocamera) is an adjunct to barium meal studies. Cytologic studies of gastric washings may reveal suspicious malignant cells. Palpation of the stomach may reveal a mass. Laboratory studies of the blood show a hypochromic, microcytic anemia in the majority of patients. Fecal studies show occult blood in about 45% of the patients.

Carcinoma of the esophagus.[13, 22] Carcinoma of the esophagus (Fig. 6-5) ranks next to carcinoma of the colon and rectum and carcinoma of the stomach in frequency among the gastrointestinal malignancies. In the United States and the United Kingdom it comprises about 2% of all cancer deaths. It is about twice as common in men than in women, and the great majority of the patients are over 50 years of age. The etiology is unknown, but a correlation has been suggested between sideropenic dysphagia (for example, Plummer-Vinson disease in which a web is formed that bridges the lumen in the proximal esophagus) and carcinoma of the esophagus.[22] More than half the esophageal carcinomas arise in the midthird portion of the esophagus. They usually extend by local invasion and lymphatic spread. Tumors in the lower third may extend into the stomach; those in the upper third may invade the trachea; those in the middle third may extend into the bronchi, lungs, and major vessels and nerves. The lymph nodes' involvement includes those in the mediastinum and in the left gastric and celiac groups. Hematogenous spread may involve the liver, lungs, bones, and kidneys.

One of the most prominent clinical manifestations is dysphagia, which is caused by full circumferential involvement of the esophagus. Pain is not remarkable in the early stages, but later it may be dull or burning in the xiphoid and epigastric areas. Patients also complain of bad taste, bad breath, and constant thirst. When the esophagus is obstructed, regurgitation of food and liquids may occur. Severe bouts of coughing occur when the tumor has extended into the trachea or bronchi. When the phrenic nerve and diaphragm are involved by metastases, there may be unremitting hiccups.

The diagnosis is made chiefly by radiographic techniques using barium swallow and fluoroscopic observation (Fig. 6-5). Esophagoscopy may be performed to obtain a biopsy of the mucosal lesion. Cytologic studies may be made of esophageal washings. The 5-year survival rate after surgery is low. The carcinoma is usually well established before discovery.

Cancer of accessory digestive organs

Carcinoma of the liver.[7, 14] There is a striking difference in the incidence of hepatic carcinoma (Fig. 6-6) in various parts of the world. It is not as prevalent in the United States and Europe as it is in Southeast Asia and some areas of Africa.[14] In Europe and the United States it is more prevalent in the age group between 40 and 60 years, with males predominating.[14]

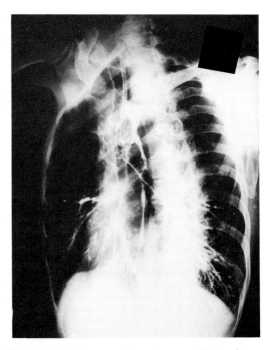

Fig. 6-5. Carcinoma of esophagus with tracheoesophageal fistula (oblique view). Carcinomas of the esophagus usually extend to involve the full circumference of the esophagus and often invade the trachea. (From Young, C. G., and Likos, J. J.: Medical specialty terminology, x-ray and nuclear medicine, St. Louis, 1972, The C. V. Mosby Co.)

In Africa the average group is nearer to 30 years.[14] It may occur in infancy. This type of cancer rarely arises in the absence of cirrhosis, but it is not known how cirrhosis predisposes to carcinoma of the liver. When it does occur in the absence of cirrhosis, women are affected equally with men, but their life expectancy is usually less than 6 months. Carcinoma of the liver has also been found in association with hemochromatosis.

Hepatic carcinoma usually arises from hepatic cells, but it may be of bile duct origin. Primary carcinoma of the liver is either massive, nodular, or diffuse. The right lobe is more often affected in the massive and nodular types. In infants and children, liver cell carcinomas with rare exceptions arise in noncirrhotic livers, and

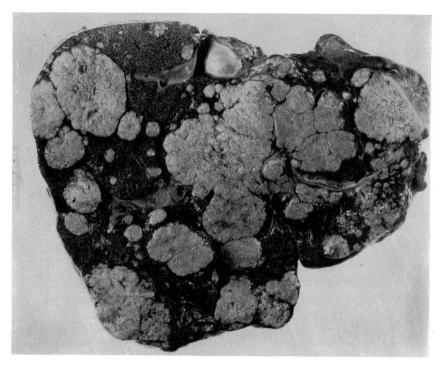

Fig. 6-6. Carcinoma of liver—large metastatic nodules from primary carcinoma of stomach. (From Edmondson, H. A., and Peters, R. L.: In Anderson, W. A. D., editor: Pathology, ed. 6, St. Louis, 1971, The C. V. Mosby Co.)

a high percentage of the patients have congenital defects.[7] Bile duct carcinoma is known to occur in patients who have had Thorotrast injections for liver studies.[7]

Clinically there is an enlarging abdominal mass, pain in the right upper quadrant, loss of weight, ascites, and a vascular bruit heard over the tumor. Hypoglycemia may be a manifestation. The changes in liver function include an elevation of serum alkaline phosphatase level and sulfobromophthalein retention.

Secondary carcinomas of the liver are as a rule metastatic from primary sources in the lung, gastrointestinal tract, and breast (Fig. 6-6). The metastatic cancer usually involves both lobes of the liver, which is enlarged and easily palpable. Abdominal pain and jaundice are presenting symptoms. Jaundice, however, does not usually develop until there has been massive enlargement of the liver.

Diagnosis is made by angiograms after injection of an iodine compound into the hepatic artery, by needle biopsy, and by scintiscans following injection of colloidal gold.[41] Needle biopsy is particularly useful in diagnosis of secondary carcinoma (metastatic) of the liver.

Carcinoma of the pancreas.[15, 17] Carcinoma of the pancreas is not a common neoplasm, but it ranks fourth among fatalities from malignancies in the United States. It is rare before the age of 40 years, and most patients are over 60 years. It is more prevalent in men. Most of the carcinomas of the pancreas arise in the ductal epithelium, with the head of the pancreas being involved more often than the body and tail. The tumor may extend directly to invade the duodenum. Carcinomas of the head of the pancreas may invade the common bile duct, producing obstruction. Obstruction of the common bile duct is a late complication in carcinoma of the body or tail of the pancreas. Metastases occur most frequently in the regional lymph nodes, liver, lungs, peritoneum, and adrenals.

Pain is the most common symptom.[15] (See Fig. 18-22, *F*.) It may be colicky and located in the upper right quadrant of the abdomen, or it may be a steady, dull pain in the midepigastric region radiating to the back, or it may be paroxysmal near the umbilicus and extending over the back, anterior chest, and abdomen. The invasion of the perineural lymphatics accounts for the abdominal pain.[15] Jaundice is the next most common symptom, particularly in patients with carcinoma of the head of the pancreas with obstruction of the common bile duct. Complaints include anorexia, weight loss, nausea, and vomiting. When the lesion has extended to involve the stomach or duodenum, occult blood may be found in the feces. Multiple venous thromboses may be associated with carcinoma of the pancreas, with the iliac and femoral veins being most often involved. The course of the disease is usually one of swift progression to death after onset of symptoms, with the majority dying within a year after discovery of the carcinoma.

Physical examination discloses a hard liver, distended gallbladder, jaundice, tenderness or resistance in the upper part of the abdomen, and a mass in the region of the pancreas. Roentgenologic studies may reveal abnormalities of the upper gastrointestinal tract caused by the tumor. Percutaneous transhepatic cholangiography is an aid to diagnosis in obstructive jaundice.[41] Serum lipase and amylase may occasionally be elevated in early obstruction of the pancreas. Radioactive photoscanning is another diagnostic tool, as well as pancreatic angiography.[41] Glucose tolerance tests are performed in patients suspected of having a pancreatic tumor, since about 25% of the patients develop diabetes.[15]

Carcinoma of the gallbladder.[10, 26] Carcinoma of the gallbladder (Fig. 6-7) is the most common tumor of the biliary system.

A

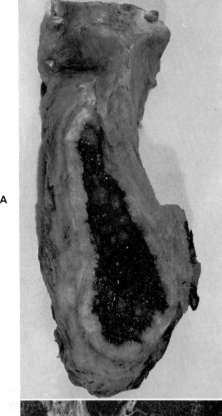

B

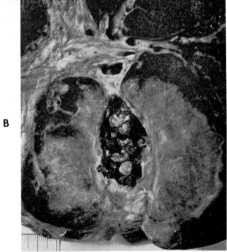

Fig. 6-7. Carcinoma of gallbladder. **A,** Entire wall diffusely involved with multiple areas of ulceration in mucosa. Viscus contained no calculi (39-year-old man). **B,** Lumen filled with mixed gallstones that are faceted. Wall of viscus blends with neoplastic tissue that forms crust several centimeters thick about gallbladder (55-year-old man). (From Halpert, B.: In Anderson, W. A. D., editor: Pathology, ed. 6, St. Louis, 1971, The C. V. Mosby Co.)

It occurs more often in women, and the age incidence is during the sixth and seventh decades. An association with gallstones is believed to be a factor in etiology, with the carcinoma developing because of chronic irritation from stones and infection. The spread of the tumor is governed by its location. Those in the fundus frequently extend through the wall of the gallbladder and invade the liver and peritoneum. Those that occur in the body and neck of the gallbladder are prone to infiltrate the cystic, hepatic, and common bile ducts. As the carcinoma spreads down the common bile duct, it involves the pancreas and duodenum. The liver is involved by direct extension or by lymphatic drainage into the porta hepatis.

The early signs and symptoms of carcinoma of the gallbladder are indistinguishable from those of other diseases of the gallbladder (for example, cholecystitis and cholelithiasis). Late symptoms are anorexia, weight loss, weakness, abdominal pain, a palpable mass, and hepatomegaly. These symptoms are usually evident after local or distant spread of the carcinoma. About 90% of the carcinomas of the gallbladder are associated with cholelithiasis.[10] Acute cholecystitis may develop from obstruction in the cystic duct. Obstructive jaundice is a late development after hepatic or common bile duct involvement.

A diagnosis is made after early investigation of symptoms by roentgenographic special procedures. A palpable mass may be present in the region of the gallbladder. The tumor may be discovered unexpectedly during operations for cholelithiasis or acute cholecystitis.

Lung cancer[19, 32]

Fifty years ago lung cancer was uncommon; however, it is the most common cause of death from cancer today among American men. There is a higher risk for men than women, and the incidence is increasing in other countries.

The search for the cause, which is still unknown, is extensive. A number of studies have implicated cigarette smoking as a direct cause in lung cancer, or they have shown at least a strong association between the two. Other factors under study are occupational hazards, particularly air pollution, since cancer of the lung occurs more commonly among the urban population than in rural areas.

The most common type of cancer arising in the lungs is *bronchogenic carcinoma* (Fig. 6-8). The squamous cell type grossly resembles caseating tuberculosis, and when partially necrotic often has a broad, gray, ill-defined area resembling lobar or tuberculous pneumonia or diffuse bronchiolar carcinoma.

The first symptoms of lung cancer are cough, wheeze, and vague chest pains, which rarely motivate a person to consult a physician for investigation. The cough may be persistent, since the tumor seems to act like a foreign body or obstruction within the lung, which the person tries to expel. The chest pains are usually per-

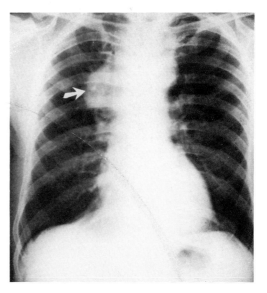

Fig. 6-8. Bronchogenic carcinoma of lung. Arrow points to the malignant mass, which is demarcated. (From Young, C. G., and Likos, J. J.: Medical specialty terminology, x-ray and nuclear medicine, St. Louis, 1972, The C. V. Mosby Co.)

sistent and unrelated to cough and are most often on the side on which the tumor is located. The appearance of blood-streaked sputum is usually the first symptom that prompts the patient to consult a doctor. The subsequent chest x-ray examination may show an abnormal shadow, which can be interpreted by the radiologists as a suspected malignancy. Such examinations can then be followed by bronchoscopy, biopsy, thoracotomy, or exfoliative cytologic examination of the sputum for presence of malignant or suspicious cells. Unfortunately all too often the symptoms appear only after the disease has spread to other parts of the body. Some cancers of the lung grow slowly and remain localized so that if they are diagnosed early enough, there is a chance of longer survival.

The local effect of lung cancer is obstruction of the lumen caused by intraluminal growth or stenosis encircling the wall. The obstruction usually becomes complete. Obstructions often lead to emphysema, infection or retained secretions, bronchiectasis, abscess, or even gangrene. Chronic pneumonitis or an abscess, which is commonly the first sign of carcinoma, may cause death.

The tumor may compress a pulmonary artery or vein. Growth around the superior vena cava occurs most often when the tumor is in the right main bronchus. Venous distention of the head, neck, and upper arm causes edema and cyanosis of these areas. Fatal bleeding can result from erosion of a large blood vessel in the wall of the bronchus. A hilar tumor may destroy nerves on the side of the trachea. When the tumor invades the pericardium and pleura, there is serous or sanguineous effusion, often responsible for empyema. Growth of the tumor can extend into the chest wall or the adjacent lung lobe. Hilar lymph node involvement is present in a great many cases. The tumor may extend through the diaphragm and involve the lymph nodes along the abdominal aorta. Involvement of the scalene lymph nodes renders a grave outlook. With invasion and obstruction of the thoracic duct, chylothorax develops. Cancer of the lung can spread to any part of the body by the bloodstream. Extrathoracic metastases are usual, caused in part by invasion of the pulmonary veins. The organs involved are the liver, brain, adrenals, skeletal system, kidneys, and spleen. Metastases are more frequent in these organs or tissues, but the skin, pancreas, myocardium, intestine, and posterior lobe of the pituitary gland may also be involved.

Adenocarcinomas of the lung are more common in women than are bronchogenic types of cancer. This type of carcinoma has been variously named alveolar, bronchiolar, and bronchioalveolar. The organs most often involved in metastasis are similar to those of bronchogenic carcinoma.

Metastatic carcinoma in the lung is common, the lungs being involved in about 20% to 40% of all cases of carcinoma. Metastases are carried mostly by the pulmonary arteries, and less often by the lymphatics, but the lungs may also be invaded from adjacent carcinomatous structures.

Renal carcinoma[1, 24]

Two forms of renal carcinoma will be discussed—the renal carcinoma occurring in adults and the Wilms' tumor or embryoma occurring in children.

The renal carcinoma as a rule occurs in individuals past 40 years, with a peak incidence in the sixth and seventh decades.[1] It is twice as common in males as in females. The renal carcinomas are variously known as hypernephromas, hypernephroid tumors, Grawitz tumors, clear cell carcinomas, and renal cell carcinomas (Fig. 6-9).

Carcinomas in any part of the kidney cause atrophy and fibrosis of adjacent tissues, and in the later stages, they invade the renal substance extensively, with the tumor cells tending to invade veins and grow along the blood vessels. They metastasize by the lymphatics and bloodstream to the lungs, liver, and brain, the most common sites of secondary tumor.

The tumor may attain a relatively large size with only painless hematuria as a symptom.[24] Occasionally the metastatic lesion in the bones or lungs is the first indication of a carcinoma of the kidney. Renal carcinoma may mimic a prolonged septic disease.[24] As a rule the classic triad of hematuria, pain, and a mass occurs in the later stages.[24] The most common symptoms are leukocytosis, fever, evidence of metastases, abdominal and flank pain, albuminuria, anorexia, weight loss, nausea, and vomiting. Both Wilms' tumor and renal carcinoma in the adult have been associated with erythema and polycythemia. Renal carcinomas are usually accompanied by an elevated urinary alkaline phosphate activity and elevated lactic dehydrogenase (LDH).[1] These changes in

enzymes are not specific, but they are helpful in diagnosing a mass in the kidney.[1]

Early diagnosis is achieved by way of accidental or routine diagnostic studies, since generally no initial symptoms are present. A spherical mass may be palpated, and roentgenographic studies may reveal a mass. Metastases may be observed in the lungs, and osteolytic lesions may be found in the long bones (femur and humerus), or there may be involvement of lymph nodes, liver, adrenals, and contralateral kidney. Distant metastases may be the first sign of the cancer. Renal tomography, renal arteriography, and radioactive renal scans are techniques that contribute to an earlier diagnosis.[41]

Embryonal or *Wilms' tumor* may occur in the fetus or later in childhood, with 70% occurring before the age of 5 years. The average age is 3 years.[1] The tumor grows rapidly and may attain the weight of the rest of the body.[24] Wilms' tumor is believed to originate from mesodermal cells displaced during development. These displaced cells retain their capacity to grow and differentiate into various types of tissue. The tumor is originally encapsulated, but eventually the capsule breaks and the tumor extends to the omentum and adjacent viscera, with blood-borne metastases commonly found in the lungs and brain. The liver and regional lymph nodes are also frequently involved. The symptoms in children are generally the same as those for adults with renal carcinoma.

Bone neoplasms[2, 32]

Cancer of the bone is relatively rare but is one of the more common types of cancer in children and young people.

Osteogenic sarcomas (Fig. 6-10), which are primary tumors arising in the bone, cartilage, and fibrous tissue, occur mainly in those between the ages of 10 and 25 years.[23] Males are affected twice as often as females. Although this tumor often occurs after trauma, it is impossible in any given case to prove an etiologic relationship.

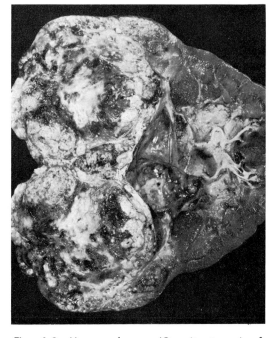

Fig. 6-9. Hypernephroma (Grawitz tumor) of kidney. (From Anderson, W. A. D., and Jones, D. B.: In Anderson, W. A. D., editor: Pathology, ed. 6, St. Louis, 1972, The C. V. Mosby Co.)

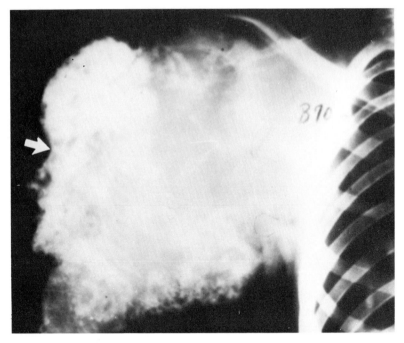

Fig. 6-10. Osteogenic sarcoma of bone. A large soft tissue mass is present from extension of the lesion through the cortex. The cancellous bone and cortex are destroyed in osteogenic sarcoma. (From Young, C. G., and Likos, J. J.: Medical specialty terminology, x-ray and nuclear medicine, St. Louis, 1972, The C. V. Mosby Co.)

The tumor arises most often in the metaphyseal ends of shafts of long bones, particularly the lower end of the femur and upper ends of the radius or humerus. They involve the interior of the bone, extending through the cortex and elevating the periosteum for some distance along the shaft before being recognized. They are usually classified according to their pattern of growth and destruction as sclerosing osteogenic sarcoma or osteolytic osteogenic sarcoma.

The symptoms are bone pain in the area of the tumor and swelling. Fever is usually not an initial sign but develops later in the course of the disease.

Metastasis is chiefly by way of the bloodstream, with the lung being most frequently involved. By the time the disease has run its course, metastases may have occurred in the liver, heart, and other organs.[2]

Ewing's sarcoma is another malignant tumor occurring in young people. It is more prone to begin in the shafts of long tubular bones and bones of the pelvis, but may have its origin in any bone. It mimics osteomyelitis in some respects, since usually the temperature is slightly elevated, there is pain in the bones, and the leukocyte count may be slightly or moderately elevated. As the disease progresses, metastasis to other skeletal bones and lungs occurs.

Multiple myelomas or *plasma cell myelomas* are bone marrow tumors occurring in middle-aged and older people.[23] The symptoms are pain, anemia, weakness, weight loss, and fractures of bones, particularly bodies of the vertebrae. The extensive bone destruction produces punched-out areas in the bones. This tumor may run its fatal course in any time from a few months to a few years.

Metastatic bone tumors (Fig. 6-11) often arise from a primary cancer elsewhere in the body. They reach the skeleton through the circulatory system or by extension from an adjacent organ or tissue involved in can-

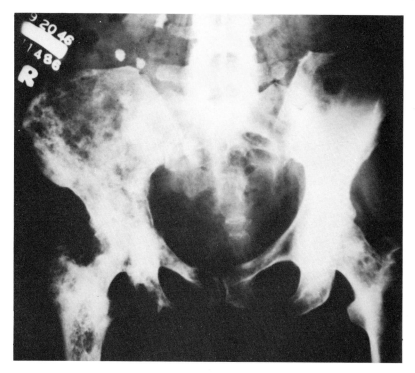

Fig. 6-11. Metastatic carcinoma from the breast, showing bone destruction. (From Young, C. G., and Likos, J. J.: Medical specialty terminology, x-ray and nuclear medicine, St. Louis, 1972, The C. V. Mosby Co.)

cer. The metastatic tumors are more prevalent than the primary bone tumors and usually occur in middle-aged and older people who have primary cancer of the kidneys, thyroid, prostate, or breast.

Diagnosis of a bone tumor is made from roentgenographic changes in the bone, from surgical or needle biopsy, and from investigation with radioisotopes. Since the bones are favorite sites for metastases from primary carcinoma elsewhere, multiple lesions in a patient known to have a primary carcinoma of an organ present no diagnostic problem. It is the single bone lesion in a patient without evidence of a primary carcinoma elsewhere that presents a diagnostic problem.

Cancer of the prostate[4, 25, 34]

Cancer of the prostate is the second most frequent cause of death in men 55 to 75 years of age in the United States. In the United States it is more prevalent among blacks than among whites, and apparently it occurs more frequently among married men than among single men, which is in contrast to almost all other forms of cancer.

Carcinoma of the prostate is a slow-growing lesion, and because of its relatively late start in the lives of its victims, many men do not die of the disease itself. Its presence may be an incidental finding, or it may be discovered as the major contributing cause of death at postmortem examinations.

The cancer is likely to arise in the posterior lobe and in areas just beneath the prostatic capsule. For this reason the rectal examination provides a method of detecting some of these early lesions. The areas of malignant change may be small, no more than 1 centimeter in diameter, but any area of increased consistency in the prostate may represent a malignant change. The areas of involvement may have a stony consistency in contrast to firm or boggy areas palpated in chronic prostatitis. The rectal examination plus a biopsy of suspicious cases provides a reasonable and effective means for detection of carcinoma of the prostate.

A number of symptoms relating to urinary difficulty may be indicative of malignancy of the prostate. These include weak or interrupted flow of urine, frequency of urination, inability to urinate or difficulty in starting a stream, painful or burning urination, and, later, blood in the urine. These symptoms may occur because of obstruction of the bladder neck, but they may also be caused by a noncancerous enlargement of the prostate called benign prostatic hypertrophy. Other symptoms are pain in the pelvis, lower back, or upper thighs. Pain in these areas may be the first symptom, since obstructive symptoms are often late manifestations of the disease. About half the patients with prostatic carcinoma, whose tumor has been diagnosed in the early localized stage, are alive and well 5 years after treatment.

The cause of prostatic carcinoma is unknown.

Most cancers of the prostate gland eventually metastasize, generally to bones, showing a predilection for the vertebrae and pelvic bones. The routes of metastasis may be lymphatic and systemic circulation. Lymphatic spread involves the inguinal, periaortic, mediastinal, and supraclavicular lymph nodes. The lungs and liver may also be involved, but this is infrequent.

Cytologic examination of prostatic smears may reveal neoplastic cells. Demonstration of an elevated total serum acid phosphatase and prostatic acid phosphatase is a useful tool for detecting bone metastases. Since carcinoma of the prostate is prone to metastasize to bones, roentgenographic examinations are made for bone metastases. Diagnosis of carcinoma is also made after pathologic examination of tissue removed by needle or surgical biopsy.

Carcinoma of the prostate is a slow-growing tumor, and with proper therapy the patients may live for many years.

Neoplasia of endocrine glands

Pheochromocytoma.[12, 28] This tumor is a rare catecholamine-secreting tumor of the adrenal medulla, but can also arise in other neural crest–derived tissues. On the average this type of tumor weighes about 90 grams, but may become a mass of over 2 kilograms.[28] Symptoms evidenced with pheochromocytoma are persistent or episodic hypertension associated with tachycardia, cardiac arrhythmias, sweating, and flushing. An episode of acute hypertension may be triggered by exercise, external pressure on the tumor, anesthesia, bone surgery, or ingestion of tyramine-containing compounds, or use of monamine oxidase inhibitor drugs. The majority of the patients also have hyperglycemia.[12] Symptoms include throbbing headaches, blurring of vision, anxiety, polydipsia, and polyuria. A diagnosis is made by a confirmation of elevation of urine levels of vanillylmandelic acid, metanephrines, and catecholamines.[12]

Carcinoma of the thyroid.[6, 28] Carcinomas of the thyroid are usually designated as Hürthle cell, medullary, papillary, follicular, mixed, or anaplastic. This classification is made on histologic examination. The etiology is unknown, but exposure in early childhood of the pharyngeal or thymic area to irradiation or x-rays has been associated with subsequent development of carcinoma.[6, 28] This is particularly true of patients who develop thyroid carcinoma before the age of 20 years.[6]

The most common thyroid carcinoma is the papillary type, comprising about 60% of all carcinomas of the thyroid.[28] Most affected children and adolescents give a history of exposure to ionizing radiation. Metastasis may be prominent in the cervical lymph nodes, and it may be confined in this area for a long period of time. It may also invade the strap muscles and the larynx and metastasize to the lungs. When the papillary carcinoma is massive and spreads into extrathyroid tissues and lymph nodes, it is fatal in about one third of the patients within 20 years.[6] The 10-year survival rate with various forms of therapy is 80% to 90%.[6] The disease is less aggressive in patients under 40 years.

The follicular type metastasizes early to the lungs and bone through the bloodstream. The 10-year survival rate is approximately 50%.[6] Hürthle cell types tend to invade and metastasize locally in the neck. Their 10-year survival is about equal to that of the follicular type.[6]

Symptoms include hoarseness, pain, difficulty in swallowing, and enlarged cervical lymph nodes. Surgery is usually performed, unless otherwise contraindicated, in patients with a neck mass thought to be caused by thyroid cancer or in those with a thyroid mass plus cervical adenopathy.

Diagnosis is aided by radioisotope-uptake and scanning studies.[40] Clinical examination and radioisotope scanning cannot segregate carcinomas from benign adenomas.[6] If the nodule is firm, fixed to the trachea, and is known to have recently grown, and the cervical nodes are palpable, there is the likelihood of malignancy.[6] Frozen sections are made of adenomas removed at surgery and examined for malignancy.[28] (See Fig. 17-3, *B*.)

Craniopharyngiomas. These are pituitary tumors that appear to arise from squamous cell remnants of Rathke's pouch.[5] (See Fig. 17-2, *C*.) Craniopharyngiomas comprise about 3% of all intracranial tumors. They may occur at any age, but the two peaks of incidence are in late childhood and early adulthood and again in the fifth decade.[3] They are usually suprasellar but may occur in the sella.[5] The clinical effects depend on the size and site of the tumor. Symptoms and signs may be those of a space-occupying lesion or of pressure on the pituitary gland and destruction of the hypothalamic nuclei, resulting in pituitary dwarfism or diabetes insipidus.[8] Pressure on the optic chiasm may result in optic atrophy. Since these tumors tend to have areas of calcification, this has radiodiagnostic value.

Intracranial tumors[3, 8, 37, 38]

Intracranial tumors (Fig. 6-12), like other tumors, may be either benign or malignant. Among the various forms are such space-occupying lesions of chronic inflammatory origin as the granulomas and parasitic cysts (see Figs. 18-20, 18-22, and 18-32). The tumors may develop in the brain, meninges, or bones of the skull. Brain tumors may occur in all age groups. But an estimated 85% occur in adults with a peak at ages 50 to 60 years.[37] The remaining affect infants or children and differ by location and type from adult brain tumors. The age peak for children is 5 to 10 years.[37] About 50% of brain tumors are inevitably fatal. Both sexes are about equally affected by many kinds of brain tumors, but a few types show a predilection for male and female.

Brain tumors may be classified as either benign or malignant. Unlike benign tumors in other parts of the body, however, a benign tumor of the brain may expand inside the closed bony skull until it strangles vital nerve centers. Benign tumors of the brain like those in other parts of the body often have a capsule and frequently may be removed completely by surgery. A malignant brain tumor may have roots like a plant, which invade surrounding brain tissue and cannot be removed completely by surgery and hence will grow again from the remaining portion.

About 30% of brain tumors are metastatic, originating from an extracranial primary tumor, most commonly from carcinoma of the lungs, breast, kidneys, skin (melanoma), gastrointestinal tract, and prostate, in that order of frequency.[3] Metastatic tumors in the brain may seed secondary tumors in several areas of the brain. The tumor emboli reach the brain in most cases by way of the arteries.

The largest group of primary brain tumors are the *gliomas,* which include the

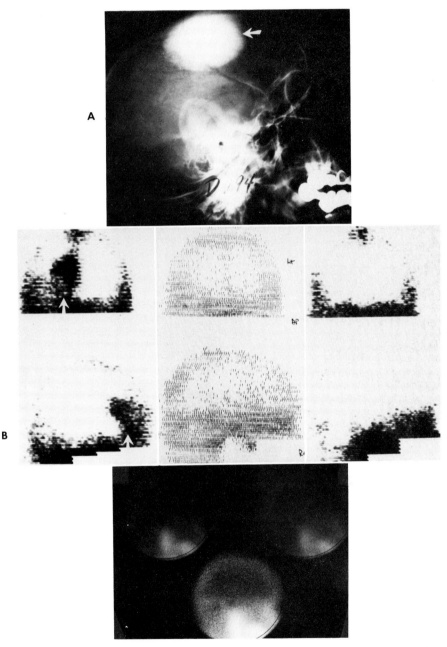

Fig. 6-12. Intracranial tumors. **A,** Meningioma. **B,** Brain scans with radioisotopes showing tumor. (From Young, C. G., and Likos, J. J.: Medical specialty terminology, x-ray and nuclear medicine, St. Louis, 1972, The C. V. Mosby Co.)

glioblastomas, astrocytomas, ependymomas, oligodendrogliomas, medulloblastomas, and pinealomas. All of these are composed of malignant glial cells.

The *glioblastomas* are among the most malignant of all brain tumors. (See Fig. 18-20, *B*.) The various types of this tumor are classified as grade III or grade IV (astrocytic series) on a histologic basis, and they constitute about 50% to 60% of all gliomas.[3] They are more common in adults than in the younger age group. They grow rapidly and are characterized by tissue necrosis and brain edema. Complete surgical removal is impossible, and the average life expectancy is about 1 year.

The *grade I astrocytomas* constitute about 15% of all gliomas.[3] In adults they occur in one of the cerebral hemispheres, but in young adults and children they are more often found in the pons and cerebellum. They are a relatively slow-growing tumor. The average survival is in excess of three years following onset of symptoms. The *grade II astrocytomas* (formerly called astroblastomas) are uncommon tumors, comprising only about 1% of all gliomas.[3] They are more common in young adults than in children. The average survival is approximately 2 years following surgery. Complete excision, however, may be impossible because of marked invasion of brain tissue.

The *ependymomas* constitute approximately 5% of intracranial gliomas and usually arise in the posterior fossa. They are also found in the spinal cord, arising at every level.[3] These malignant tumors in an intracranial site originate from cells lining the ventricles or choroid plexus. They may fill or obstruct the ventricles and invade the adjacent tissue. They may involve the subarachnoid space and the cerebrum. Death usually occurs within 3 years.

The *oligodendrogliomas* constitute about 5% of all gliomas.[3] They are slow growing and are found in the cerebral hemisphere of an adult, usually during the fourth or fifth decade of life. Most patients have a life expectancy of more than 4 years after clinical onset.

Medulloblastomas are highly malignant tumors and are uniformly fatal. They are restricted to the cerebellum. They represent about 8% of all neuroglial tumors and occur predominantly in children,[3] with a peak incidence between the ages of 5 and 9 years.[8] There is another increase in incidence between the ages of 20 and 24 years.[8] Males are affected more than twice as frequently as females. Familial occurrence has been reported, including tumors in identical twins.[8] In children most of them originate in the cerebellar vermis, and in older patients they may arise in one of the hemispheres. The fourth ventricle is almost always occupied by the rapidly growing tumor. They frequently metastasize through the subarachnoid space and involve the cerebrum or spinal cord.

Meningiomas (Fig. 6-12) are benign, slow-growing tumors. They comprise approximately 15% of all classified symptom-producing intracranial tumors.[3] They are slightly more common in women. Meningiomas arise in the meninges, and they may invade the adjacent bone as well as compress and distort the brain tissues. Unless critical structures are invaded, a complete removal may be possible.[8]

Acoustic neuroma.[38] An acoustic (Fig. 18-18) neuroma is a tumor involving the nerve of hearing or balance—the eighth cranial nerve. This nerve is actually two different nerves: one, the vestibular, for balance and the other, the cochlear, for hearing. The acoustic neuroma originates more often from the balance nerve than from the hearing nerve. These nerves course through the bony internal auditory canal between the inner ear and the brain.

Acoustic neuromas have been found in all age groups, and at times they are found only at autopsy, having been too small to cause disabling symptoms. Both sexes are equally affected, and most often the tumors are diagnosed and removed when a man or woman is in the age group of 30 to 50 years.[38]

Acoustic neuromas are not cancers, and they do not metastasize to other parts of the body. In general, the cause or causes of acoustic neuroma are unknown, but there is one rare known cause: heredity. The inheritable type of acoustic neuroma generally develops on both the right and left acoustic nerves between the brain and the inner ear. This contrasts with the typical one-sided neuroma. It is a dominant hereditary trait, and each child of an affected parent has a 50% risk of developing an acoustic neuroma like that of the parent.[38]

Symptoms of acoustic neuroma are dizziness or other balance problems as well as interference with hearing, but often there is a loss of skin sensation or movement around the ear. If an acoustic tumor is removed while it is tiny, perhaps about the size of a pea or less, and if it has merely squeezed the blood supply to the ear, hearing may be improved and dizziness cured. If a section of the nerve must be removed in order to remove the tumor, nerve function will be lost. If the acoustic tumor is not removed, it will continue to grow, sometimes very rapidly, and as it grows it presses against the brain and causes damage to some essential brain tissue. When a tumor is pressing on the brain, the symptoms progress from dizziness and some hearing loss to headache, difficulty in walking steadily, trouble with vision, facial muscle weakness, numbness of head or face, difficulty in swallowing, and clumsiness of arm movement.

Brain tumors give rise to focal disturbances in brain function and to increased intracranial pressure.[8] The focal manifestations occur when the brain is compressed or infiltrated by tumor, when the blood supply is compromised resulting in tissue necrosis, or when there is cerebral edema. Some intracranial tumors have distinctive signs and symptoms, but on the whole, brain tumors are characterized by an insidious onset and progression of focal or general neurologic signs and symptoms. A wide variety of neurologic diseases simulates brain tumor, because they too are characterized by neurologic signs and symptoms. The clinical manifestations of brain tumor vary according to the tumor's location and rate of growth. Headache is a major symptom, but not an invariable one.

Headaches occur from many causes. They are associated with high blood pressure, tension muscle contraction, migraine, various infections, and defects of blood vessels.[33] Some are psychogenic, brought on by emotional conflicts or anxiety. Although recurrent headaches may be a major sign of brain tumor, only the doctor can establish the basis for this symptom.

Personality changes may be an early symptom, particularly of masses in the cerebral hemispheres. The personality changes may be confusioned states and at times bizarre behavior, but the most common mental changes are impairment of memory and judgment and a shortened attention span. With increasing intracranial pressure, there is drowsiness progressing to stupor and coma. With intracranial pressure, there may also be characteristic ophthalmoscopic appearance of papilledema. Diplopia is caused by involvement of either or both of the sixth cranial nerves by tumor or indirectly by increasing intracranial pressure. When the visual pathways are involved there may be blindness in one half of the field of vision in one or both eyes (hemianopia).[8] Disturbances of speech also occur. Ataxia or unsteadiness of gait occurs from tumors in various intracranial sites. Contralateral spastic hemiparesis is characteristic of tumors of the cerebral hemispheres.[8] When the tumor involves the thalamus or the ascending spinothalamic pathways, there may be sensory disturbances, affecting touch, pain, temperature, and proprioception.[8] Tumors involving the thalamus may cause episodes of pain affecting the contralateral side of the face or body. Focal sensory seizures may be the result of tumors of the cortex. When tumors affect the base of the skull, particularly those arising in the nasopharynx and sinuses, there is facial pain. Seizures may be the first manifestation of a brain tumor, or they may occur at any time during the course of the tumor growth. Seizures resemble the classic grand mal type. They may be focal motor and sensory seizures and limited to one region of the body, or they may progress as jacksonian seizures and involve the entire body. When convulsions occur in any person over 20 years who does not have a previous history of convulsions, there is a possibility of an expanding lesion.[8] Nausea and vomiting may also occur, particularly in association with intracranial pressure and displacement of the brainstem caused by herniation or bleeding into the cerebrospinal fluid. The vomiting may be projectile. Dizziness or vertigo may be another symptom. Meningeal irritation may be manifested by a stiff neck. Bradycardia and hypertension, apnea and fever occur as late signs. Hyperthermia may occur just prior to death.

Although signs and symptoms may point toward the diagnosis of a brain tumor, a search is usually made to discover if they are the result of other systemic disease or a primary neoplasm in some other part of the body. Diagnostic procedures include skull roentgenogram; roentgenographic contrast studies (pneumoencephalography, ventriculography, and arteriography), electroencephalography,[41] and examination of the cerebrospinal fluid. Various scanning techniques with radioisotopes (Fig. 6-12) are also employed in diagnosis. Ancillary laboratory tests are made that include audiometry and vestibular tests, and visual tests.[8]

Neuroblastomas[28]

These are highly malignant tumors occurring in infancy and childhood. They are the most common congenital tumor next to the retinoblastoma (a retinal malignant neoplasm) and are second only to Wilms' tumor as the most common retroperitoneal neoplasm of childhood. They usually arise from the medulla of the adrenal gland, but may also arise retroperitoneally and retropleurally from sympathetic nerve endings. The Hutchinson type is characterized by profuse osseous metastases, particularly to the skull and orbit, with resulting exophthalmos. The Pepper syndrome is characterized by hepatic metastases. Metastases occur early and widely either by permeation or embolic spread to regional lymph nodes and abdominal organs, in addition to the metastases discussed above.[28]

The signs and symptoms are abdominal enlargement (Pepper syndrome), vomiting, pain, fever, loss of weight, and anemia. Ecchymosis of the eyelids and proptosis of the eye occur with the Hutchinson syndrome. If the tumor is confined to the abdomen, a high percentage of cures is achieved by surgery and therapy. There is elevation of the urinary VMA (vanillylmandelic acid).

Diagnosis is made by x-ray examination showing evidence of metastases and downward and lateral displacement of the kidney.

Hodgkin's disease[35]

Hodgkin's disease was first described in 1932 by an English physician, Thomas Hodgkin. This is not strictly a neoplasm but is considered to be a malignant disorder of the lymphatic tissues of the body.[35] Clinically it is characterized by swollen lymph nodes and often a swollen spleen. (See Fig. 18-31.) It is much more common in men than in women, and it occurs mostly in the age group of 20 to 40 years. Any lymph node group may be involved, but the most common site is in the cervical region. Other lymph nodes that may also be involved include the inguinal, the axillary, the mediastinal, the abdominal, and the substernal. The earliest recognizable signs are enlargement and proliferation of the reticuloendothelial cells of the lymphoid tissues in microscopic examinations. Biopsy offers the only method of diagnosis that will show distinctive, abnormal cells known as the Reed-Sternberg cells.

The initial symptom may be a painless swollen lymph gland, usually in the neck. Other symptoms are pain in the abdomen, back, or legs, with fatigue, fever, loss of weight, and itching sensations. A persistent sore throat may also be a symptom. Symptoms are variable from case to case.

The cause is unknown. With the improved therapy, patients with this disease often lead normal, productive lives for a number of years.

Responses

Step 1: 1. neoplasm or tumor; 2. malignant; benign; 3. malignant; benign
Step 2: oma
Step 3: 1. osteoma; 2. myoma; 3. neuroma; 4. fibroma; 5. lipoma; 6. angioma; 7. lymphoma
Step 4: 1. fibrosarcoma; 2. leiomyoma; 3. chondrosarcoma; 4. osteochondroma; 5. osteosarcoma; 6. lymphosarcoma; 7. adenocarcinoma; 8. osteoblastoma; 9. retinoblastoma; 10. melanoblastoma; 11. angiofibroma; 12. cystadenoma
Step 5: 1. malignant; 2. benign; 3. benign; 4. malignant; 5. benign; 6. malignant; 7. malignant; 8. benign
Step 6: 1. metastasis; 2. metastases; 3. benign; 4. malignant
Step 7: 1. venous; 2. lymphatic; 3. emboli
Step 8: 1. Papanicolaou smear; 2. frozen section; 3. biopsy; 4. Papanicolaou or cytologic smear; biopsy; 5. Papanicolaou or cytologic examination
Step 9: 1. are not; 2. can; 3. has; 4. can; 5. can
Step 10: 1. X; 2. X; 5. X
Step 11: 1. contrast medium or equivalent response; 2. radioisotopes

REFERENCES

1. Anderson, W. A. D., and Jones, D. B.: In Anderson, W. A. D., editor: Pathology, ed. 6, St. Louis, 1971, The C. V. Mosby Co. (renal carcinoma).
2. Bennett, G. A.: In Anderson, W. A. D., editor: Pathology, ed. 6, St. Louis, 1971, The C. V. Mosby Co. (tumors of bone).
3. Chason, J. L.: In Anderson, W. A. D., editor: Pathology, ed. 6, St. Louis, 1971, The C. V. Mosby Co. (brain tumors).
4. Colby, F. H.: Essential urology, ed. 2, Baltimore, 1953, The Williams & Wilkins Co. (prostatic carcinoma).
5. Currie, A. R.: In Anderson, W. A. D., editor: Pathology, ed. 6, St. Louis, 1971, The C. V. Mosby Co. (craniopharyngioma).
6. DeGroot, L. J.: In Beeson, P. B., and McDermott, W., editors: Cecil-Loeb textbook of medicine, ed. 13, Philadelphia, 1971, W. B. Saunders Co. (thyroid carcinoma).
7. Edmondson, H. A.: In Anderson, W. A. D., editor: Pathology, ed. 6, St. Louis, 1971, The C. V. Mosby Co. (liver carcinoma).
8. Fishman, R. A.: In Beeson, P. B., and McDermott, W., editors: Cecil-Loeb textbook of medicine, ed. 13, Philadelphia, 1971, W. B. Saunders Co. (intracranial tumors).
9. Geschickter, C. F.: Diseases of the breast, ed. 2, Philadelphia, 1945, J. B. Lippincott Co.
10. Halpert, B.: In Anderson, W. A. D., editor: Pathology, ed. 6, St. Louis, 1971, The C. V. Mosby Co. (gallbladder carcinoma).
11. Hertig, A. T., and Gore, H.: In Anderson, W. A. D., editor: Pathology, ed. 6, St. Louis, 1971, The C. V. Mosby Co. (uterine and cervical carcinoma).
12. Himathengkam, T., and others: Pheochromocytoma, J.A.M.A. 230:1692-1693, 1974.
13. Horn, R. C., Jr.: In Anderson, W. A. D., editor: Pathology, ed. 6, St. Louis, 1971, The C. V. Mosby Co. (alimentary tract tumors).
14. Jeffries, G. H.: In Beeson, P. B., and McDermott, W., editors: Cecil-Loeb textbook of medicine, ed. 13, Philadelphia, 1971, W. B. Saunders Co. (liver carcinoma).
15. Kowlessar, O. D.: In Beeson, P. B., and McDermott, W., editors: Cecil-Loeb textbook of medicine, ed. 13, Philadelphia, 1971, W. B. Saunders Co. (pancreas carcinoma).
16. Kuzma, J. F.: In Anderson, W. A. D., editor: Pathology, ed. 6, St. Louis, 1971, The C. V. Mosby Co. (breast cancer).
17. Lacy, P. E., and Kissane, J. M.: In Anderson, W. A. D., editor: Pathology, ed. 6, St. Louis, 1971, The C. V. Mosby Co. (pancreatic carcinoma).
18. Meissner, W. A. and Warren, S.: In Anderson, W. A. D., editor: Pathology, ed. 6, St. Louis, 1971, The C. V. Mosby Co. (neoplasms).
19. Millard, M.: In Anderson, W. A. D., editor: Pathology, ed. 6, St. Louis, 1971, The C. V. Mosby Co. (lung cancer).
20. Miller, R.: Detection of colon carcinoma and the barium enema, J.A.M.A. 230:1195-1198, 1974.
21. Papanicolaou, G. N., and Traut, H. F.: Diagnosis of uterine cancer by vaginal smear, New York, 1943, The Commonwealth Fund.

22. Peterson, M. L.: In Beeson, P. B. and McDermott, W., editors: Cecil-Loeb textbook of medicine, ed. 13, Philadelphia, 1971, W. B. Saunders Co. (neoplastic disease of the alimentary tract).

23. Robbins, S. L.: Pathology, ed. 3, Philadelphia, 1967, W. B. Saunders Co. (neoplasia).

24. Schreiner, G. E.: In Beeson, P. B., and McDermott, W., editors: Cecil-Loeb textbook of medicine, ed. 13, Philadelphia, 1971, W. B. Saunders Co. (renal carcinoma).

25. Scott, W. W.: In Campbell, M., editor: Urology, Philadelphia, 1954, W. B. Saunders Co. (carcinoma of the prostate).

26. Sleisenger, M. H.: In Beeson, P. B., and McDermott, W., editors: Cecil-Loeb textbook of medicine, ed. 13, Philadelphia, 1971, W. B. Saunders Co. (carcinoma of gallbladder).

27. Smith, E. H., and Bartum, R. J., Jr.: Ultrasonic evaluation of pararenal masses, J.A.M.A. **231:**51-55, 1975.

28. Sommers, S. C.: In Anderson, W. A. D., editor: Pathology, ed. 6, St. Louis, 1971, The C. V. Mosby Co. (neuroblastoma; thyroid carcinoma, pheochromocytoma).

29. U.S. Department of Health, Education, and Welfare, National Cancer Institute, Public Health Service Publication No. 1057, Health Information Series 109, revised 1967 (cancer of the uterus).

30. U.S. Department of Health, Education, and Welfare, National Cancer Institute, Public Health Service Publication No. 1304, Health Information Series 124, revised 1966 (cancer of the colon and rectum).

31. U.S. Department of Health, Education, and Welfare, National Cancer Institute, Public Health Service Publication No. 1237, Health Information Series 102, 1964 (cancer of the stomach).

32. U.S. Department of Health, Education, and Welfare, National Cancer Institute, Public Health Service Publication No. 1173, Health Information Series 115, revised 1966 (cancer of the lung).

33. U.S. Department of Health, Education, and Welfare, National Cancer Institute, Public Health Service Publication No. 1070, Health Information Series 110, revised 1967 (cancer of the bone).

34. U.S. Department of Health, Education, and Welfare, National Cancer Institute, Public Health Service Publication No. 1352, Health Information Series 127, 1965 (cancer of the prostate).

35. U.S. Department of Health, Education, and Welfare, National Cancer Institute, Public Health Service Publication No. 864, Health Information Series 102, 1966 (Hodgkin's disease).

36. U.S. Department of Health, Education, and Welfare, Public Health Service, Public Health Service Publication No. 905, Health Information Series 104, revised 1966 (headaches).

37. U.S. Department of Health, Education, and Welfare, National Institute of Neurological Diseases and Strokes, Public Health Service Bulletin, 1970 (brain tumors and spinal cord tumors).

38. U.S. Department of Health, Education, and Welfare, National Institute of Neurological Diseases and Strokes, DHEW Publication No. (NIH) 73-201, 1973 (acoustic neuroma).

39. U.S. Department of Health, Education, and Welfare, National Cancer Institute, DHEW Publication No. (NIH) 74-232, revised 1973 (the cancer story).

40. Willis, R. A.: Pathology of tumors, ed. 4, London, 1967, Butterworth & Co. Ltd.

41. Young, C. G., and Likos, J. J.: Medical speciality terminology, vol. 2, x-ray and nuclear medicine, St. Louis, 1972, The C. V. Mosby Co.

CHAPTER 7

Metabolic derangements

Metabolism is the sum of processes in the living body by which a particular substance is handled to maintain and promote life, growth, maturation, and reproduction. Foods must first be digested and absorbed before they can be metabolized or utilized by the body. The body uses, that is, metabolizes, proteins, fats, carbohydrates, vitamins, mineral salts (for example, calcium and phosphorus), and water in two general ways, catabolism and anabolism.[2] *Catabolism* is the breaking down of food compounds or of protoplasm into simple compounds, thereby making their stored energy available for cellular work. *Anabolism* is the opposite of catabolism. It is the synthesis of complex compounds, such as protoplasm and hormones, from simple compounds, such as amino acids, simple sugars, fats, and minerals.

A number of the systemic diseases that affect the body as a whole are the result of malfunction in metabolism. Most of these diseases are caused by an isolated defect in the metabolism of one of three major foodstuffs—the carbohydrates, fats, and proteins. These defects are cellular derangements that usually take the form of excesses or deficiencies of metabolites. Metabolic diseases also occur as the result of faulty utilization of minerals, water, and pigments, but these are discussed in later chapters.

The energy of the body is derived from the carbohydrates and fats. The proteins use this energy to build and repair the tissues. The chemical reactions within the cells are responsible for the proper utilization of the carbohydrates, fats, and proteins.[1] No attempt will be made here to review the normal chemistry or metabolism of these substances, since it is a complex subject and available in detail in a number of textbooks of biochemistry and physiology.

Many of the metabolic diseases are hereditary or inborn errors of metabolism. These represent biochemical disorders that modify normal function because of an alteration in the genetic process. The discovery of the molecular structure of DNA (deoxyribonucleic acid) and the unravelling of the genetic code with the understanding of the biochemistry of protein and enzyme synthesis have contributed immensely to the understanding of metabolic defects.[2] The diseases caused by faulty metabolism are of particular interest, since many of them are responsible for mental retardation. Many of the metabolic diseases are rare, and some are of such slight significance that the affected person suffers very few if any ill effects. Others may be debilitating and even fatal.

The metabolic diseases tend to involve many organs, and each disease evokes its own pattern of symptoms and derangements of function of the cells. Identification of a specific metabolic defect may be accomplished by chemical means. The clinical manifestations of a specific metabolic defect may be so pronounced and characteristic that exact diagnosis is not a problem. In the case of suspected inborn errors of metabolism a family history of similar defective metabolism is a valuable diagnostic aid.

CARBOHYDRATE METABOLISM[1, 2, 13]

The carbohydrates are the body's preferred fuel for energy. The body cells burn or catabolize carbohydrates to carry on many functions in the body. They are the chief source of glucose, which is found in all the body tissues. If the stores of carbohydrates are inadequate, as might occur in some prolonged chronic diseases, the fats and proteins are mobilized as secondary or supplementary energy or fuel sources. Thus the metabolism of carbohydrates is intimately interrelated with that of fat and protein.

Carbohydrate metabolism starts with the transport of glucose through the cell membranes. Glucose is the most important carbohydrate since it can be used as food immediately after a meal. It can pass unchanged from the small intestine into the blood, whereas other more complex carbohydrates must first be changed before they can be absorbed into the blood for use by the tissues. The temporary excess of carbohydrates is changed into glycogen, in a process called *glycogenesis,* by the liver cells in the presence of insulin (the famous sugar-regulating hormone secreted by the islands of Langerhans in the pancreas). Glycogen is then stored in the liver and skeletal muscles until it is needed, at which time it is changed back into glucose by a process called *glycogenolysis.* Both these processes are a part of the homeostatic mechanisms of the body for maintaining a suitable physiologic environment for survival. When glucose is inadequate to meet the body's demands, it is produced from fats or proteins (amino acids) and diffused out of the liver cells into the blood; this is called *gluconeogenesis.* When blood glucose remains higher than normal after glycogenesis and catabolism in the presence of adequate blood insulin, the excess glucose is converted into fat, mainly by the liver cells, and is stored in the adipose tissues of the body. This is why you gain weight when your intake of carbohydrates far exceeds the output of energy. The carbohydrates and fats are stored in the adipose tissues instead of being burned for energy.

One of the most notable diseases in which defective carbohydrate metabolism is involved is diabetes mellitus, in which the body's normal ability to utilize carbohydrates and fats is believed to be impaired because of varying degrees of insulin insufficiency. Other congenital metabolic errors in carbohydrate metabolism occur in the defective hydrolysis and intestinal absorption of the carbohydrates—lactose, sucrose, galactose, and isomaltose. Still others result from defective mucopolysaccharide metabolism, defective monosaccharide metabolism, and disorders of glycogen metabolism *(glycogenosis).* The monosaccharides are carbohydrates that cannot be decomposed by hydrolysis. These include galactose, fructose, glucose, and pentose. The mucopolysaccharides are a group of polysaccharides that may or may not be combined with protein and which when dispersed in water form many of the mucins. There are a group of genetic disorders that appear to be related to defective metabolism of the mucopolysaccharides. These are manifested by skeletal abnormalities caused by heritable disorders of connective tissue in most instances. The diseases caused by glycogenosis are related to accumulation of glycogen in the tissues.

Several of the diseases resulting from defective carbohydrate metabolism have been selected for review at the end of this chapter.

PROTEIN METABOLISM[1, 2, 13]

The proteins are an essential and distinctive constituent of all living tissues. The functions of protein are many and diverse. Many of the hormones, all of the known enzymes, collagen and the oxygen-carrying substances of the blood, antibodies, and the chemical units of hereditary transmission are the property of protein. The growth of body tissue in the young and the repair of protein structure of the adult depend upon protein (amino acids) content of the diet. Protein given as food, however, differs from that of the tissues. Food as a rule must be completely broken down into its separate amino acids before it can be utilized by the body cells. The effects of excess or deficiency of various amino acids and proteins may be manifest in disease processes when there is faulty metabolism of these substances. Certain diseases show disturbances of the condition or quantity of intracellular protein substances or show the appearance of abnormal protein materials in tissue spaces or cells. Defective protein metabolism is of particular interest because congenital errors of protein metabolism often result in mental retardation.

FAT METABOLISM[1, 2, 9, 13]

Fatty substances form a considerable part of all cells and tissues and, in addition, are stored in fat reserves or depots constituting the body's largest reserve energy source. The adipose tissues are principally the storage depots. Adipose tissue is found mainly in the subcutaneous tissue, omentum, mesentery, perirenal tissue, and bone marrow. In obesity there is an abnormally large amount of fat accumulation in the adipose tissues, which is invariably the result of an energy intake (carbohydrates and fats) greater than the output in work, play, or exercise. In some endocrine disturbances, however, there may be an accumulation of fat in adipose tissue, but the endocrine factors are believed to be more important in determining the distribution of the fat than in causing a change in metabolic energy balance.[1] Excessive adipose tissue also forms localized tumors, called lipomas. In some diseases when cells are injured or the metabolic processes are depressed, fat can no longer be handled at the normal rate and it accumulates in the tissues. The liver is an important organ in the metabolism of fat, and metabolic disturbances are often reflected in this organ by accumulation of fat in the liver cells. Fatty accumulations or changes are found in the liver in starvation, in wasting diseases, and in chronic alcoholism, as well as in obesity. Fatty depositions in the cells may also result from anoxia, which deprives the cells of energy transfer mechanisms. In other instances fatty accumulations in the liver may result from infections associated with high toxicity or high temperature or from intoxications by chemicals (carbon tetrachloride, benzol, ether, and phosphorus). Fatty infiltration also occurs in the heart muscle (myocardium) and in and around the pancreas. Fatty degeneration of cells occurs most frequently in the kidneys, heart, and liver but may affect other organs. It represents a rather severe injury to the cells and is often associated with disturbance in functional efficiency of the involved organs. Injury to the cells themselves through fatty degeneration may develop in severe anemias, anoxemias, chemical poisons, and many infections.[1, 13]

The term "lipid" represents a variety of naturally occurring esters, sterols, and fatty acids, all of which have the solubility properties of fat (low solubility in water and high solubility in solvents such as ether, chloroform, and petroleum ether). The principal lipids found in human serum are free and esterfied cholesterol, phospholipids, triglycerides (neutral fat), and fatty acids. Interest in these compounds has increased because of their link with diseases such as atherosclerosis (arteriosclerosis), diabetes, and heart ailments. Cholesterol is one we particularly hear about in connection with its deposition in the intima of the large blood vessels in atherosclerosis. Cholesterol also forms an important constituent of gallstones, and cholesterol deposits are common in the lining of the gallbladder in a condition called cholesterolosis. Hypercholesterolemia (increased cholesterol levels in the blood) occurs in a number of disorders, and its determination is of diagnostic aid in conditions such as hepatic disease, hypothyroidism, and xanthomatosis. Triglycerides are usually elevated in glycogen storage disease (von Gierke's disease). The lipids form a large source of calories, which can be available either for immediate use or for storage in depots or reserves. The lipids also assist in the absorption of fat-soluble vitamins.

Some disturbances of fat metabolism that result in an increase of lipids in the brain are the so-called lipidoses of the central nervous system.[8] These include infantile amaurotic idiocy (Tay-Sachs disease), Neimann-Pick disease, Gaucher's disease, and Hurler's disease (gargoylism). Some of these are discussed in the following sections.

ROLE OF THE PITUITARY IN METABOLISM[10]

The hormones of the pars distalis of the hypophysis (anterior pituitary) play a regulatory role in the different aspects of carbohydrate, protein, and fat metabolism. Between them profound relations and repercussions are constantly in action. The pars distalis of the hypophysis is one of the most important factors in the endocrine balance, which regulates metabolism. Somatotropin (growth hormone) is important in protein metabolism. Important hormones under the control of the pars distalis help to keep the level of glucose constant in the blood. These hormones are ACTH of the pituitary, epinephrine from the adrenal glands, thyroxine from the thyroid, and insulin from the pancreas. Each has a specific function in maintaining the glucose level. Thyroxine speeds up the burning of food for energy. ACTH tends to stimulate the liver cells to add to the blood glucose concentration. Epinephrine accelerates both liver and muscle glycogenolysis, thereby causing more glucose to enter the blood. The islands of Langerhans in the pancreas secrete the insulin hormone, as mentioned previously.

In summary, it can be stated that such mistakes in body chemistry as failing to manufacture a certain enzyme (as in heredity), ordering a wrong protein, speeding up or slowing down enzyme production, or failure to properly utilize substances (carbohydrates, fats, and proteins) within the cells can result in metabolic diseases. The secret of all the chemical reactions that run the body efficiently lies in the protoplasm of the cell. The fundamental components of protoplasm are the proteins, which are the mediators of the metabolic and genetic functions of the living organism. In the productions of disease and in the genetic transmission of metabolic defects, even a minute change in the structure of a protein can have profound effects.

STEP-BY-STEP EXERCISES

Step 1. Complete the blanks in the following statements.

1. The sum of processes in the living body by which a particular substance is handled to maintain and promote life, growth, maturation, and reproduction is called _____.
2. The breaking down of food compounds or of protoplasm into simple compounds, thereby making their stored energy available for cellular work, is called _____.
3. The synthesis of complex compounds, such as protoplasm and hormones, from simple compounds, such as amino acids, simple sugars, fats, and minerals, is called _____.

Step 2. Metabolic diseases are the result of cellular derangements. These may be manifested by excesses or deficiencies of metabolites or inborn errors of metabolism.

Indicate in the spaces provided the conditions responsible for metabolic diseases or defects.

1. Deficiencies of metabolites __
2. Excesses of metabolites __
3. Inherited errors of metabolism __
4. Normal cellular metabolic activities __

Step 3. Metabolic defects are largely the result of deficiencies or excesses of metabolites affecting the three major foodstuffs of the body—the carbohydrates, fats, and proteins. The fats and carbohydrates supply energy; proteins are needed for growth and repair of tissue.

Complete the blanks in the following statements.

1. Energy-producing foods are _____

   and _____.

2. Tissue-building foods are _____.

Step 4. Metabolic diseases tend to involve many organs, and each disease may represent a distinct entity in that it evokes its own patterns of symptoms and derangements of function of the cells. Diseases that are the result of faulty metabolism of protein may differ widely in symptoms and effects from those produced by defective carbohydrate and fat metabolism, but all are interrelated when it comes to the production of energy to run the body. If carbohydrate metabolism is faulty and cannot supply the energy, the fats and proteins may be mobilized as secondary or supplementary energy sources.

Mark the following statements T for true or F for false.

1. The patterns of symptoms and metabolic derangements are the same for all metabolic diseases. ___
2. If through faulty carbohydrate metabolism more energy is needed to run the body, fats and proteins are mobilized as energy sources. ___

Step 5. In the following statements you are asked to identify certain substances and define some phases in carbohydrate metabolism. Refer to the text, if necessary.

1. One of the chief carbohydrates of the body found in all body tissues is

   called _____.

2. The sugar-regulating hormone secreted by the islands of Langerhans

   in the pancreas is called _____.

3. The disease in which the hormone referred to in No. 2 is insufficient is

   called _____ _____.

4. The temporary excess of carbohydrates is changed into _____

   in a process called _____.

5. _____ is stored in the liver and skeletal muscles until it is needed, at which time, it is changed back into

   _____ in a process called

   _____.

6. When _____ is inadequate to meet the body's demands, it is produced from fats or proteins and diffused out of the liver cells into the

   blood in a process called _____.

Step 6. You usually gain weight when your intake of carbohydrates and fats far exceeds the output of energy. These are stored in the adipose tissues instead of being burned for energy.

1. If your diet is high in carbohydrates and fats and you get very little or no exercise, would you tend to gain weight ___ or would your weight remain at or near normal ___?
2. If you are working very hard at manual labor but your diet is inadequate to meet the increased demands for energy, would you be likely to lose weight ___ or gain weight ___?
3. If you are overweight and you reduce the carbohydrates in your diet as well as the fats and you start exercising vigorously and regularly, would you be likely to lose weight ___, or would the burning of the stored fats and a reduction of intake of carbohydrates make no difference in your weight ___?

Step 7. Complete the blanks in the following statements.

1. _____ are tissue-building foods.
2. Protein as food differs from that of the tissues, for it has to be completely

broken down into its separate _____

_____ before it can be utilized by the body cells.

Step 8. Fatty substances or lipids form a large part of all the cells and tissues and are also stored in reserves or depots, particularly in the adipose tissue. Fats constitute the body's largest reserve energy source.

Complete the blanks in the following statements.

1. The main depots for storage of fats in

   the body are the _____

   _____.

2. In obesity there is an abnormally large amount of fatty accumulation

   in the _____ tissues. This is invariably the result of an energy intake of carbohydrates and fats greater than the output.

Step 9. Fatty accumulations, infiltrations, and degenerations in some organs, particularly the liver, are common findings in a number of diseases or conditions. Fatty accumulations or changes are found in the liver in chronic alcoholism, wasting diseases, and starvation. Fatty infiltrations and degeneration of cells occur most frequently in the kidneys, heart, and liver, in infections with high toxicity, intoxications from chemicals, severe anemias, and anoxia.

Indicate in the spaces provided those conditions in which you might expect to find fatty accumulations, infiltrations, and degenerations reflected in the cells.

1. Poisoning with carbon tetrachloride __
2. Reduction of oxygen content of blood below physiologic level __
3. Cirrhosis of the liver as an expression of chronic alcoholism __
4. Balanced diet with adequate nutrients __
5. Wasting of the muscles in starvation __

Step 10. The lipids form a large source of calories, which can be made available either for immediate use or for storage in deposits or reserves. Lipids also assist in the absorption of fat-soluble vitamins and furnish essential fatty acids.

Mark the following statements *T* for true or *F* for false.

1. If there were an inability to absorb fat-soluble vitamins, this would be a possible fault of fat metabolism. __
2. Lipids constitute the sole source of calories. __

Step 11. Important hormones under the control of the anterior pituitary gland help to keep glucose at a fairly constant level.

Give the name of the gland responsible for the secretion of the following hormones.

1. Thyroxine _____

2. ACTH _____

3. Epinephrine _____

4. Insulin _____

REPRESENTATIVE METABOLIC DISEASES
Gaucher's disease[4, 12, 13]

Gaucher's disease is a relatively common familial disorder in which there is abnormal accumulation of lipid (glucocerebrosides) in reticuloendothelial (RE) cells caused by deficiency of an enzyme necessary for degradation of the glycolipids. Three types of Gaucher's disease have been recognized. The chronic non-neuronopathic type is the most common and occurs at any age and in both sexes equally. It is characterized by hypersplenism, skin pigmentation, and bone lesions. From 50% to 75% of the patients have roentgenographic bone changes, the common one being expansion of the cortex of the lower end of the femur, producing the characteristic radiolucent area with the configuration of the Erlenmeyer flask. The phalanges, long bones, vertebrae, ribs, and pelvis may be involved more commonly than the skull. Pathologic fractures may occur in affected bones at the site of the lesion. Pingueculae (brownish, wedge-shaped lesions) tend to develop first on the nasal and later on the temporal side. The bases of the wedges are near the cornea and the apices point toward the inner or outer canthi. Patients with Gaucher's disease are likely to develop hemolytic anemia, leukopenia, thrombocytopenia, or any combination of these during the course of the disease.

The acute neuronopathic type is an infantile form, and as a rule, it is evident by the time the infant is 3 months, but symptoms may appear at any time between birth and 18 months. This type is characterized by splenomegaly (see Fig. 18-31), chronic cough, and psychomotor retardation. Neurologic signs are retroflexion of the head, retraction of lips, and often spastic extremities held in flexion. The disease is fatal within 3 years. This type is believed to be transmitted as an autosomal recessive gene in a homozygous person.

In the juvenile type (subacute neuronopathic), there is splenomegaly, hypersplenism, bone lesions, mental retardation, and at times, strabismus.

Diagnosis is made by detection of Gaucher cells in bone marrow aspirates, and by liver biopsy in which glucocerebroside accumulation and deficient glucocerebrosidase activity are demonstrated. Assay of cerebrosidase activity in white cells or fibroblasts in tissue culture is another diagnostic measure.

Galactosemia[5, 8]

"Classic galactosemia" is caused by a marked deficiency of the enzyme galactose-l-phosphate uridyl transferase. In a rarer type of galactosemia there is a deficiency of the enzyme galactokinase. Both types are the result of inborn errors of carbohydrate metabolism in which the infants are unable to metabolize galactose. In both types, galactose accumulates in the body. In the classic type the toxic effects of galactose accumulation are noted in the liver, eye, and brain, and there is mental retardation. Cataracts may be present at birth or may develop within the first few weeks or months of life. The symptoms are hepatomegaly, ascites, jaundice, vomiting, and diarrhea. The only clinical manifestations

of galactokinase deficiency are cataracts and galactose intolerance.

Diagnosis of galactokinase deficiency is established by assaying galactokinase activity of the red blood cells. The classic galactosemia is diagnosed by the absence of galactose-l-phosphate uridyl transferase activity from erythrocytes. With early diagnosis and the institution of a galactose-free diet, the development of the child may be normal or nearly so, but if there is a delay in diagnosis and treatment, mental retardation may occur and cataracts may be irreversible. Galactokinase deficiency is a relatively harmless disorder, except for cataracts.

Galactosemia can be prevented through genetic counseling. Procedures are available to detect the monozygous individual, but identification of the heterozygous galactosemic person is difficult since he is usually asymptomatic. Family studies of transferase levels in red blood cells may reveal the presence of hereditary galactosemia and have been used to confirm the suspected heterozygotes.

Gargoylism (Hurler's disease; mucopolysaccharidosis)[3, 4, 8]

Hurler's syndrome is caused by a disturbance in carbohydrate metabolism and appears to be the result of an absence of one or more of a group of enzymes that degrade mucopolysaccharides. The mucopolysaccharides accumulate in many cells of the nervous system, reticuloendothelial system, liver, endocrine glands, heart muscles, and in bone and cartilage cells. It has been divided into two types. The classic and most prevalent type is an autosomally inherited abnormality of mucopolysaccharides. The milder type is inherited as an X-linked recessive. Both types resemble each other in clinical manifestations, except that in the milder type, corneal clouding is minimal or absent and mental deterioration is slower in development.

The classic type occurs in about 1 in 40,000 individuals. It is characterized by skeletal deformities, hepatosplenomegaly, corneal clouding, and mental retardation. The clinical manifestations are usually evident during the first year or two of life, but the infant may appear normal at birth. The head is large and facial features are coarse, with a broad saddle nose, wide nostrils, thick lips, large tongue, and an open-mouth expression. The neck is short, and the patient has a short stature with dorsal and lumbar kyphosis. Joint deformities include genu valgus, coxa valga, pes planus, and talipes equinovarus. There may be nodular thickenings of the skin over the thorax and upper extremities. Coarse hair may be profuse over the extremities. The abdomen is large and protruding.

Diagnosis of the classic type of gargoylism is made from characteristic clinical manifestations, x-ray studies of skeleton, biopsy of tissues, blood and bone marrow studies, and examination of the urine for increased mucopolysaccharide excretion. In classic Hurler's syndrome, both parents are obligatory heterozygotes and yield metachromatic cultures; in the X-linked type, the cultured fibroblasts from the mother are metachromatic, but the cells from the father are normal.

Phenylketonuria[7, 15]

The classic type of phenylketonuria is caused by an inborn error of metabolism, inherited as an autosomal recessive. The condition results from complete absence of phenylalanine hydroxylase activity. It is manifested by hyperphenylalaninemia, mental retardation in most cases, and excessive urinary excretion of phenylpyruvic acid and other phenylalanine derivatives. The finding of hyperphenylalaninemia is not always diagnostic of phenylketonuria, since in recent years the mass screening of newborn infants has disclosed that there are several types of hyperphenylalaninemia. These types behave as independent autosomal recessive traits, and the manifestations of the disorder are atypical, mild, transient, or benign. Their recognition and differentiation from the classic type are important, since the latter is responsible for mental retardation.

The phenylketones can cross the placental barrier and affect the mental development of the fetus in utero. Successfully treated females not only continue to transmit phenylketonuria in their heredity but also continue to accumulate phenylketones. It is imperative that these women be traced or redetected and during their period of child-bearing be placed on a low-phenylalanine diet.

The infants with this defect are usually normal at birth, and physical development is normal. Later, however, there are eczematous lesions of the skin and decreased pigmentation, excessive perspiration, irritability, and vomiting. The urine has a characteristic mousy odor. The symptoms of the central nervous system predominate and include, tremor, ataxia, convulsions, retardation, and schizoid changes. The lack of melanin gives these infants the characteristic blue color of eyes, blond hair, and decreased pigmentation of the skin, and it accounts for the eczematous lesions. This is because phenylalanine is not converted to tyrosine, a precursor of melanin. Mental deficiency accompanies an accumulation of phenylalanine in the serum, but the mechanism is obscure. The brain and spinal cord are structurally damaged by demyelination. The myelin or fatlike substance forming a sheath around nerve tissue is destroyed.

The diagnostic aids include tests for phenylpyruvic acid in the urine, tests for serum elevation of phenylalanine, and other tests for screening the neonate for phenylketonuria. A ferric chloride urine test is positive based on a reaction with phenylpyruvic acid, which is present in the urine in this disease after the third to sixth week of life. The x-ray examinations show metaphyseal cupping of bones.

Maple syrup urine disease[15, 17]

Maple syrup urine disease derives its name from the characteristic odor of the urine of the patient with branched-chain ketoaciduria and aminoacidopathy. It is caused by an inborn error of amino acid metabolism, in which leucine, isoleucine, alloisoleucine, and valine are elevated in the plasma and urine. The abnormal enzymatic defect is primarily a block in decarboxylation of branched-chain α-keto acids. The disease is autosomal recessive.

The urinary maple syrup odor, often occurring toward the end of the first week of life, is the prominent symptom. There is failure to thrive, anorexia, convulsions, semicomatose condition, and hypertonicity. The Moro reflex is inactive in these infants. (The Moro reflex is elicited by placing an infant on a table and then forcibly striking the table on either side of the child. His arms are suddenly thrown out in an embrace attitude as a normal response.) When the branched-chain amino acids are eliminated from the diet along with other therapeutic measures, maple syrup odor disappears from the urine, and the Moro reflex becomes more active. The almost uniform mortality and disability previously associated with this disorder are prevented if treatment is begun sufficiently early in life and strictly maintained. The mental retardation is progressive in untreated patients, with a fatal outcome, but in treated patients it is believed the mental retardation can be prevented or held to a moderate level.[17]

The diagnosis is made by detection of aminoacidopathy in the blood and urine within the first week of life. The enzymatic defect can be assayed in leukocytes and in cultures of skin fibroblasts.

Glycogen storage disease[1, 16]

Glycogen storage disease occurring in infancy represents a rare genetic defect of glycogen metabolism. There are several types and subtypes referred to as the glycogenoses. From available evidence, all are transmitted as a recessive trait except for type IXa (defect is phosphorylase kinase), which is sex-linked. Some types involve the striated muscle, and others are charac-

terized by accumulations of glycogen in the liver, kidney, and gastrointestinal tract. Some of the types are rare, and only the two most common types will be discussed here.

The most frequent type is type I, which was identified in 1929 by von Gierke, and hence is known by his name. It is characterized by an absence or reduction of glucose-6-phosphatase activity in hepatic and renal cells, which results in accumulation of glycogen in the tissues.

In *von Gierke's disease*, or type I, the enlargement of the liver is present at birth. This may be the only symptom for the first year of life. However, in some infants succumbing in the early neonatal period there has been dehydration, acidosis, and fatty infiltration of the liver. Other symptoms of type I are hypoglycemia, ketosis, growth disturbances, and a greater susceptibility to infections.

In type II, *Pompe's disease*, there is cardiac hypertrophy, neuromuscular involvement, and a generalized accumulation of glycogen caused by lack of the enzyme that hydrolyses maltose and glycogen to glucose. This type is fatal, usually within a few months. In some cases that come to autopsy the heart is involved with nodular or tumor-like masses, and the cardiac muscle fibers are heavily infiltrated and enlarged by the accumulation of glycogen.

A definitive diagnosis of glycogen storage disease can be made by enzymatic assay of liver or muscle biopsies or of both.

Amaurotic familial idiocy[8, 14]

The infantile form of amaurotic familial idiocy—Tay-Sachs disease—is a genetically determined lipid-storage disease. It is caused by absence of the enzyme, hexosaminidase A, which a faulty gene is unable to produce. Tay-Sachs disease occurs primarily among Jews of Eastern and Central European ancestry.

The onset of Tay-Sachs disease occurs at any time during the first years of life, and it terminates fatally, usually by the third year. There is progressive muscular weakness, blindness, and mental deterioration. A characteristic sign is a cherry red spot that appears in the macula of both eyes. Reflexes are hyperactive. There is progressive motor loss and increasing atony of muscles, with intense spasticity. Blindness is progressive. Megalencephaly occurs in the patients with prolonged survival, but the entire brain may be small and atrophic in those dying early in the course of the disease.

Other types of this disease, referred to as juvenile, adult, and late infantile, also occur. In all there is mental deterioration and progressive blindness, but in the late juvenile or adult form, the span of life is longer, ranging from 5 to 10 years after onset.

Diagnosis in all types depends upon the characteristic clinical combination of dementia and blindness, plus in the infantile and juvenile types a cherry red or red-purple discoloration in the macula of both eyes.

A blood test of persons at risk will reveal the presence or absence of the enzyme hexosaminidase A, and in an effort to stamp out Tay-Sachs disease, screening tests are made from time to time in Jewish communities to discover the carriers of the faulty gene. In pregnant women a test of the amniotic fluid can reveal the presence of the disease in an unborn child, so that an abortion can be performed to prevent the birth of an affected child if the test proves positive.

Diabetes mellitus[6, 11, 18]

Diabetes mellitus is a generalized chronic disease resulting from a disorder of carbohydrate metabolism. It is believed that it is probably caused by inadequate secretion of insulin (sugar-regulating hormone) by the beta cells of the islands of Langerhans in the pancreas. Diabetes is considered to be transmitted as an autosomal recessive trait or to involve a hereditary predisposition. The known clinical elements that serve to characterize the disease, hyperglycemia and glycosuria, are thought to be secondary to a genetic defect or defects. Intensive investigations are now being made to elucidate the genetic abnormality.

The American Diabetes Association has recommended that the course of diabetes (assuming that it has a genetic basis) be divided into the four stages of prediabetes, suspected diabetes, chemical or latent diabetes, and overt diabetes. The prediabetics are offspring of diabetic parents, and it is assumed that these individuals will subsequently develop diabetes. Suspected diabetics means that the patient has developed an abnormal glucose tolerance test or has diabetic symptoms influenced by obesity, pregnancy, infections, trauma, or pharmaceutical and hormonal agents. These patients are normal in all respects, and when the precipitating agent is removed, the metabolism returns to normal limits. The chemical or latent diabetics have no signs or symptoms of the disease, but have an abnormal glucose tolerance test or an elevated fasting blood glucose independent of stress. The overt diabetics have symptoms of diabetes.

Although diabetes may develop at any time from a few months after birth to eight or nine decades later, some investigators have subdivided diabetes into two types—the juvenile and the maturity-onset diabetes. This subdivision is based upon the time of onset of diabetes. The juvenile type occurs in patients under 25 years of age, the average being 11 years. The adult type develops mainly in obese people over 40 years.

The most common signs of diabetes mellitus are polyuria (increased urinary output), polydipsia (increased thirst), polyphagia (excessive appetite), and loss of weight and strength. These symptoms are particularly prominent in the juvenile type. In the adult type, however, the first presenting symptom may be polyuria, followed by polydipsia as a compensatory mechanism. Polyuria develops because large amounts of water are mobilized from the tissues to dilute the sugar brought to the kidneys so that it can be eliminated. Sugar is an energy food, and when the body is unable to utilize carbohydrates, the patient becomes weak or loses strength. The loss of nutrients for energy causes the polyphagia.

The complications of diabetes mellitus involve the vascular, endocrine, and nervous systems, but other systems may also be involved. The degenerative disorder of arteriosclerosis is likely to be more progressive in the diabetic than in the nondiabetic and also appears at an earlier age. Gangrene is frequently a result of infection when there are circulatory disturbances of the lower extremities. Diabetics have an increased susceptibility to infection. Coronary artery disease may also develop. The retina may be damaged, with impaired vision and sometimes blindness occurring. Kidney symptoms are edema, albuminuria, hypertension, and even renal failure. When the peripheral nerves are involved, there may be paresthesia, muscular weakness, loss of reflexes, and atrophy. These symptoms are not necessarily caused by the diabetic condition but develop in these patients as complications, since they are more susceptible to disease than are nondiabetics.

In pregnancy, abortions occur three times more often in the diabetic than in the nondiabetic. Diabetes is not easy to control during pregnancy.

The most serious complication of diabetes mellitus is diabetic acidosis or coma. It usually occurs when there is poor control of diabetes or loss of ability to metabolize carbohydrates and fats properly. As precipitating factors there may be gross dietary excesses, insufficient insulin or omission of insulin, infections, or vomiting and diarrhea from any cause. Diabetic acidosis may also develop in thyrotoxicosis, pregnancy, and toxemias of pregnancy. The diabetic coma may range from drowsiness to deep unconsciousness.

The cycle of events leading to acidosis or coma is as follows: The glucose level in the blood is higher than can be tolerated by the body and is therefore excreted in the urine. The kidneys in order to handle the excess sugar must draw fluid from the blood, and this causes dehydration. Protein and fat are metabolized to produce energy. The fatty acids, the products of fat metabolism, form in excess of the body's ability to utilize them and are thus carried to the liver and converted into ketone bodies. The liver attempts to neutralize the excess fatty acids through chemical reactions that result in drawing more fluid from the body and sodium and other electrolytes from the blood, resulting in dehydration, loss of blood base and chloride, and a shift in the normal alkaline level of the blood to the acid side. If the process is not reversed, the blood pressure falls, and there is circulatory collapse and depression of renal activity leading to death. The breath will have an acetone odor in acidosis, glycosuria will be present, and the blood sugar level will almost always be very high.

Hypoglycemia is a condition in which the blood sugar falls below normal levels. The precipitating cause may be hyperinsulinism, which is known as insulin shock or insulin reaction when the patient is a known diabetic. It can occur as a result of overdose of insulin but is usually the result of factors that reduce insulin, such as inadequate food intake or long delay in eating following an insulin injection, vigorous exercise with increased energy requirements, or vomiting and diarrhea that interfere with absorption of food. The reaction of shock is usually of sudden onset, with a feeling of weakness and nervousness. In the absence of a quick-acting carbohydrate, headache, drowsiness, nausea, and paresthesia or extremities occur. Irritability may be followed by confusion, with visual disturbances, ataxia, and eventually unconsciousness. Hypoglycemia occurs more often in juvenile diabetes mellitus than in the adult type.

Diagnostic aids are urine and blood sugar determinations. The blood sugar determinations may be made on fasting blood specimens. Glucose tolerance tests or postprandial blood tests are necessary to detect the mild or very early cases. A family history of diabetes mellitus is also helpful in diagnosis.

Responses

Step 1: metabolism; catabolism; anabolism
Step 2: 1. X; 2. X; 3. X
Step 3: 1. fats; carbohydrates; 2. proteins
Step 4: 1. F; 2. T
Step 5: 1. glucose; 2. insulin; 3. diabetes mellitus; 4. glycogen; glycogenesis; 5. glycogen; glucose; glycogenolysis; 6. glucose; gluconeogenesis
Step 6: 1. gain weight; 2. lose weight; 3. lose weight
Step 7: 1. proteins; 2. amino acids
Step 8: 1. adipose tissues; 2. adipose
Step 9: 1. X; 2. X; 3. X; 5. X
Step 10: 1. T; 2. F
Step 11: 1. thyroid; 2. pituitary; 3. adrenals; 4. pancreas

REFERENCES

1. Anderson, W. A. D.: In Anderson, W. A. D., editor: Pathology, ed. 6, St. Louis, 1971, The C. V. Mosby Co. (degenerative changes and disturbances of metabolism).
2. Anthony, C. P., and Kolthoff, N. J.: Textbook of anatomy and physiology, ed. 9, St. Louis, 1975, The C. V. Mosby Co.
3. Bearn, A. G.: In Beeson, P. B., and McDermott, W., editors: Cecil-Loeb textbook of medicine, ed. 13, Philadelphia, 1971, W. B. Saunders Co. (mucopolysaccharidoses, Hurler syndrome).
4. Bennett, G. A.: In Anderson, W. A. D., editor: Pathology, ed. 6, St. Louis, 1971, The C. V. Mosby Co. (bones).
5. Beutler, E.: In Beeson, P. B., and McDermott, W. editors: Cecil-Loeb textbook of medicine, ed. 13, Philadelphia, 1971, W. B. Saunders Co. (galactosemia).
6. Bondy, P. K.: In Beeson, P. B., and McDermott, W. editors: Cecil-Loeb textbook of medicine, ed. 13, 1971, Philadelphia, W. B. Saunders Co. (diabetes).
7. Centerwell, W. R., and Centerwell, S. A.: Phenylketonuria, Children's Bureau Publication No. 388, Washington, D.C., 1965, U.S. Department of Health, Education, and Welfare.
8. Chason, J. L.: Anderson, W. A. D., editor: Pathology, ed. 6, St. Louis, 1971, The C. V. Mosby Co. (neuronal lipid-storage diseases).
9. Havel, R. J.: In Beeson, P. B., and McDermott, W., editors: Cecil-Loeb textbook of medicine, ed. 13, Philadelphia, 1971, W. B. Saunders Co. (disorders of lipid metabolism).
10. Houssay, B. A.: International forum (vol. 11, no. 3), Therap. Notes **70:**181, July-Aug., 1963 (role of pituitary gland in metabolism).
11. Lacy, P. E., and Kissane, J. M.: In Anderson, W. A. D., editor: Pathology, ed. 6, St. Louis, 1971, The C. V. Mosby Co. (diabetes mellitus).
12. Miale, J. B.: In Anderson, W. A. D., editor: Pathology, ed. 6, St. Louis, 1971, The C. V. Mosby Co. (Gaucher's disease).
13. Robbins, S. L.: Pathology, ed. 3, Philadelphia, 1967, W. B. Saunders Co. (metabolic diseases).
14. Schienberg, L. C.: In Beeson, P. B., and McDermott, W., editors: Cecil-Loeb textbook of medicine, ed. 13, 1971, Philadelphia, W. B. Saunders Co. (amaurotic idiocy).
15. Scriver, C. R.: In Beeson, P. B., and McDermott, W., editors: Cecil-Loeb textbook of medicine, ed. 13, 1971, Philadelphia, W. B. Saunders Co. (inborn errors of amino acid metabolism).
16. Sidbury, J. B., Jr.: In Beeson, P. B., and McDermott, W., editors: Cecil-Loeb textbook of medicine, ed. 13, 1971, Philadelphia, W. B. Saunders Co. (glycogen storage disease).
17. Snyderman, S. E.: Pediatrics **34:**454, 1964 (maple syrup urine disease).
18. U.S. Department of Health, Education, and Welfare, Division of Chronic Diseases, Public Health Service Publication No. 137, Health Information Series 70, 1965 (diabetes).

CHAPTER 8

Disturbances of body water and electrolytes

A group of disorders that occur as a result of disturbances or abnormalities of body water and electrolytes are outstanding signs of a number of major diseases. The values of electrolytes are measured in many laboratory examinations, and their excesses or deficiencies may indicate or help to pinpoint the contributing underlying defect in many diseases. Many of the disorders are considered only as symptoms, for example, edema, dehydration, and excesses or deficiencies of sodium, potassium, chloride, and magnesium.

ABNORMALITIES OF WATER DISTRIBUTION[8, 9]

Water constitutes the major part of the weight of the body, amounting to about 50% to 71% (average 60%) of the total body weight in a normal young adult male. The ratio of water to total body weight is somewhat less in the female and is greater in the newborn infant. The importance of this constituent of the body cannot be overemphasized, since death occurs when water loss amounts to approximately 15% of the body weight, which is about 7 to 10 days after complete deprivation of water.[1] All the chemical reactions that take place within the body are dependent upon water.

The total body water is divided into intracellular fluid and extracellular fluid. The extracellular fluid is subdivided into intravascular fluid or blood plasma; interstitial and lymph fluid; dense connective tissue, cartilage, and bone water; and transcellular fluid.[9] There is a constant exchange of fluid and electrolytes between the plasma and interstitial spaces across the semipermeable capillary endothelium.[8]

In a healthy person there is a balance between the intake and the output of water by the body as well as a normal distribution and balance of the body fluids and their electrolytes. Water intake from fluids and foods is by way of the gastrointestinal tract. Water is eliminated by the kidneys, gastrointestinal tract, skin, and lungs. Small amounts of water are also lost through the secretions from the nose, the mouth, the tear ducts, and from the mammary glands (milk).

Maintenance of an adequate intake of water is largely regulated by thirst when there is free access to water. Normal renal function is necessary in the regulation of water and electrolyte balance. When water is lost by evaporation, hyperventilation, marked sweating, or vomiting and diarrhea, the water balance is maintained by renal compensatory mechanisms. The kidneys can either conserve or excrete water and electrolytes to maintain a normal distribution and balance of body fluids. The regulatory activity of the renal tubules is influenced by the posterior pituitary antidiuretic and adrenal cortical hormones. When there is an excessive loss of water, the posterior pituitary causes an increased secretion of the antidiuretic hormone (ADH), allowing more water to be absorbed by the kidney tubules and returned to the concentrated body fluids. Another pathway through which fluid regulation is attained is the excretion or retention of extracellular sodium by the kidneys. Increased sodium excretion is accompanied by an increase in urinary output. Thus the body gets rid of excess water. Sodium retention and excessive secretion are discussed under electrolyte disturbances.

Edema[8, 9]

Edema generally refers to excessive accumulation of fluid within tissue spaces or body cavities, giving the clinical picture of swelling of a part or parts when it is manifested outwardly. It is not a disease but a symptom in that it is always provoked by a primary lesion or by a disturbance in the function of an organ or organs. The terminology referring to edema indicates the type and location. It is called hydrothorax (*hydro* meaning water) in the thoracic cavity; hydroperitoneum or ascites in the peritoneal cavity; and hydropericardium in the pericardial cavity. When the body cavities and subcutaneous tissue as a whole are affected, it is called anasarca or dropsy.

Edema is caused by a number of conditions that interfere with the normal movement of blood, tissue fluid, and lymph. All these disturb the mechanism of fluid balance. Swelling created by an obstruction to the lymph flow is called lymphedema. An outstanding example of this is the edema of the arm that occurs following surgical removal of the breast and axillary lymph nodes for cancer. The edema in this instance can also be caused by obstruction of the axillary lymph nodes by malignant neoplasm. In filariasis (infestation with nematode worms) the flow of lymph from the inguinal lymph nodes may be obstructed. The resulting chronic edema of the scrotum and legs is called elephantiasis. (The term "elephantiasis" is often applied to hypertrophy and thickening of tissues from any cause.) When the abdominal or thoracic lymph channels are blocked by tumor or infection, there may be large accumulations of fluid in the pleural or peri-

toneal cavities. If the thoracic or pleural intraductal pressure of lymph channels is increased or if they rupture, there is effusion of a milky chyle. These conditions are called chylothorax and chyloperitoneum or chylous ascites, respectively. A hereditary form of edema called congenital edema may affect a number of family members. This form is chronic and persistent, involving the lower extremities. It is attributed to faulty development of the lymphatic vessels.

Increased capillary permeability is a common cause of edema. An intact capillary endothelium is necessary to maintain a fairly constant blood volume. The capillary endothelium acts as a semipermeable membrane for the exchange of water and electrolytes between the vascular system and tissue spaces. Plasma proteins, however, are allowed to pass through this membrane only in small amounts. In any condition in which the endothelial lining of the capillaries is injured, proteins are allowed to escape into the interstitial fluid. There is a consequent imbalance between the osmotic pressure of the blood and that of the interstitial fluid, resulting in the escape of fluid into the interstitial tissues, which produces edema unless the lymph drainage is sufficient to remove the excess fluid. This type of edema occurs in many conditions, notably inflammatory response to wounds, severe infections, anaphylactic reactions (in allergies), poisonings from various drugs and chemicals, and anoxia from any cause. In inflammatory edema there is an immediate response to increased permeability of the capillary endothelium; this is seen in wheals, urticaria, and other allergic reactions as well as in bites of spiders and snakes, burns, infections, and any type of mechanical injury. A good example of inflammatory edema is seen in blisters produced by burns. Angioneurotic edema, which possibly has an allergic or neurogenic basis for increased vascular permeability, usually is sudden, with swelling of the eyelids, lips, tongue, larynx, lungs, and sometimes the extremities. Individuals subject to angioneurotic edema usually have a variety of allergies.[8, 9]

Edema may also result from a reduction in plasma proteins (hypoproteinemia) or more particularly from a decrease in plasma albumin (hypoalbuminemia). The nephrotic syndrome is an example of a condition in which profuse proteinuria, hypoproteinemia, and hyperlipemia (excessive lipids in the blood) cause renal edema. Renal edema, however, may be brought on by many factors. It may be caused by sodium retention, by increased capillary permeability resulting from toxic factors, as well as by loss of plasma proteins through injured glomerular filtration membranes. This type of edema is found not only in the nephrotic syndrome but in those diseases that particularly affect the glomeruli, such as glomerulonephritis, amyloidosis, and nodular glomerulosclerosis. In renal edema there is a classic swelling of the face, most noticeable in the eyelids.

Nutritional or starvation edema may occur from a decrease in plasma proteins, although a disturbance in the metabolism of sodium has also been implicated. In liver disease, hypoproteinemic edema occurs from a faulty synthesis of proteins.

When venous pressure is increased, edema may occur. This is seen in thrombosis of the veins of the lower extremities (for example, the iliacs) when they are obstructed by tumor or by pressure or a pregnant uterus. Cardiac edema is basically the result of increased venous pressures that are most elevated in the dependent portions of the body and by the generalized tendency to edema caused by retention of salt and water. Portal venous obstruction, as occurs in hepatic cirrhosis, leads to portal venous hypertension and a transudation of fluids into the peritoneal cavity (ascites).[8]

Individuals whose occupations require standing for long periods of time often develop postural edema, which is swelling of the legs and particularly the ankles. It seldom develops when an individual is active in walking or moving about, since the escaping fluid in the interstitial spaces is drained by the action of the muscles. Postural edema is transient and disappears after rest in a horizontal position.

Sodium retention occurs when its intake exceeds that of its excretion in the urine. This leads to water retention. When retention of sodium and water is progressive, the extracellular fluid is expanded and edema results. Retention of sodium and water occurs in a number of edematous states, including congestive heart faliure, cirrhosis of the liver, nephrotic syndrome referred to previously, and possibly in acute glomerulonephritis. Aldosterone, a potent adrenocortical hormone that regulates tubular reabsorption causing retention of sodium and excretion of potassium, is found in increased amounts in the urine of patients with congestive heart failure, hepatic cirrhosis, and the nephrotic syndrome. The mechanism of hypersecretion of aldosterone in these conditions is not entirely clear. Retention of water in edematous states has also been attributed to increased secretion of antidiuretic hormones.

Edema is more marked in those tissues that have a loose connective tissue matrix, such as the subcutaneous tissues. This is noted particularly in the soft parts about the eyes and external genitalia, where tissue tension is low. It is also noted in tissues overlying bone, as that in the legs and ankles, which sometimes show pitting edema on digital pressure.

Local edema may cause interference with physiologic functions. Fluid in the pericardial or pleural spaces may hamper cardiac or respiratory movements. Abdominal ascites also may make breathing difficult. Cerebral edema creates increased intracranial pressure and interferes with cerebral function. If the pharynx or glottis is swollen, breathing may be hampered by obstruction of the airway, which can produce asphyxia if severe. Rapid pulmonary edema obstructs alveoli and interferes with the normal exchange of gaseous elements (oxygen and carbon dioxide), which may eventuate in anoxia and even death. Fluid in lungs also furnishes a culture medium with the potential hazard of pneumonia.

Dehydration[1, 8, 9]

Dehydration is the result of water imbalance, in which the output exceeds the intake, causing a reduction of body water below normal. Not only is water lost, but sodium is depleted.

Dehydration can result from a number of conditions and in a number of diseases. It can be caused by restriction of water intake. This can occur in many conditions, such as in mental patients who refuse to drink water; patients with lesions that interfere with swallowing; patients who are in a coma; and particularly those who find themselves in a hazardous position with no access to water, such as lost in the desert or adrift on ocean rafts. Dehydration also occurs in diabetic acidosis. Excessive water loss occurs in profuse sweating when there is inadequate water to replenish thirst. A high body temperature also results in a loss of fluids.

ELECTROLYTE DISTURBANCES[1, 8, 9]

The electrolytes considered in this discussion are sodium, potassium, chloride, and magnesium.

Sodium

Sodium is available in drinking water and food, particularly when salt is added to food. Normally the output of sodium almost equals the intake. Sodium is excreted mainly in the urine, with small amounts eliminated in sweat and feces. Sodium is present chiefly in the extracellular fluids, but a small amount is also present within the cells. The chief function of sodium is to maintain osmotic equilibrium in extracellular fluids. Most of the sodium lost in acute cases of depletion is derived from the combined plasma-interstitial-lymph fluids.

The discussion of sodium overlaps that of water, and certain phases therefore will not be repeated.

A decreased sodium concentration in the plasma is called hyponatremia (*natremia* referring to sodium in the blood). This may be caused by sodium depletion (depletional hyponatremia) or retention of water over and above sodium retention (dilutional hyponatremia). Sodium retention has been previously discussed under retention of water. Dilutional hyponatremia is seen in water intoxication, congestive heart failure, and cirrhosis of the liver or diseases attributed to an excessive secretion of the antidiuretic hormone. The symptoms are muscular twitching and cramps, listlessness, fatigue, confusion, and even stupor. Circulatory failure and disturbances of renal function may also occur. Many of these symptoms may be absent in hyponatremia in salt-wasting or sodium-losing syndrome, in some cerebral disorders, in tuberculosis, and in bronchogenic carcinoma.

Hypernatremia is an increased sodium concentration in the blood, occurring when there is either an output of water in excess of sodium or severe restriction of water intake, as in dehydration discussed previously. It occurs in patients with cerebral lesions (for example, encephalomalacia, hemorrhage, wounds, malignancy, and meningitis). The mechanism in these cases is believed to be interference with the production of antidiuretic hormone, causing an acute diabetes insipidus (excessive urinary loss of water and electrolytes) that is not compensated for by water intake. Hypernatremia may also occur in diabetic coma when patients are treated solely with insulin and saline solutions.

Potassium

Potassium is concentrated within the cell in much greater amounts than in the extracellular fluids. It is essential to cellular metabolic processes, and its functions are concerned with the conduction of nerve impulses, cardiac muscular contraction, and the maintenance of normal irritability of skeletal muscle. Even small amounts above or below the normal in the serum can produce significant disturbances. Potassium also helps to maintain osmotic equilibrium between cell water and extracellular fluids. Most of it is excreted in the urine, but some is eliminated in the feces and a very little in perspiration.

Hypopotassemia and hypokalemia are terms associated with deficiency of potassium. This condition may occur as a result of inadequate intake (for example, starvation) or as a result of excessive loss from the body (for example, vomiting, diarrhea, diuresis), adrenal cortical hyperactivity, and surgical trauma.

Hyperpotassemia and hyperkalemia are terms applied to an increase in serum potassium, which is not as frequent as hypopotassemia. This condition sometimes occurs in patients who receive excessive parenteral or oral administration of potassium and are unable because of oliguria or renal functional impairment to eliminate the excess. It also may occur in untreated cases of chronic renal disease with failure and in adrenal insufficiency. The symptoms are paresthesia, flaccid paralysis, listlessness, mental confusion, and hypotension.

Chloride

Changes in chloride plasma concentration usually accompany those of sodium. An increase in chloride concentration is termed hyperchloremia. It may occur in patients receiving parenteral administrations of hypertonic sodium chloride solution and in dehydration caused by water depletion. It is also associated with decreased bicarbonate (an electrolyte) concentration and metabolic acidosis. Hypochloremia is a decrease in concentration of chloride in the plasma. It occurs in prolonged vomiting, adrenal insufficiency, dehydration from sodium depletion, acute infections, and renal failure.

Magnesium

Magnesium is principally an intracellular cation concerned with protein and carbohydrate metabolism and neuromuscular conduction. Magnesium is present in all foods and does not occur as a dietary deficiency except in starvation. Hypomagnesemia is decreased magnesium concentration, and it may be observed in chronic alcoholism, diabetic acidosis, starvation, and prolonged diuresis in congestive heart failure. Symptoms are muscular twitching, choreiform movements, convulsions, and coma. Hypermagnesemia is increased magnesium concentration, and it may occur in severe dehydration, untreated diabetic acidosis, renal failure, and excess administration of magnesium. The symptoms include lethargy, coma, and respiratory failure.

STEP-BY-STEP EXERCISES

Step 1. The vital physiologic values in the body that must be kept at a constant level include the normal circulation of the blood, a normal balance and distribution of the body fluids, and the preservation of a normal concentration of their electrolytes. The normal state and function of all the bodily tissues are dependent upon the normal maintenance of these values. Any major deviations from the normal may significantly affect the tissues, organs, and functions of the body as a whole.

Which of the following conditions are concerned with homeostasis (maintenance of a stable internal environment)?

1. Normal circulation of blood ___
2. Normal balance and distribution of water ___
3. Normal concentration of electrolytes ___
4. Normal balance of water but preservation of normal concentration of electrolytes not important ___

Step 2. The total body water is divided into compartments called intracellular and extracellular. The extracellular water is further divided into that which is contained in the plasma and that which is contained in the interstitial spaces (between tissue spaces).

Complete the blanks in the following statements.

1. Fluid within the cells is called _____.

2. Fluid outside the cells is called _____.

3. Fluid in the plasma is _____.

4. Fluid found in interstitial spaces is _____.

Step 3. Water is the single largest constituent of the body and is vital to health. To maintain health there must be a balance between the intake and output of water of the body. Water is taken into the body by way of the gastrointestinal tract and excreted by the kidneys, skin, lungs, and intestinal tract. Excess losses or drastically curtailed intake of water have a harmful effect on the body, since the normal balance is upset.

Which of the following would be likely to upset the normal balance of intake and output of water?

1. Excessive perspiration without replenishment of water lost ___

2. Excessive perspiration with replenishment by drinking water ___

3. Excessive loss through kidneys without replenishment of body water ___

4. Prolonged vomiting and diarrhea ___

Step 4. Maintenance of an adequate intake of water is largely regulated by thirst when there is free access to water. Regulation of water and electrolyte balance depends upon normal renal function. The kidneys can either conserve or excrete water and electrolytes to maintain a normal distribution and balance of body fluids. However, if the kidneys are involved primarily or secondarily in a disease process, normal renal function may break down, and the kidneys may excrete too much water, or water may be retained in excess of the body's needs.

Complete the blanks in the following statements.

1. Regulation of water and electrolyte balance depends upon _____ _____ _____.

2. Kidney diseases or diseases of other bodily systems may affect the secretion or retention of fluids. This would be a breakdown of _____ _____ _____.

Step 5. The fluid excreted by the kidneys is called urine. It is largely water, but it also contains other solid matter—urea, sodium chloride, phosphoric acid, sulfuric acids, uric acid, and other organic salts. In certain diseases the output of urine is an important symptom. A scanty urinary output is referred to as oliguria. Anuria is cessation of urinary output. Excessive urinary output is called polyuria.

Complete the blanks in the following statements.

1. Scanty or abnormally small output of urine is referred to as _____.

2. Excessive urination is referred to as _____.

3. Cessation of urinary output is called _____.

Step 6. Excessive accumulation of fluid within tissue spaces or body cavities is referred to as edema. The terminology indicates the type and location of the accumulation of fluid. If necessary, you may refer to the text to complete the blanks in the following statements.

1. Excessive accumulation of fluid in the thoracic cavity is called _____.

2. Excessive accumulation of fluid in the peritoneal cavity is called _____.

3. Excessive accumulation of fluid in the pericardial cavity is called _____.

4. When there is excessive accumulation of fluid in the subcutaneous tissues and body cavities as a whole, it is referred to as _____.

Step 7. Edema is caused by a number of conditions that interfere with the normal movement of blood, tissue fluid, and lymph. Refer to the text if necessary and complete the blanks with the type of edema described.

1. Obstruction of lymph flow _____
2. Increased venous pressure with heart

   involvement _____

3. After long period of standing _____
4. Swelling of eyelids and lips, in particular, with an allergic or neurogenic

   basis _____ _____

5. In the nephrotic syndrome or in diseases particularly affecting the glomeruli _____ _____

Step 8. Dehydration results when the output of water exceeds the intake, thereby reducing the body water to below normal values. Water depletion may be primary or secondary. When primary, it results from restriction of intake of water. When secondary, it refers to loss from the body of electrolyte-containing fluids, often called sodium depletion, since this is the significant ion concerned with maintenance of extracellular fluid volume.

Complete the blanks in the following statements.

1. When body water is reduced below normal values because output exceeds

   intake, it is called _____.

2. If there is inability to swallow, this might result in dehydration, which

   would be ___ _____.

3. Electrolyte-containing fluids are lost in vomiting and diarrhea; this would

   be _____ dehydration.

Step 9. Electrolytes are important in the maintenance of osmotic pressures and of normal balance and distribution of body fluids. They are also important for preservation of acid-base balance and normal neuromuscular irritability.

On the basis of this statement would you say that electrolytes contribute to the vital physiologic values that must be maintained at a normal level for good health?

Yes ___ No ___

Step 10. Sodium is a cation that occurs chiefly in the extracellular fluids, but it is also present in low concentration within the cells. Its chief function is to maintain osmotic equilibrium in extracellular fluids. We get sodium from drinking water and from eating food and salt. When we are in good health, the sodium output almost equals the intake.

Complete the blanks in the following statements.

1. A cation occurring chiefly in the extracellular fluid whose chief function is to maintain osmotic equilibrium of

   this fluid is called _____.

2. The principal sources of sodium are

   _____, _____, and _____
   added to food.

Step 11. Sodium is the principal ion in circulating fluid volume, and of all the body organs involved in the regulation of water (lungs, kidneys, small intestine, colon, and skin), the kidneys are primarily responsible for maintaining normal sodium levels in the body.

Which of the following organs are *not* primarily responsible for maintaining normal sodium levels?

1. Kidneys ___   3. Skin ___
2. Colon ___   4. Lungs ___

Step 12. Refer to the text if necessary and complete the blanks in the following statements.

1. Decreased sodium concentration in

   the plasma is called _____.

2. Increased sodium concentration in the

   plasma is called _____.

3. Decreased sodium concentration brought about by sodium depletion

   is called _____ _____.

4. Decreased sodium concentration

caused by retention of water over and above the retention of sodium is called _____ _____.

Step 13. Potassium is the intracellular cation that is essential to cellular metabolic processes. It is concerned with the conduction of nerve impulses, the contraction of cardiac muscle, and the maintenance of normal irritability of skeletal muscle. Unlike sodium, which can be conserved by the kidneys in the absence of sodium intake, potassium continues to be lost in the urine when there is no potassium in the diet.

Which of the following functions are properties of potassium?

1. Normal functioning of the muscles ___
2. Normal functioning of the nerves ___
3. Normal functioning of the lungs ___

Step 14. Refer to the text if necessary to complete the blanks in the following statements.

1. Deficiency of cell potassium is referred to as _____ or _____.
2. Increase in serum potassium is referred to as _____ or _____.

Step 15. Considering the main functions of sodium and potassium, complete the blanks with whichever one is *more likely* to be involved in the following diseases or disorders:

1. Flaccid paralysis _____

2. Familial periodic paralysis _____

3. Involvement of heart muscle _____

4. Salt-wasting syndrome _____

5. Overhydration or water intoxication

_____

6. Impaired water diuresis _____

Step 16. On the basis of what you have learned about regulation and balance of fluids in the body, particularly extracellular, which is the most important electrolyte in this connection?

1. Sodium ___   3. Magnesium ___
2. Potassium ___

DISTURBANCES IN EXCRETION OF URINE

Two symptoms commonly present in kidney disturbances are anuria (cessation of urinary secretion) and polyuria (excessive excretion of urine). Either may be a complication of many diseases or a direct result of renal disorders.

Anuria[2, 8]

Anuria (see Fig. 18-5) is the cessation of urinary secretion. It is manifested clinically by a production of less than 100 ml. of urine per day. Any urine output of 100 to 400 ml. of urine per day is called oliguria (scanty urine). When anuria exists, there is resulting hypokalemia (deficiency of potassium), azotemia (urea or other nitrogenous bodies in the blood), or overhydration. It is caused by prerenal, renal, and postrenal disorders.

Anuria may be caused by inadequate water intake, dehydration from excessive loss of water through profuse sweating, severe diarrheal or febrile illness, decreased cardiac output, or shock. Renal failure can also be caused by narrowing of the renal arteries from atherosclerosis, occlusion by a thrombus or embolus, and bilateral renal vein thrombosis. All these vascular disorders would cause impairment of blood flow to the kidney. Injury to the tubules is a common cause of acute renal failure; it has been called lower nephron nephrosis and acute tubular necrosis. This type of renal failure may be precipitated by hemoglobinuria, the result of intravascular hemolysis, and by myoglobinuria, often seen after severe injury, extensive surgery, and in the crush syndrome. Poisoning may cause acute renal failure in tubular injury by damaging the proximal portion of the tubules. The agents are notably the heavy metals.[8]

Acute glomerulonephritis decreases the amount of urinary filtrate resulting in anuria. Acute pyelonephritis may also produce anuria, especially when there is papillary necrosis. Preeclampsia, purpuric affections, and hypersensitivity reactions can cause oliguria or anuria.

The obstructive lesions that produce anuria are bilateral. If they are unilateral, they are associated with absence of a kidney or a diseased kidney that is functioning poorly. Calculi, renal or ureteral, can cause anuria, but simultaneous blockage is rare. Carcinoma of the urinary bladder may block the ureteral orifices. Pressure directly on the ureters by uterine fibromyomas, ovarian cysts, and visceral tumors may cause suppression of urine.[8, 9]

Anuria is a feature in acute renal failure. The artificial kidney was first developed to give temporary relief to patients with reversible acute renal failure,[5] but it is now used often in acute renal failure from a variety of causes.[7] Dialysis is discussed in Chapter 18. (See Fig. 18-6.)

Polyuria[4]

Polyuria results from the inability of the kidney to produce concentrated urine. This may be caused by an insufficient production or release of vasopression (the antidiuretic hormone [ADH]) or by an inability of the kidney to respond to this hormone.[4] When ADH is present, the convoluted segment of the distal tubule and the collecting duct are permeable to water. The water is reabsorbed into the interstitial space with sodium. If ADH is absent, the entire distal tubule and the collecting duct are impermeable to water but not to sodium. Thus osmotic equilibrium with the interstitial space is not achieved, and hypotonic urine is excreted.[4] More than one abnormality may be present in a given case of clinical polyuria. In diminished circulating ADH there may be impaired ability to secrete ADH, with the primary defect being diabetes insipidus (discussed later), but some patients may develop an acquired renal resistance to ADH when it is supplied. There may be a diminished need to secrete ADH, such as occurs in potassium deficiency, hypercalcemia and hypercalciuria (these relate to calcium), and compulsive water drinking,

as well as lesions of thirst centers in the brain. In polyuria, when there is adequate circulating ADH, the defect may be in impaired ability of the tubule to respond to ADH. This occurs in some congenital diseases and may also be acquired, as in compulsive water drinking, potassium deficiency, diabetes insipidus, and again in hypercalcemia and hypercalciuria. Adequate circulating ADH may be present, but there may be faulty mechanism for producing hypertonic interstitial fluid in the medulla of the kidney, such as occurs in partial renal artery occlusion, chronic pyelonephritis, and destruction of the nephrons in chronic renal failure. Adequate circulating ADH may be present, but there may be increased solute output per nephron (osmotic diuresis).[4] This occurs when there is a normal number of nephrons but a glycosuria or a salt diuresis following relief of urinary obstruction. Osmotic diuresis also occurs when there is a greatly reduced number of functioning nephrons, as occurs in chronic renal failure.[4]

Diabetes insipidus[3, 6]

Diabetes insipidus is customarily divided into two categories—false diabetes insipidus, or psychogenic polydipsia (excessive thirst), and true diabetes insipidus caused by deficiency of vasopressin, an antidiuretic hormone. Both types are characterized by polyuria and polydipsia. Other than the annoyance of these two conditions, there may be no evidence of ill health or of other physiologic causes, unless the patient has an underlying local or systemic disease that has destroyed the neurohypophyseal system. The latter might be the result of primary or metastatic tumors in or near the sella turcica or surgical attempts to remove these lesions.

The polyuria in diabetes insipidus usually begins abruptly. Thirst is pronounced, but this compensatory polydipsia is essential to survival. In postoperative patients or those with central nervous system disease, who because of confusion or coma are unable to be aware of the need for water, dehydration accompanied by severe hypernatremia and hyperchloremia may develop rapidly. A dry skin and mucous membrane, soft eyeballs, and circulatory collapse are symptoms in these patients. In diabetes insipidus the large volume of urine is usually fairly constant. If there is a variation to any marked degree, compulsive drinking or primary polydipsia (not caused by diabetes isipidus) is probably the precipitating cause of the variation in urine output. True diabetes insipidus involves a lack of circulating vasopressin to the kidneys, which are capable of responding to it. The specific gravity in diabetes insipidus is usually below 1.003, whereas in polyuria of renal origin it will be higher, being fixed close to 1.010. Nephrogenic diabetes insipidus, which is rare, results from a failure of the renal tubule to respond to vasopressin.[6]

In patients with persistent polyuria and a urine of low concentration, differential diagnosis is aimed at determining if there is inability of the kidney to elaborate a concentrated urine despite adequate vasopressin, or if there is deficient vasopressin, or if there is persistent excessive water intake.[6] Several special procedures test the ability of the kidneys to respond to osmotic stimuli by elaboration of a concentrated urine, whether failure to do so is the consequence of a lack of endogenous vasopressin or of an inability of the renal tubules to respond to vasopressin.[6] The simplest test is water restriction with observation of urine volume and concentration. Another test is the infusion of hypertonic solutions to reduce urine flow. If these tests fail to reduce urine flow or to increase urine concentration, a test involving exogenous vasopressin is used to separate nephrogenic causes from hormone deficiency.[6] Compulsive water drinking to such a degree that it is confused with diabetes insipidus is a severe psychogenic disorder requiring clinical evaluation.[6]

Responses

Step 1: 1. X; 2. X; 3. X
Step 2: 1. intracellular; 2. extracellular; 3. extracellular; 4. extracellular
Step 3: 1. X; 3. X; 4. X
Step 4: 1. normal renal function; 2. normal renal function
Step 5: 1. oliguria; 2. polyuria; 3. anuria
Step 6: 1. hydrothorax; 2. hydroperitoneum or ascites; 3. hydropericardium; 4. dropsy or anasarca
Step 7: 1. lymphedema; 2. cardiac; 3. postural; 4. angioneurotic edema; 5. renal edema
Step 8: 1. dehydration; 2. primary; 3. secondary
Step 9: Yes
Step 10: 1. sodium; 2. water; food; salt
Step 11: 2. X; 3. X; 4. X
Step 12: 1. hyponatremia; 2. hypernatremia; 3. depletional hyponatremia; 4. dilutional hyponatremia
Step 13: 1. X; 2. X
Step 14: 1. hypopotassemia; hypokalemia; 2. hyperpotassemia; hyperkalemia
Step 15: 1. potassium; 2. potassium; 3. potassium; 4. sodium; 5. sodium; 6. sodium
Step 16: 1. X

REFERENCES

1. Bland, J. H.: Clinical metabolism of body water and electrolytes, Philadelphia, 1963, W. B. Saunders Co.
2. Chromographs of clinical symptomatology, Detroit, 1965, Parke, Davis & Co. (anuria).
3. Currie, A. R.: In Anderson, W. A. D., editor: Pathology, ed. 6, St. Louis, 1971, The C. V. Mosby Co. (diabetes insipidus).
4. de Wardener, H. E.: J. Chronic Dis. 11:199, 1960 (polyuria).
5. Kincaid-Smith, P.: In Beeson, P. B., and McDermott, W., editors: Cecil-Loeb textbook of medicine, ed. 13, Philadelphia, 1971, W. B. Saunders Co. (dialysis).
6. Leaf, A.: In Beeson, P. B., and McDermott, W., editors: Cecil-Loeb textbook of medicine, ed., 13, Philadelphia, 1971, W. B. Saunders Co. (diabetes insipidus).
7. Maher, J. F.: Ohio State Med. J. 60:235, 1964 (dialysis).
8. Robbins, S. L.: Pathology, ed. 3, Philadelphia, 1967, W. B. Saunders Co. (metabolism).
9. Scotti, T. M.: In Anderson, W. A. D., editor: Pathology, ed. 6, St. Louis, 1971, The C. V. Mosby Co. (disturbances of body water, electrolytes, and circulation of blood).

CHAPTER 9

Disturbances in circulation of blood

The normal circulation of the blood is imperative for maintenance of the body in health. Many of the major diseases and disorders are characterized by disturbances in the circulation of the blood. These may be obstructive and are of paramount importance as the leading symptom of some underlying major disease or malfunction of organs. They include thrombosis, embolism, ischemia, and infarction.

The entire circulatory system transports all the substances used and produced by the cells. These include oxygen, carbon dioxide, water, salt, nutritional substances, metabolites, hormones, and waste products. Although the blood itself is contained in vascular channels (arteries, veins, capillaries, venules), through the endothelial lining of the capillary walls there is a constant exchange between the blood and the tissues of all these substances. The interstitial or intercellular fluid, discussed in Chapter 8, is the intermediary that serves as the distributor and collector of the materials within the tissues. The cells contain a considerable amount of water but are surrounded and separated from the bloodstream by the tissue fluid.[21, 22]

DISTURBANCES OF BLOOD VOLUME

Hyperemia or congestion is defined as an increased volume of blood in dilated vessels in an organ or part. It may be arteriolar dilatation with an increased flow of blood into capillaries, called active hyperemia or active congestion. It may be caused by decreased venous outflow secondary to venous stasis, called chronic passive congestion. The flushed appearance that follows muscular exercise is an example of active hyperemia, as are the local vascular dilatations in inflammatory conditions and blushing. The latter may result from neurogenic conditions.[21]

Passive hyperemia or passive congestion of abdominal viscera and extremities is usually systemic in origin, such as occurs in cardiac failure, chiefly of the right ventricle, producing so-called backward failure in which there is progressive venous stasis involving the systemic circuit. In left ventricular failure or insufficient cardiac output, which is the so-called forward failure, the pulmonary venous circuit is congested because the left ventricle fails to pump out all the blood that enters from the right heart. However, both right and left cardiac decompensation occur together and cause generalized congestion.[21]

Local venous congestion occurs when there is obstruction to the venous return of blood, as in tumors, thrombosis, and external pressures (tight bandages, tourniquet, hernia, constricting scar tissue).[21] There may be localized vascular obstruction in the portal venous drainage in cirrhosis of the liver, which causes passive congestion in abdominal viscera. Varicosities of the extremities are causes of local venous congestion.

Congestion and edema usually occur together, since congestion of the capillary bed is related to the development of edema. When congestion is slight, there may be only slightly increased redness and vascularity, but in severe congestion there is also edema, producing increases in weight and size of the organs, as in the lung, liver, and spleen in chronic passive congestion.[22] Chronic congestion of the lungs with pulmonary edema is encountered in all forms of heart failure.

HEMORRHAGE

The escape of blood from a blood vessel, which implies a defect in its wall, is known as hemorrhage. If the released blood accumulates in the tissues and produces a large massive clot, this is a hematoma. (See Fig. 18-20, A.) Collection of blood (usually massive) in the body serous cavities is known as hemothorax (within thoracic cavity), hemopericardium (within pericardial cavity), and hemoperitoneum (within peritoneal cavity). The small hemorrhages in the skin, in the mucous membranes, and on serosal surfaces are known as petechiae (which means minute). If somewhat larger, they are known as purpura, and when large and blotchy, as seen in bruises, as ecchymoses.[21]

Hemorrhages are usually the result of trauma to a vessel causing a rupture of the wall, but rupture may also be spontaneous, as occurs in cerebral hemorrhage in hypertensive patients. (See Figs. 18-20, E, and 18-28, B.) Other conditions that may produce spontaneous hemorrhage are aneurysms (blood-filled sacs formed by dilatation of walls of arteries or veins) and inflammatory and degenerative disorders affecting the vascular system, such as cardiovascular syphilis, polyarteritis nodosa, arteriosclerosis, and medial necrosis of the aorta. Some systemic bacterial diseases, such as meningococcemia and rickettsial infections, may be characterized by multiple hemorrhages (small), which are presumably caused by vascular toxins that damage the vessel walls. (See Fig. 14-1.)

A number of hematologic disorders are characterized by defects in the clotting mechanism that cause serious hemorrhage.

This type of hemorrhage may be spontaneous or traumatic. The outstanding example of a defect in the clotting mechanism is hemophilia, an inherited disorder, which is discussed in Chapter 16. A number of substances are involved in coagulation of the blood; they are termed coagulation factors and are designated by Roman numerals, such as factors II, V, VII, VIII, IX, X, XI, and XII.[17, 27] The basic steps in the formation of a blood clot are the formation of thromboplastin, the conversion of prothrombin to thrombin, and the conversion of fibrinogen to fibrin. This explanation of the formation of a blood clot is an oversimplification, since, as mentioned previously, there are other coagulation factors involved. The mechanisms of deficiencies in the blood factors in producing disease are complicated and are of prime concern to physicians and to hematologists in particular. In a discussion of limited scope it is not possible to elaborate on these factors, but if interested, the student should refer to textbooks on hematology or blood diseases. Some bleeding disorders, such as hypofibrinogenemia or afibrinogenemia and thrombocytopenia, are discussed at the end of this chapter.

In all cases of defective clotting of the blood the patient is likely to bleed profusely from relatively trivial traumatic damages to vessels. This increased tendency to bleed in certain disorders is known as hemorrhagic diathesis.

The effects of hemorrhage may be local or systemic, and the clinical significance depends upon the amount of blood lost, its rate of escape, and the site of hemorrhage. Small hemorrhages may have no clinical significance unless the hemorrhage involves the brain or pericardial sac, where it may produce sufficient increases of pressure to cause death. External bleeding, bleeding into the gastrointestinal tract, bleeding hemorrhoids, and menstrual irregularities represent a permanent loss of vital iron, causing an iron-deficiency anemia of the hypochromic type. (See Fig. 18-29, F.)

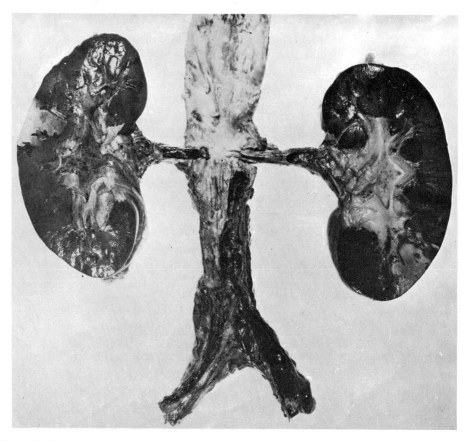

Fig. 9-1. Thrombosis of common iliac and renal arteries in patient with acute periarteritis. Note infarcts in kidneys. (From Gore, I.: In Anderson, W. A. D., editor: Pathology, ed. 6, St. Louis, 1971, The C. V. Mosby Co.)

If bleeding occurs in a body space or tissue where blood cannot escape, the progressive breakdown of hemoglobin permits the reabsorption of the iron pigment, which is reutilized to form new red cells. This, of course, does not pertain to massive internal hemorrhages.[23, 27]

Significant hemorrhage may be followed by shock, a condition in which the circulation of the blood is seriously disturbed. This is discussed at the end of this chapter.

THROMBOSIS[15, 21, 28]

The formation of a blood clot (thrombus) within a vessel or the heart is known as thrombosis (Fig. 9-1). As a physiologic response to injury, the formation of a blood clot may be a lifesaving device, but it can be serious when it occurs under abnormal circumstances. These circumstances are alterations in the blood and its channels, including the heart itself. To understand abnormal blood clotting, it is necessary to review the normal integrity of the vascular system, which maintains the fluidity of the blood, and to relate this to abnormal conditions conducive to clot formation.

The entire cardiovascular system has a completely smooth, uninterrupted endothelial lining, which is vital to the maintenance of the fluidity of blood and its laminar flow. Since it is nonwettable, this lining or surface normally provides no place for adherence of platelets or fibrin, which are necessary ingredients of blood clot formation. However, if the endothelial lining has been damaged, as from sclerosis or hardening of the walls, a favorable nidus is provided for clot formation. This occurs in arteriosclerotic vessels when they develop intravascular clots.

The fluidity of the blood normally is influenced by the thickness of the walls of the blood vessels and their manner of branching as well as by the normal cardiac structure and functions of the heart. In the arteries the flow of blood is rapid, which repels the settling of the formed elements and formation of adherent masses in the walls. The slower somewhat sluggish flow of the venous blood, however, predisposes to thrombosis.

The thickness of the walls of vessels is also a factor in clotting. Arteries have thick muscular walls that resist abnormal dilatation and at the same time serve to keep the lumen distended and more resistant to compression or invasion by tumors or inflammatory processes. The thick walls, however, which serve as a protective enclosure for the blood column, can narrow the lumen by means of contraction when they are injured or irritated. When the lumen is narrowed, there is resistance to arterial blood flow, resulting in stasis or slowing, which facilitates the formation of a clot. Except for the vena cava and its main branches, veins do not have extensive musculature in their walls. The forward flow of the blood to the heart is much slower and is regulated by valves along the route. Veins are therefore subject to abnormal dilatation from internal sources and to pressure from external neighboring lesions.[21] The slower flow of blood when it encounters obstructions in its pathway becomes turbulent (eddying currents), resulting in platelets adhering to the vessel walls. The thinner walls of the veins are also more vulnerable to penetration by inflammations and tumors, which create a nidus for platelet adherence and clotting.[21]

Thrombosis is a potentially serious disorder, especially if it occludes vessels of vital tissues and organs. (See Figs. 9-1, 18-1, 18-8, and 18-20.) It is the parent of the embolus in many instances. The very beginning of a thrombus formation is a minute mass projecting into the lumen of a vessel or from the lining of the heart. Called a plaque, this is initiated by the platelets adhering to the wall. The ruptured and intact platelets in this minute mass culminate in the precipitation of fibrin and the accumulation of all the formed blood elements within the fibrinous coagulum, now known as a mural thrombus. When a mural thrombus occurs in a vascular channel of large diameter, such as the aorta or major aortic branches, or in the chambers of the heart, it remains stationary as a clot. (See Figs. 18-1, 18-7, and 18-8.) A mural thrombus in the heart is particularly hazardous, since it may become pedunculated and project into the cardiac chamber, dislodging small fragments that accumulate at valvular orifices. These small fragments may pass through the heart valves, gaining entrance to the systemic bloodstream as emboli. Since mural thrombi may not totally obstruct the blood flow, in some blood vessels the passing bloodstream tends to sweep away the entire clot or at least some fragments.[21, 22]

In small blood vessels if there is sufficient stasis from injury to permit formation of a thrombus, complete occlusion of the vessel may occur. An occlusive thrombus may continue to elongate from the deposition of more platelets and formed blood elements and give rise to a propagating thrombus. This type of thrombus has an advancing head that may eventually reach a bifurcation of major vessels where parts of it may break off and be carried away by the faster bloodstream in the major vessel, creating an embolus. The propagating thrombus is prone to occur in the large veins (femoral veins) of the lower extremities, from the extension of an occlusive clot in a smaller vein. From the femoral vein it may extend into the inferior vena cava, where it has a direct pathway leading to the heart and to the pulmonary arteries.[15, 21, 28]

Among the highly important factors favoring thrombus formation are the inflammations arising from without blood vessels, such as abscesses or tumors. Bacterial diseases of the heart damage the endocardium, providing favorable sites for clot formation. These are friable masses of precipitated blood clot on heart valves with colonies of bacteria and are called vegetations. There are also many microorganisms, such as the rickettsiae and meningococci, and toxins and chemical poisons that cause changes of blood vessels leading to thrombus formation. Physical trauma, extremes of cold, burns, and electrical injuries are all potential antecedents to thrombosis. Penetrating malignancies are another source.[21]

EMBOLISM[15, 21, 22]

An embolus is composed of material that is carried by the blood to a site distant from the point of origin. Here it lodges in a vessel too small to permit further passage and partially or totally obstructs the lumen. Most emboli are the result of fragmentations of a thrombus, as previously described under thrombosis. Emboli are classified by whether they are from preexisting thrombi, from fat globules entering the circulation (fat embolism), from air or other gases (gas embolism), from amniotic fluid embolism, from tumor cells, or from aggregates of bacteria or parasites.

By far the most common type of embolus is the venous or arterial fragmentation from thrombotic accumulation. (See Fig. 18-8, F.) The arterial emboli most often arise from mural intracardiac thrombi or from vegetative masses on the heart valves, as in bacterial endocarditis, and less commonly from atheromatous plaques or from aortic aneurysms. The vascular occlusions occur most often in the spleen, kidneys, brain and lower extremities. (See Fig. 18-25.) Venous emboli usually arise from thrombosis within the veins of the leg, especially those of the deep calf muscles. Other sites are the veins of the pelvis and the right side of the heart, particularly the atrium. On reaching the heart, if the embolus is small enough, it may pass through the heart and enter the pulmonary circulation, where it may occlude a major pulmonary vessel or lodge at the bifurcation of the main pulmonary artery, creating a saddle embolus. Smaller emboli may reach the periphery of the lung tissue, occluding small vessels and causing pulmonary hemorrhage or infarcts. Death usually results from the larger pulmonary embolus.

Fat embolism[6, 22]

In fat embolism, globules of fat gain entrance to the circulation, usually venous, and cause diffuse minute emboli. In most instances the fat globules are deposited in the lungs, where the minute emboli are trapped, but when the process is severe, some pass through the lungs and reach the brain and other organs, particularly the kidneys and liver. If a fat embolus reaches the lungs, there may be a sudden onset of respiratory distress with cyanosis caused by massive obstruction to the pulmonary blood flow. Most of the deaths are from systemic lesions. In severely traumatized patients with cerebral emboli there may be immediate loss of consciousness with rapidly progressing, central nervous system disturbances. Clinical manifestations, however, may be delayed in traumatized cases for latent periods of 12 to 48 hours and become manifest with an onset of pyrexia, tachycardia, respiratory distress, and cerebral signs of restlessness and irritability, progressing to drowsiness and confusion and finally to death.[5]

Fat globules enter the systemic circulation from many sources, such as fractures of long bones, severe burns, soft tissue trauma, decompression sickness, fatty changes in the liver, sickle cell crisis with bone marrow infarction, and iatrogenic causes such as orthopedic procedures and inadvertent intravenous injections of oily radiographic media.[5]

Air or gas embolism[21, 22]

Bubbles of air may gain access to either the venous or arterial circulation in a number of ways. They may be sucked into veins or arteries or they may be introduced accidentally. Air may be forced into a large ruptured uterine venous sinus by increased intrauterine pressure during contractions of labor.[21] Venous air embolism may occur as a complication in chest surgery, artificial pneumothorax and pneumoperitoneum, cardiac operations, thorascopic and peritoneoscopic procedures, angiographic procedures, neck surgery, radical mastectomy, cesarean section, intravenous therapy, or during collection of blood from a donor.[22] Death results from an air-trap blockage in the outward tract of the right ventricle at the mouth of the pulmonary artery. The amount of air necessary to cause death is uncertain; some have estimated that 100 to 150 ml. is fatal, but others have reported that an excess of 300 ml. is required. There are mitigating factors, however, such as the general health of the patient and the rate and rapidity of entry of the air. Arterial air embolism occurs when air enters a pulmonary vein or one of its tributaries. This can occur during chest surgery, pneumothorax, thoracocentesis, penetrating wounds of the lung or rupture of the lung.[22] Air embolism occurs in scuba divers who, after breathing the denser air at depths, do not release the air from their lungs during ascent and the pressure builds up sufficiently to cause rupture of lung tissue.[9, 23] Air embolism can also occur in divers even when they vent excess air during ascent.[23] This occurs when the lung tissue distal to a poorly communicating diseased bronchial passage is ruptured.[9] The symptom of lung rupture is a frothy, bloody sputum.

A special type of air embolism occurs in decompression sickness or caisson disease, which occurs in divers or other persons exposed to increased atmospheric pressure. The gas emboli are seen in individuals decompressed from high atmospheric pressures to a normal level or from normal level to the low atmospheric pressure of high altitudes.[9] They are caused by formation of nitrogen bubbles in body tissues and fluids. They can arise in a diver whose tissues are saturated with nitrogen and who surfaces rapidly from a depth in excess of 33 feet, or in a flier who rapidly ascends from sea level to an altitude higher than 18,000 feet.[7] Gas emboli can occur in those exposed to simulated high altitudes (at or over 30,000 feet) in decompression chambers. The term *aeroembolism* is used in this form of decompression sickness, but it is applied by some to any variety of gas or air embolism.[9]

In decompression sickness the embolic occlusions or interstitial gas about joints and muscles causes pain, which is called the "bends."[9] This pain is deep and boring and in most cases occurs within 30 minutes after decompression, that is, after reaching a critical altitude or after surfacing following a dive that exceeded the depth-time factor.[9] Other symptoms include prickling or burning sensation of the skin and what is termed chokes. Chokes consist of burning retrosternal pain and cough, which progresses in severity until it is paroxysmal and uncontrollable. Partial relief is gained by recompression by descent, but symptoms may linger for several days. All the manifestations of decompression sickness usually respond to early and adequate recompression treatment.

Diagnosis of air embolism during life is made by observing certain characteristic signs.[22] These include marbling of the skin caused by embolism of cutaneous vessels, pallor of a part of the tongue, called Leibermeister's sign, caused by an obstructed branch of a lingual artery, and bubbles of air in retinal vessels on ophthalmoscopic examination. Air bubbles may also be seen in blood escaping through a small incision in the upper part of the body.[22]

Amniotic embolism[11, 22]

Amniotic embolism is a potentially fatal obstetric complication, but it is relatively rare. There is sudden respiratory distress, cyanosis, and shock. Death of the mother may occur during or immediately after parturition. In this type of embolism the pulmonary circulation may be blocked by amniotic debris, causing death. The precise mechanism by which the amniotic fluid gains entrance to the maternal blood is not known. Some believe it escapes through a rupture of a uterine sinus during labor; others think that it may be accomplished through tears or surgical incisions in the myometrium or endocervix.[11]

INFARCTION[21, 22]

Infarcts are localized areas of ischemic necrosis caused by partial or complete obstruction to the arterial supply or to the venous drainage of the part. The most common causes, as mentioned previously, are thrombosis and embolism. Other causes include the cutting off of venous drainage or arterial supply of blood to an organ by the twisting of a mobile viscus, such as an ovary, a testis, or a loop of bowel. Segments of the bowel may be trapped in hernial sacs, with circulation of blood severely taxed. Compression of arteries or veins may also impede circulation. Any alteration in blood vessels that reduces the oxygen-carrying capacity of the blood or the speed of its flow through an organ or tissue is a predisposing factor in developing infarction. Severe anemia can also cause anoxia of tissues or organs. All the organs and tissues are dependent upon a supply of oxygen for life, and if this is cut off for any reason, the result may be infarction, necrosis, or complete death of the organ or tissue. Some organs, however, are more susceptible to ischemic anoxia than others. The brain is dependent upon oxygen, and complete anoxia of the brain for only a few minutes can produce irreversible ischemic necrosis of the neurons. The renal tubules are likewise dependent on oxygen and may suffer ischemic necrosis in anoxia.

Some organs have a double blood supply, and if one vessel is injured, the other can carry the load. This is true of the radial and ulnar arteries of the arm and the tibial and fibular vessels of the leg. Some blood vessels have numerous anastomoses in organs, such as the skeletal muscles, bone, uterus, thyroid, and skin; because of this branching and rebranching with bridging of channels, infarction is less likely to occur from injury of any type. Some organs, however, are served with a single vessel that may branch but does not have bridging channels. These are referred to as end arteries. An example of this type of blood supply exists in the kidneys and spleen. When the vessels of these organs are occluded, infarction almost inevitably occurs, unless minute neighboring capillaries from surrounding vessels can maintain nutrition of the affected zone.

Arterial infarcts are much more common than venous for several reasons. Venous thrombi from veins cause pulmonary arterial embolization, whereas thrombi from the left side of the heart and the aorta give rise to arterial occlusion. Therefore venous infarction is almost entirely dependent upon intravascular venous thrombosis without embolization. Since the arteries carry the oxygen, interruption of this supply to an organ or tissue is much more likely to cause ischemic necrosis than is venous obstruction. Further, the anastomotic shunts through increased venous pressure or collateral circulation develop in areas of venous obstruction, causing only stasis of blood flow for a brief period of time until vascular supply to the affected tissue is restored. Collateral circulation is much more likely to carry the blood flow in young people than in the elderly who have weakened or diseased vascular channels. Collateral circulation is an important lifesaving factor in myocardial infarction, which is one of the most common and serious forms of heart disease. (See Fig. 18-29, C.) Myocardial infarction is discussed at the end of this chapter.

The clinical significance of infarction depends on its size and most importantly on its site. For example, a small infarct in the brain is much more serious than a larger one in some other organ, like the spleen. As causes of clinical morbidity and mortality the infarctions rank with malignancies and infectious diseases. This is because ischemic infarction occurs rather frequently in many vascular or other diseases in the vital organs, including the brain, heart, lungs, and kidneys. Pulmonary infarction (Fig. 9-2) is often the cause of death in postoperative and postpartum patients as well as in illnesses necessitating long-term bed rest. The gangrene or ischemic necrosis of the lower extremities in diabetic patients is a constant possibility, although rare. Cerebral infarction, called encephalomalacia, is a serious condition. Occlusion of a cerebral artery usually results in infarction of the region supplied by the vessel; the size and extent of the infarction depend upon the availability of collaterals and upon the state of the vessels. (See Fig. 18-8, *E.*) The damage is permanent since neurons cannot regenerate.[21]

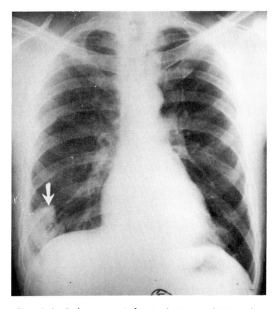

Fig. 9-2. Pulmonary infarct. Arrow points to infarct (area of increased shadow). (From Young, C. G., and Likos, J. J.: Medical specialty terminology, x-ray and nuclear medicine, St. Louis, 1972, The C. V. Mosby Co.)

STEP-BY-STEP EXERCISES

Step 1. An increased volume of blood in dilated vessels in an organ or part is called hyperemia. The morbid red color seen with the naked eye in the skin is called erythema; this is caused by the congestion of the capillaries.

Identify the following conditions.
1. Congestion of blood at the site of a wound _____
2. Morbid red color of skin around a wound _____

Step 2. Hyperemia caused by an increased blood flow into the capillaries from arteriolar dilatation is called active hyperemia or active congestion. It might be neurogenic (as in blushing); it might be in response to a call for more blood (as in muscular exercise); or it might be in response to a slight local injury.

In a superficial skin burn there would be some capillary congestion in response to the injury; this would be _____.

Step 3. A decreased outflow of venous blood caused by stasis obstructing the escape of blood is referred to as passive congestion or passive hyperemia.

If there is obstruction to the outflow of blood from the liver, this might be called _____ _____.

Step 4. Identify the following types of congestion.
1. Muscular exercise with an increase in blood flow to muscles _____

_____
2. Congestion of the liver with progressive venous stasis resulting from heart failure _____ _____
3. Blushing _____ _____
4. Congestion of visceral organs or extremities occurring in heart failure

_____ _____
5. Congestion of capillaries at the site of a superficial injury _____

_____

Step 5. A tourniquet or tight bandage applied to a part of the body obstructs the venous blood, and it accumulates as local venous congestion. Local venous congestion also occurs where there is pressure from a tumor or when there is thrombosis.

Identify the following type of congestion.

1. A bandage has been applied too tightly around the arm, and the return of blood to the heart has been temporarily impeded; this would be

   _____ _____ _____ .

2. A tumor is compressing a large vein in an organ and impeding the blood

   flow; this would be _____

   _____ _____ .

Step 6. Congestion and edema usually go hand in hand. When there is severe congestion, there is also edema with an increase in the weight and size of an organ. The dilatation of the capillary bed is related to the development of edema. When congestion is slight, however, there may be only slightly increased redness and vascularity but no edema (see below).

Step 7. The escape of blood from a perforated or ruptured vessel is referred to as hemorrhage. It implies a free flow of blood.

Indicate which is a hemorrhage and which is hyperemia.

1. Bleeding from a penetrating wound

   with severed blood vessels _____

2. Accumulation of blood at the site of an injury with no rupture of blood

   vessels _____

Step 8. A massive blood clot in the tissues formed at the site of injury from blood accumulating as it escapes from ruptured vessel wall is called a hematoma.

If you had injured your wrist with a massive blow and there suddenly appeared a large blood clot underneath

the skin, this would be a _____ .

Step 9. In the following blanks identify the medical term for the type of hemorrhage described.

1. An accumulation of blood in the thoracic cavity _____

2. An accumulation of blood in the peritoneal cavity _____

3. An accumulation of blood in the pericardial cavity _____

4. Small hemorrhages in the skin or mucous membranes _____

5. Accumulation of blood as in a bruise

   _____

Step 10. Hemorrhages resulting from blood vessels rupturing because of preexisting disease or damage to the blood vessel wall, are called spontaneous hemorrhages. On the other hand, ruptures of normal vessel walls caused by a sudden blow or other type of exogenous injury are called traumatic hemorrhages.

Identify the type of hemorrhage that would result in the following conditions.

1. Rupture of a blood vessel in the lung with hemorrhage in a tuberculous patient _____

2. Rupture of a blood vessel in the spleen from an impact _____

Step 11. The tendency to bleed freely either from injury or disease results from

---

Indicate the probable findings in the following conditions.

	Severe congestion	Slight congestion	Edema
1. Lungs in heart failure	—	—	—
2. Liver in heart failure	—	—	—
3. Superficial skin injury	—	—	—
4. Severely infected abdominal wound	—	—	—

a defective blood-clotting mechanism called hemorrhagic diathesis, which in Greek means disposition.

Which of the following people would have a tendency to hemorrhage from injury or spontaneously from disease?

1. People with hemophilia ___
2. People with normal blood-clotting mechanism ___
3. People with inherited defects in the blood-clotting mechanisms ___

Step 12. The effects of hemorrhage may be local or systemic. A hemorrhage's severity or even life-threatening capability depends on the location, the rate of escape, and the amount of blood lost.

Indicate whether the following conditions pose an immediate threat to life or whether they will lead to an iron-deficiency anemia.

	Threat to life	Iron-deficiency anemia
1. Cerebral hemorrhage	___	___
2. Chronic loss of blood from hemorrhoids	___	___
3. Massive hemorrhage from a ruptured aneurysm	___	___
4. Slow gastrointestinal bleeding over a period of time from ulcers	___	___

Step 13. A blood clot within a vessel is called a thrombus, and the condition is referred to as thrombosis. The inherent danger from a thrombus is that a part of it will fragment or break off and be carried to another part of the body through the circulatory system, creating an obstruction called an embolus.

Complete the blanks by indicating whether the clot is a thrombus or an embolus.

1. A stationary clot within a blood vessel _____
2. A fragment of a clot lodging in a blood vessel at some distance from its original source _____

Step 14. Emboli may be made up of air bubbles, fat droplets, amniotic fluid, tumor cells, or bacteria, but these are much rarer than the embolus originating from a thrombus in an artery or vein.

Complete the blanks by identifying the type of obstruction.

1. A fragment of a blood clot from a vein in the lower extremities that has lodged in the inferior vena cava is a _____ _____.
2. During a pneumothorax a vessel has been accidentally ruptured, allowing the entrance of _____ and thus creating an _____ _____.
3. Emboli entering the circulation from a trauma, such as fracture of a long bone, or from inadvertent intravenous injections of oily radiographic media would be _____ _____.

Step 15. A thrombus forms from a plaque, which is initiated by platelets adhering to a vessel wall. As this minute nidus grows with the accumulation of formed blood elements, it becomes known as a mural thrombus. A mural thrombus remains stationary. If a thrombus in a vessel elongates and advances from deposition of more platelets and formed blood elements, it becomes a propagating thrombus.

Complete the blanks by identifying the type of thrombus.

1. An extension of an occlusive clot in the iliac vein into the inferior vena cava _____ _____
2. A clot in the iliac vein that remains stationary _____ _____

Step 16. Infarctions are localized areas of ischemic necrosis caused by partial or complete obstruction to the arterial supply or the venous drainage of an organ or part. They are usually the result of an embolus or thrombus but may occur after the cutting off of blood supply or drainage of an organ, as when a testis becomes twisted on its pedicle, when an intestinal loop is caught in a hernial sac with strangulation, or when vessels of an organ are compressed by tumor.

Which of the following would be likely to cause infarction of an organ?
1. Occlusion of a cerebral artery ___
2. Occlusion of a renal vein ___
3. Intestinal loop caught in a hernial sac with strangulation ___
4. Occlusion of a coronary artery ___
5. Compression of the spleen by an adjacent tumor ___
6. Hematoma on the forehead from an impact ___
7. Chronic bronchitis ___
8. Pulmonary circulation occluded by an embolus ___

REPRESENTATIVE DISEASES
Conditions or defects associated with abnormal bleeding tendency

Hypofibrinogenemia or *afibrinogenemia*[19, 22] is a deficiency of fibrinogen in the blood, resulting from lack of formation, depletion of the circulating levels, or as a result of fibrinolysis (enzymatic lytic destruction of fibrinogen). These defects in clotting are associated with excessive bleeding usually following trauma. The lack of formation or depletion of fibrinogen in the circulating blood, called fibrinopenia, may occur as an inherited defect or in an acquired form. The acquired form may occur in certain obstetric conditions because of widespread intravascular clotting induced by the infusion of thromboplastin-rich amniotic fluid. The fibrinolytic type is particularly encountered in bacterial infections, such as streptococcus, as well as in trauma.

Hypothrombinemia[13, 19] is a deficiency of prothrombin in the blood associated with a slow, oozing type of hemorrhage rather than with one that is massive. This type of hemorrhage is encountered in association with vitamin K deficiency or diffuse liver disease. (Vitamin K deficiency is discussed in Chapter 10.) Deficient prothrombin may also be caused by uncontrolled use of anticoagulants or large doses of salicylates.

Thrombocytopenia is caused by a platelet deficiency in the blood. In this condition the deficiency of platelets restricts the quantity of thromboplastin formed in a given time and leads to abnormal bleeding tendencies because there are too few platelets to agglutinate and serve as a core for clot formation.[8]

Phlebothrombosis and thrombophlebitis[15, 21, 22]

Thrombosis, which occurs in the veins, particularly those of the lower extremities, from stasis is called *phlebothrombosis*. This implies no inflammatory injury to the veins. When, however, the thrombosis is superimposed upon a preexisting inflammatory condition of the veins, it is called *thrombophlebitis*. Phlebothrombosis is much more likely to precipitate emboli, since the clots are not so firmly attached to the walls. Cardiac failure and shock are predisposing factors to peripheral vascular stasis and phlebothrombosis. The risk of portal vein thrombosis in the liver is a likelihood in cirrhosis, since there may be stasis in the portal system. Phlebothrombosis occurs with relative frequency in the pelvic and muscular veins of the lower extremities in elderly, bedridden cardiac patients. This is because of stasis of the failing circulation and stagnation of blood in the lower extremities caused by inactivity of muscles. Also there is the added hazard of compression of veins of the calf muscles.

Varicosities[21, 22, 24]

Varicose veins are enlarged, tortuous dilated vessels resulting from venous insufficiency usually in the lower extremities. (See Fig. 18-25, *D*.) They are more common in people over 40 years of age and affect women more often than men.

Varicose veins are found most frequently on the inner side and back of the calf and on the inner side of the thigh. The long saphenous vein is most often involved with primary varicosities, but the short saphenous vein as well as the perforating veins may also be incompetent.

The superficial saphenous system and the deep femoral veins drain the lower extremities. The superficial veins are relatively unsupported, since they are surrounded only by superficial fascia and subcutaneous fat. The femoral veins, however, are located deep in the muscles of the thigh. The saphenous and femoral veins are connected at a junction in the groin and at the knee in the popliteal space. There are, however, numerous additional venous connections. Semilunar valves located irregularly along the veins allow the blood to flow toward the heart during muscular contraction but prevent backflow during muscular relaxation. Valves are also located at anastomoses between the deep and superficial systems. In normal veins with competent valves, blood flows from the superficial to the deep systems, and in walking, the venous pressure drops while the pressure in the deep veins remains relatively high. With incompetent valves, as in varicose veins, the standing pressures are higher than normal, and exercise or walking causes little or no drop. The venous blood accumulates at the periphery, and stasis and edema follow. This is because the backflow of blood under high pressure is from the deep system into the relatively unsupported superficial veins. It is this transmitted pressure that leads to dilatation of the superficial veins, with elongation, tortuosity, loss of elasticity, and eventual destruction of the valves. The typical brownish tan to bluish discoloration of the skin is caused by the breakdown of red blood cells, with the release of hemosiderin. The red blood cells escape into the tissue spaces because of the progressive increase in capillary permeability resulting from the persistent venous hypertension. Tissue fluid clots in the lymphatic channels, producing lymph stasis. The areas of lymph and venous stasis are most susceptible to bacterial and fungal infection. Even a slight trauma can precipitate a chronic ulcer. (See Fig. 18-25, *D*.)

Humans' unique upright position is a contributing cause of varicosities. Varicosities do not appear in quadrupeds. Weaknesses in the structure of the veins and phlebitis as well as abdominal pressure from stomach muscles are contributing causes. Obesity and increasing age are other factors. In old age there is loss of tone of the skin and tissues that surround the veins and help to support them. Pressures on veins during pregnancy are also factors that predispose to development of varicosities. Heredity is believed to be an important factor, since a significant number of cases occur in persons with a family history of varicosities.

Shock[21, 22]

Shock is a condition in which the circulation of the blood is seriously disturbed; it is characterized by a reduction in the effective circulating volume and the blood pressure. If over 40% of the blood volume is lost, vascular collapse or shock is almost inevitable, sometimes leading to death. When between 10% and 40% of the blood volume is lost, the full-blown picture of shock may or may not occur, depending upon the rapidity of the loss.[21] Any damage to the body may be accompanied or followed by some degree of shock.

In shock the whole body reacts as if injured, and a series of changes occur to restore the body to normal. These changes, although directed at defense, may in themselves cause further damage to the body. The general mechanisms of the development of shock are as follows: When a person is injured, the blood flow in the entire body is disturbed. To compensate, the heart beats faster and the blood vessels near the skin and in the arms and legs contract, sending most of the blood to the vital organs and to the nerve centers in the brain that control all body functions. Blood diverted to vital organs robs other body cells of enough blood, thus depleting their oxygen and nutrients. Eventually the blood vessels themselves lose their ability to contract, and when this occurs, the vital organs are deprived of their blood supply, and the patient loses consciousness. With progressive shock, despite adequate therapy, a point may be reached from which there is no recovery. This is known as irreversible shock.

Primary or initial shock may occur following pain from any injury or other causes of acute pain, or it may even be precipitated by emotional reactions, such as fear, grief, and the sight of blood as in violence. The reaction of shock may be out of all proportion to the initiating factors, since it can occur after trivial injuries. The symptoms are prostration, unconsciousness, pallor, weak, rapid pulse, and low blood pressure. Usually primary or initial shock is transient, and in many cases recovery occurs naturally and rather quickly. However, the initial shock may be followed by secondary or delayed shock, which is much more profound.

Secondary or delayed shock occurs as a result of major injury or after primary shock, as mentioned previously. It can result from crush injuries, fractures, burns, hemorrhage, poisoning, surgical operations, bacterial infections, drug toxicity, irradiation, intestinal obstruction, perforated viscera, dehydration, cardiac insufficiency, and a number of other causes. In practically all conditions in which breathing is interrupted from any cause, shock almost inevitably occurs. The symptoms may develop gradually. The signs are weakness, cold moist skin, shallow respiration, rapid weak pulse, low blood pressure, collapse of superficial veins, oliguria, and even anuria. As shock progresses, the patient is less and less responsive to what is going on around him and may even be oblivious to pain. Finally there is stupor, coma, and even death in some cases where despite adequate therapy the shock was irreversible.

A number of factors influence the seriousness of shock in different individuals. Very young children and very old people do not have as much resistance to shock as young or middle-aged adults. People who have been starved, dehydrated, or exposed to extremes of cold or heat go into shock easily. Excessive fatigue can increase the severity of shock, as can extreme pain. Generally people wtih chronic illnesses are more likely to go into shock from injuries than are healthy individuals.

Myocardial infarction[1, 10, 16, 21, 22]

An infarction is a localized area of ischemic neurosis caused by lack of oxygen to a part or organ whose blood supply has been cut off by an obstruction, such as an embolus or thrombus in the blood vessels. (See Fig. 18-29, C.)

An infarction of the myocardium, the heart's muscle, is one of the most common and serious forms of heart disease (Fig. 9-3). Several names are given to this type of heart attack. Since it is caused by a blocking of one of the coronary arteries or a branch, usually the left anterior descending branch, it is called myocardial infarction with coronary thrombosis, but it is also called a coronary occlusion, coronary closure, myocardial infarction, or just a coronary. All have the same meaning. A myocardial infarction simply means that a portion of the heart muscle has died because the coronary artery or one of its branches has been closed and the oxygen supply is diminished or absent. This does not imply that the patient will die because of the infarction or that he will even suffer a severe heart attack. The myocardium is sensitive to anoxia and cannot tolerate loss of oxygen very long. Acute ischemia of the myocardium may cause sudden death, in which case there is no muscle necrosis or infarction. However, if the patient survives the initial attack, as most do with modern therapy, the muscle will first become necrotic and later there will be healing and repair as occurs in all the body's tissue in response to injury. The white blood cells arrive first to clear away the muscle fibers that are dead and no longer able to contract. After this has been done, the tissue

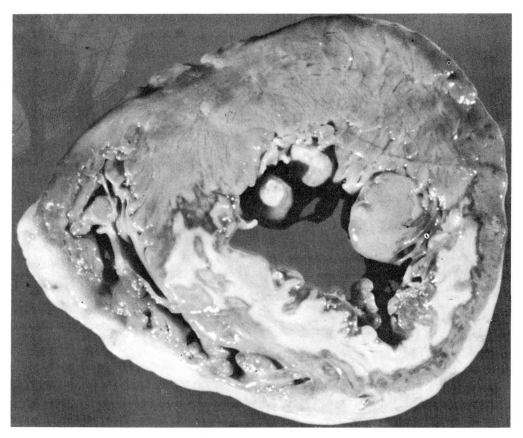

Fig. 9-3. Recent infarct of myocardium of left ventricle, anteroseptal. (From Scotti, T. M.: In Anderson, W. A. D., editor: Pathology, ed. 6, St. Louis, 1971, The C. V. Mosby Co.)

can heal and form a strong scar, which, if the patient remains under proper supervision, may cause no trouble for the remainder of his life. The survival and ultimate recovery depend to a great extent on adequate collateral circulation. The moment the obstruction occurred in the coronary vessel, other arterial branches enlarged and new branches began to form to bring a supply of blood to the area around the injury. The collateral circulation, if adequate, can compensate for the lack of oxygen normally supplied by the occluded vessel by development of bypaths for circulation. The collateral circulation, however, is usually effective only if the branches of the main arteries are narrowed. If the primary trunks, right or left main coronary artery, are occluded the anastomoses are usually in-

adequate to prevent myocardial infarction. Younger people are much more likely to have collateral circulation adequate to meet the situation than are elderly people whose vessels are diseased or weakened.

Many people have myocardial infarction with coronary thrombosis confused with other types of heart attacks, which are mainly defects or disorders of valves within the chambers of the heart, an embolus or thrombus in a ventricle with eventual occlusion of valves, or congenital abnormalities. The coronary arteries are the heart's special circulatory system, and the blood flowing through the heart proper does not pass through the coronaries on its way to systemic circulation.

Most myocardial infarctions are the result of atherosclerosis of the coronary artery or one of its branches. This is not a sudden condition, for the thickening or hardening of the walls of the arteries has been building up gradually over a period of time with the deposition of fatty material called atheromas on the inner lining. As the deposits or atheromas increase in size, they gradually narrow the channel of the vessel, and coronary thrombosis may occur. Some individuals, however, with atherosclerosis of the coronary arteries may never have thrombosis. Extensive and widespread changes in their coronary arteries may be discovered at autopsy, with death being from causes other than atherosclerosis. There may have been no indications of atherosclerosis of the coronary artery during life.

Myocardial infarction resulting from a coronary occlusion typically is characterized by agonizing, intense, prolonged pain, usually lasting for at least 1 hour and sometimes for as long as several hours. The pain is relieved only momentarily by nitroglycerine administered sublingually and responds only to administration of opiates.[10] The pain may radiate to the right or left arm, but usually to the left, and it may be felt in the elbow and even down to the fingers. It may also be felt in the jaw, in the back, and in the epigastric area. Patients with gastrointestinal diseases, such as peptic ulcer, hiatus hernia, or gallbladder disorders, may equate the pain with these conditions. The acute attack may occur after weeks or months of prodromal distress or pain of varying degree and intensity, with or without other cardiac symptoms. Prodromal symptoms are more common in patients with angina pectoris. Some cases of myocardial infarction do not manifest pain of any type; these are the so-called silent myocardial infarctions. The onset of these attacks is generally with unexplained weakness, sweating, and breathlessness.

Physical examination of a patient with an acute myocardial infarction may reveal cyanotic nailbeds, ashen face, and poor color. The skin is cool and perspiration is common. Examination of the lungs may show signs of acute pulmonary edema. The heart sounds are often distant and muffled, with a paradoxical splitting of the second sound. A third or fourth sound may be present.[10] A soft murmur suggests mitral regurgitation. The pulse may be thready and the blood pressure reduced. Laboratory findings include changes in enzymes. Glutamic-oxalacetic transaminase (GOT) and lactic dehydrogenase (LDH) may be found in the serum released from the myocardium during the first 24 hours after ischemia.[22] Elevation of the isoenzymes of LDH, alpha-hydroxybutyric dehydrogenase (HBD), and creatinine phosphokinase (CPK) suggests a recent myocardial necrosis or acute myocardial infarction.[22] Characteristic abnormalities may appear in the tracing of electrocardiograms.

Complications of myocardial infarction are arrhythmia or irregularity of heartbeat. Atrial or ventricular premature beats may appear, and when they become frequent, they may lead to rapid, forceful heart action called supraventricular tachycardia or to a totally irregular heartbeat called atrial fibrillation. Sometimes the ventricles have the same irregularities; ventricular fibrillation can lead to death in a matter of minutes without proper treatment. Heart block may appear in the conducting system of the heart. Another complication is pulmonary edema or acute congestion of the lungs, which occurs because the left ventricle is badly damaged by the injury to the heart muscle and allows blood to build up in the lungs.[16] The edema of the lung is caused by the escape of fluid from small blood vessels or capillaries in the lungs into air-bearing cells (alveoli).[16] This produces shortness of breath. Blood clots are always a hazard, for they may break away and circulate through the body causing damage to other major organs. Rupture of the heart may also occur, frequently within the first 2 weeks of infarction when the infarction is soft and prominent. The most common cause of death is congestive heart failure, usually of the left ventricle.[22]

Myocardial ischemia may be the result of factors other than thrombosis. Coronary vessels may have a diminished blood supply in shock and aortic stenosis. There may be hypertrophy of the heart in persons with hypertension and valvular heart disease in which there is an increased cardiac output without concurrent increase of coronary blood flow. The closure of the coronary vessel may not be caused by the formation of a thrombus but by the increase in size of the atheromas. The metabolic needs of the heart differ from those of other organs because the coronary flow may be reduced for compatibility with one level of energy expenditure but inadequate to permit a maximal cardiac effort when there is a greater demand, such as in strenuous exercise or emotional states when the heart is overworked.

A temporary myocardial ischemia is responsible for angina pectoris.[16] Angina pectoris is not a disease, but is a symptom of diminished blood supply to the myocardium, not an absence of blood supply as in coronary occlusion.[16] The heart is never at rest, and when it is required to perform extra work and does not receive enough extra blood with oxygen, the result may be an attack of angina. People who have angina usually have coronary arteries narrowed by atherosclerosis. The anginal pains may be mild or quite severe. They may be choking in character with a tightness and pressure in the chest. The pain is usually most marked in the center of the chest behind the sternum, but it may extend from this area to either shoulder or into either arm. It may occur with slight effort or emotional excitement, but does not often occur when at rest, and it may only rarely occur in response to vigorous exercise.

Variant angina. Prinzmetal's variant angina pectoris was first described as unprovoked by exercise or emotion. It was not accompanied by an increase in blood pressure and heart rate, and it was associated with elevated rather than depressed ST segments on the electrocardiogram. Prinzmetal attributed the cause of the syndrome to a spasm of the coronary artery. At the time this was not generally accepted. Now, however, recent arteriographic demonstrations have shown that coronary arteries can undergo spasm, which can be observed during attacks of variant angina. For this reason, some have now concluded that variant angina is a distinct dysfunction caused by transient occlusion of a major coronary artery. The mechanism is a temporary spasm and not a permanent arterial narrowing.

Rh factor[17, 18, 20, 25, 29]

Landsteiner and Wiener in 1940 discovered the Rh factor, which is inherited as a mendelian dominant character. The Rh factor derives its name from the discovery that when blood of the rhesus monkey was injected into rabbits, the rabbit's blood developed antibodies to the rhesus monkey's blood. Taking rabbit serum containing Rh antibodies and testing it against human red cells, Landsteiner and Wiener found that about 85% of the human red cells were agglutinated by the immune rabbit serum. They concluded that the blood of most people contains a substance or factor like the antigen in the monkey's blood.

Those who have the Rh factor are referred to as Rh positive; the remaining with no Rh factor are known as Rh-negative individuals. Persons in blood groups A, B, AB, or O, the basic blood groups, can be either Rh positive or Rh negative.

The majority of cases of *erythroblastosis fetalis (hemolytic disease of the newborn)* are the result of involvement of the Rh factor. The disease results from sensitization of the mother to antigens present in the red cells of the fetus. Although the Rh factor produces the disease, about 40% is caused by ABO incompatibility. The mechanism of involvement of the Rh factor is a follows: If either parent transmits the Rh-positive factor, the fetus will be Rh positive. When the mother's blood is Rh negative, the Rh factor of the fetus acts as an antigen, and the mother is immunized with the anti-Rh agglutinins being produced in her blood. These antibodies formed in the mother cross the placental barrier and bring about hemolysis of the erythrocytes of the fetus or newborn child. In a similar way, immunity may be produced by transfusion of Rh-negative individuals with Rh-positive blood, and this immunity will affect subsequent fetuses.

The three forms of hemolytic disease of the newborn represent various degrees of severity; in the first type there is congenital hydrops with effusions in serous cavities and severe edema of the organs including the placenta; in the second kernicterus (brain damage) occurs within 48 hours of birth; and in the third type there is severe anemia of the newborn infant with erythroblastosis. The initial signs are severe anemia and a failing heart. Some of the infants who live may have brain damage, accounting for a small percentage of cases of cerebral palsy. Through testing of the father's and mother's blood during pregnancy, the Rh factor can be determined. If the mother is Rh negative and the father is Rh positive, the mother's blood is tested for Rh antibodies. If the mother's Rh antibodies have hemolyzed the red blood cells of the fetus, the neonate can be given an exchange transfusion immediately after birth to prevent further damage. In carefully selected cases, intraperitoneal transfusion of the fetus in utero is given. When there have been previous erythroblastotic infants because of ABO incompatibility, during subsequent pregnancies the mother should be examined for the presence of bilirubin in the amniotic fluid, which is an indication of hemolytic disease of the newborn.

Hypertension[2, 3, 14, 22, 26]

Hypertension is not a disease per se, but it is a symptom, since it is a contributing factor in many diseases. Hypertension is a rise in blood pressure, and it is generally considered that systemic hypertension is blood pressure in adults of 90 to 95 mm. Hg diastolic and 140 to 150 mm. Hg systolic. Some, however, use the rule 100 plus the patient's age for all those over 25 years of age for systolic reading value in hypertension. An estimated 20% of the adult population in the United States has arterial hypertension with blood pressure at or above 160/95 mm. Hg in repeated examinations.[14] Blood pressure varies from day to day or from minute to minute; it also differs according to age groups and individual personalities. A rise in systolic pressure in the elderly is not uncommon, with figures of 200 systolic and 90 diastolic in millimeters of mercury. This has been attributed by some to the fact that the systolic hypertension represents the increasing rigidity of the aorta and main vessels in the elderly with a lessening effect on the arterioles. Blood pressure may rise in periods of excitement and decrease during periods of rest or sleep. These are normal changes that take place whether you have high blood pressure, low blood pressure, or blood pressure intermediate between these variables.

Hypertension is commonly divided into two types—essential and secondary. About 85% to 90% of hypertensive patients have the essential type, with 40% being over 40 years.[3] The causes of essential hypertension are unknown, but the most common form of curable or secondary hypertension is renovascular disease, which may be detected by urography and isotope renography.[14] Conditions that result in hypertension can be divided into three categories—those that raise the systolic pressure, those that raise mainly the diastolic pressure, and those that raise both systolic and diastolic pressure.[2] Systolic pressure may be elevated in hyperthyroidism, anemia, AV fistula, beriberi, malnutrition, and Paget's disease of the bone. Diastolic pressure may be increased in essential hypertension, and systolic and diastolic pressure may be elevated in essential hypertension and in certain endocrine, renal, cardiovascular, musculoskeletal and neurologic conditions, some of which are discussed below.[2]

If a diagnosis of secondary hypertension can be made, some cases are remediable, such as hypertension of unilateral renal disease, coarctation of the aorta, pheochromocytoma (tumor of the adrenals), and some acute diseases such as glomerulonephritis and some cases of Cushing's syndrome. No apparent underlying disease can be ascribed as the cause of essential hypertension. Diagnostic tests are laboratory evaluation of serum levels of glucose, potassium, cholesterol, and creatinine, urinalysis, electrocardiogram, and chest roentgenogram.[3]

In renovascular hypertension there is sudden or rapid appearance of elevated blood pressure in young people or of accelerated hypertension in the elderly. A disparity in the size of the kidneys and abdominal or flank pain prior to the elevation of the blood pressure in patients with essential hypertension are further evidences of renovascular obstruction. In patients with atrial fibrillation, a sudden rise in blood pressure may implicate a recent renal infarction and ischemia.

Several diseases of the adrenal glands are associated with hypertension. The diseases of the adrenal gland are discussed in Chapter 17.

Intracranial lesions cause both systolic and diastolic hypertension. Hyperthyroidism causes systolic hypertension accompanied by lowered diastolic pressure. Hypertension occurs after repeated acute attacks of pyelonephritis or after the disease assumes the chronic form.

In toxemia of pregnancy (eclampsia) the hypertension may be true preeclampsia, or it may be an exacerbation of antecedent hypertensive disease. Preeclampsia is a hypertensive syndrome that is peculiar to pregnancy, usually developing after the

twentieth gestational week.[12] Exceptions to the rule of its occurrence only in late pregnancy include trophoblastic disease of the placenta and Rh incompatibility.[12] In the preeclampsia stage the pregnant woman gains weight from the excessive fluid accumulation manifested as edema, excretes protein in the urine, and may have mild nervous system disorders. When convulsions or coma, or both, occur, it is called eclampsia. While adverse effects on the body usually disappear after delivery, the hypertension produced in this disorder may persist. More than half the women who recover eventually develop hypertensive cardiovascular renal disease.

In many hypertensive patients the heart involvement takes the form of left ventricular hypertrophy. Complications of the heart caused by elevation in blood pressure are a real danger to the hypertensive patient. Most complications, however, are slow in appearing, with an average of 10 to 15 years. In patients with arteriosclerotic hypertensive heart disease, elongation and dilatation of the aorta occur as the result of degenerative changes and increased pressure.

Cerebral hemorrhage is a real threat to severely hypertensive patients. The rupture of a cerebral vessel weakened by arteriosclerosis in a setting of hypertension is a common form of brain hemorrhage. (See Figs. 18-20 and 18-28.)

In hypertensive retinopathy there is mild to marked sclerosis of the retinal arterioles with exaggerated light reflex, arteriovenous compression, and irregular narrowing of the arterioles. As the blood pressure increases, numerous hemorrhages and white or gray exudates occur. In the most severe forms of the disease the optic disc becomes edematous (papilledema).

The serious form of hypertension is referred to as malignant hypertension. Some believe that this is a severe stage of the more benign or essential type, although others regard the diseases as different entities. In malignant hypertension there is retinitis with hemorrhages, exudates and papilledema, renal dysfunction, and a diastolic blood pressure of 120 mm. Hg or above. It occurs particularly in young adults, and the course is progressive, death usually resulting from renal failure in 6 months to 2 years.

In hypertension the arterioles constrict, thus narrowing the passageway of the blood to the tissues. The heart must pump blood with increased force, and the arteries must carry the blood under increased pressure. In time the walls of the blood vessels toughen and lose their elasticity, and the heart shows the strain by compensatory hypertrophy. There is no sudden breakdown in function of the blood vessels of the heart. The changes come about gradually over a period of time unless the problem is corrected.

Cor pulmonale[21, 22]

Cor pulmonale is a disease resulting from pulmonary hypertension. Any lesion or malformation that results in increased pressure in the pulmonary system produces dilatation of the pulmonary artery and hypertrophy of the right ventricle. Blood flow through the pulmonary circuit may be blocked by a pulmonary embolus or thrombus or by other obstructions such as emphysema; tuberculosis; pulmonary fibrosis resulting from pneumoconiosis; granuloma in persons working with cobalt, beryllium, and poisons; and parasitic infestations.

The sudden increase in blood pressure within the pulmonary circuit may cause the right ventricle to dilate and precipitate acute heart failure. The symptoms are venous distention in the neck blood vessels, peripheral edema, acites, pleural effusion, hepatomegaly, and splenomegaly. The right side of the heart is hypertrophied.

Arteriosclerosis[5, 21, 22]

Arteriosclerosis, commonly referred to as hardening of the arteries, is of unknown etiology, except that hypertension may be involved, and some believe that there is alteration of cholesterol metabolism. (See Fig. 18-7.) Atherosclerosis is the term used to describe the atheromatous patchy and irregularly disposed deposits that involve the intima of the large elastic and muscular distributing channels, leaving distal ramifications relatively unaffected. The accumulations may be lipids, complex carbohydrates, blood, blood products, fibrous tissue, and calcium deposits. Atherosclerosis is the most common form of arteriosclerosis. The deposits, or intimal lesions, cause the blood vessel to narrow, slowing the blood to the extent that in some instances only a trickle can get through. When scar tissue forms, there are tough fibrous plaques. A clot or thrombus can develop at the site, or an embolus can enter the bloodstream and completely occlude a vessel elsewhere.

Arterial intimal disease, through its effects on the heart, blood vessels of the brain, kidneys, mesentery, and lower extremities, accounts for more deaths and disability than does any other single cause. It is particularly a disease of the middle-aged and the elderly, although young people and even children may also be affected. Growth, maturation, and aging are all associated with intimal thickening of the vessels. In the adult, when there is no concomitant syphilitic or rheumatoid aortitis, atherosclerosis is generally more severe in the abdominal aorta than in the thoracic portion. The disease is also accentuated in the internal carotid artery, but intimal lesions are slight or absent in the pulmonary arterial tree, unless there is pulmonary hypertension. The lesions are absent in the veins. There are some predisposing factors in atherosclerosis, such as hereditary influence and the pathologic conditions of hypercholesterolemia.

Mönckeberg's sclerosis or medial calcification is related to age and is a degenerative process involving the media and internal elastic linings of muscular arteries of the head, neck, and extremities. Prolonged vasotonic influence and hypertension may be contributing factors. There is nodularity or tubelike rigidity of the vessels on palpation. The femoral, tibial, radial, and ulnar arteries are most severely affected. Calcific deposits are distributed in ringlike formations along the length of the vessel.

Arteriosclerosis obliterans is the most common form of peripheral vascular disease. In this condition luminal narrowing is severe, with frequent thrombotic obstructions in the arteries of the lower extremities. The arteries' most commonly affected are the iliac (Fig. 9-1), femoral, popliteal, and tibial. The vessels are irregularly thickened, tortuous, sclerotic, and often brittle. It is a disease of middle-aged and elderly individuals.

The symptoms are those of ischemia and include muscular cramps, intermittent claudication following exertion, and pain in the foot, calf, or hip. If gangrene of the foot or leg occurs, amputation is required. (See Figs. 18-7 and 18-25, *F.*) These patients have a high incidence of diabetes, hypertension, and other serious atherosclerotic lesions. Diagnosis may be determined in most patients by careful palpation of pulses and auscultation for bruits. The site of obstruction or stenosis is determined in this manner. Arteriography reveals the location and extent of the obstructive lesions and the collateral circulation; it is performed prior to surgery.

Aneurysms[5, 16, 21]

Aneurysm is derived from a Greek word meaning a widening. An aneurysm is a sac formed by the dilatation of a vessel wall because of structural weakness; they usually occur in the arteries (Fig. 9-4). There are a variety of etiologic factors, with most true aneurysms being the result of arteriosclerosis, syphilis, and cystic medionecrosis. Aneurysms of the smaller vessels, which are less common than those of the larger arteries, are caused by polyarteritis nodosa, trauma leading to an arteriovenous aneurysm, congenital defects such as the berry aneurysm (Fig. 9-5), and nonspecific inflammations that weaken vascular walls, causing the so-called mycotic aneurysms. Aneurysms may occur at any age but are most common after 50 years and are preponderant in males. Aneurysms may be saccular, fusiform, or cylindric in shape, or they may be dissecting.

The aorta is the vessel most often involved by aneurysms, most frequently the arch and abdominal aorta. Syphilitic aneurysms are almost always confined to the thoracic aorta and usually involve the aortic arch. They give rise to symptoms of encroachment upon thoracic structures, causing dyspnea; difficulty in swallowing because of esophageal compression; persistent cough caused by irritation or pressure on recurrent laryngeal nerves; pain from the erosion of bone, ribs, and vertebral bodies; and cardiac disease caused by dilatation of the aortic valve or narrowing of the coronary ostia. Most syphilitic aneurysms are saccular. They cause death by rupture

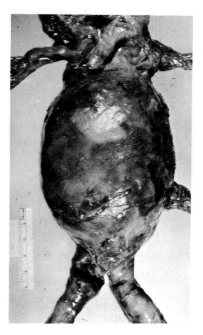

Fig. 9-4. Aneurysm of infrarenal segment of abdominal aorta. (From Gore, I.: In Anderson, W. A. D., editor: Pathology, ed. 6, St. Louis, 1971, The C. V. Mosby Co.)

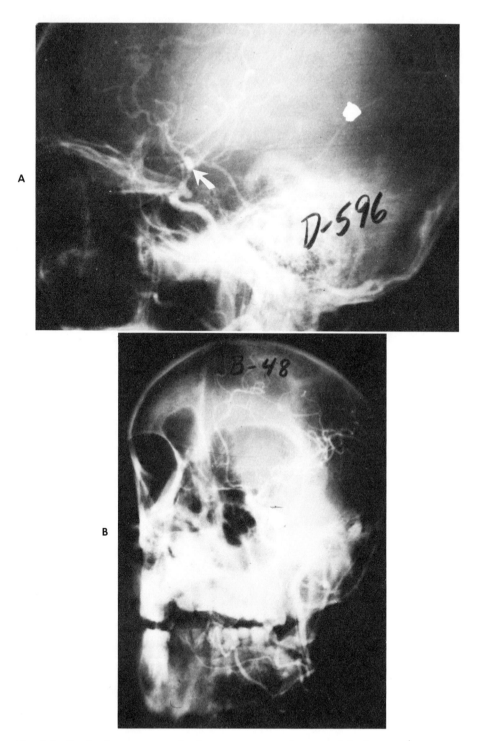

Fig. 9-5. Cerebral aneurysms. **A,** Berry aneurysm. Arrow points to saccular aneurysm (cerebral angiography). **B,** Aneurysm of posterior communicating artery (carotid angiogram). (From Young, C. G., and Likos, J. J.: Medical specialty terminology, x-ray and nuclear medicine, St. Louis, 1972, The C. V. Mosby Co.)

and hemorrhage in most cases and by compression and erosion of vital structures in the remainder.

Most arteriosclerotic aneurysms are found in the abdominal aorta or the common iliac arteries. They rarely occur in persons under 60 years of age and are more common in men. They are usually found below the renal arteries and above the bifurcation of the aorta. Severe atherosclerosis, with the atheroma extending into the media, is the cause. The fibromuscular, elastic supporting layer of the wall of the aorta is destroyed. There may be atheromatous ulcers within the aneurysm, covered by mural thrombi. Sometimes the entire aneurysmal sac is filled with thrombi, which are prime sites for emboli that invariably lodge in the arteries of the lower extremities. The aneurysm may impinge upon the common iliac arteries, with rupture into the peritoneal cavity or retroperitoneal tissues and massive hemorrhage. They may also impinge upon an adjacent structure compressing a ureter or eroding the vertebrae. The mass created by the aneurysm may simulate an abdominal tumor.

The least common form of aortic aneurysm is the dissecting one. In this type there is hemorrhage into the wall of an artery and dissection within the medial planes for variable distances. The dissection may be only a few millimeters in a spontaneous hemorrhage in the aorta or it may even extend into the iliac arteries. The abdominal aorta is involved in more than 50% of the cases. The dissecting aneurysm occurs mostly in the 40- to 60-year-old group. An intramural hematoma forms as the initial event, and as it enlarges, the tension of the vessel wall increases under the systolic thrust of the aortic blood pressure. Hypertension is present in most cases but not all. The mortality rate is high, with most victims dying from hemorrhage within a short period. The clinical symptoms are excruciating pains centered above the origin of the dissection, often mimicking angina pectoris or myocardial infarction. The pain may extend rapidly from the thoracic origin into the back and then into the lower extremities. Shock may supervene, but commonly there is no significant reduction of blood pressure. There is, however, an inequality of pulses and blood pressures between the right and left arms and legs.

The miliary aneurysms of cerebral arteries are known as berry aneurysms (Fig. 9-5, A). Generally these are considered to be congenital defects of the tunica media of the cerebral vessels, which may be aggravated by secondary conditions. Rupture and hemorrhage are frequent and are the major cause of spontaneous subarachnoid hemorrhage. Cerebral aneurysms occur with greater frequency than do all other aneurysms of extracranial arteries. (See Fig. 18-20, D.) The small berry aneurysms, which are saccular and usually multiple, involve the anterior portion of the circle of Willis twice as frequently as the posterior portion. The arteries involved are the internal carotid, the posterior communicating (Fig. 9-5, B), and the anterior cerebral. They occur in young people but are more common in those over 50 years of age. The mortality rate is high. In most patients, they are characterized by sudden onset of pain, which may be around the orbit. Headache is a common symptom. Some people have paralysis of the oculomotor nerve and involvement of other cranial nerves, with sensory and motor disturbances.

Congestive heart failure[4, 10, 16, 21, 22]

The mechanism in congestive heart failure is controversial, but the following is in line with some current concepts.

Congestive heart failure results when the heart is unable to pump forward the blood returned to it by the venous system through the inferior and superior venae cavae. The normal flow of this blood is from the right atrium to the right ventricle, through the pulmonary circuit back to the left atrium and then through the left ventricle and back to all the organs of the body. In congestive failure the usual amount of blood is emptied into the left ventricle from the left atrium, but the ventricle is unable to empty itself completely. Then when more blood flows in from the atrium, there is insufficient room to accommodate this blood in the ventricle along with that which it has retained. Blood is then dammed back into the atrium and pulmonary veins. The muscular wall of the left ventricle becomes enlarged from the extra workload and eventually becomes incapable of meeting the demands of the increased amount of blood. Through this failure of the ventricle, the blood is dammed back in the left atrium, then into the pulmonary veins and the lungs. The lungs become congested, and there is dyspnea and moist bubbling breathing.

When a similar situation occurs in the right atrium and right ventricle, there is back pressure in the inferior vena cava with damming back of the blood. This causes the dependent edema and congestion of the liver and abdominal organs. Dependent edema, however, is not always present in heart failure.

The kidney is the first organ to be affected by an insufficient blood supply. The excretory role of the kidney is significantly altered, primarily involving salt and water. These two metabolites are retained, accounting for the generalized edema, which is usually first evident in the lower extremities.

Congestive heart failure is described as being left-sided failure or right-sided failure. Left-sided failure involves the left ventricle and rarely the left atrium. The mechanisms are hypertension, various forms of ischemic coronary disease, aortic valvular disease, rheumatic endocarditis, aortic stenosis, mitral stenosis (when the atrium is involved), syphilis of the heart, congenital heart disease, and, rarely, bacterial endocarditis. Pulmonary congestion and edema are pronounced, with manifestations of orthopnea or paroxysmal dyspnea; also coughing and a blood-tinged, frothy sputum are present.

Right-sided failure is essentially a venous congestive syndrome, with the primary physiological disturbance being a damming back of blood through the systemic and portal venous circulations and a consequent inadequate flow of blood from the lungs to the left ventricle. In this type of failure there is passive congestion of the liver, congestion and anoxia of the kidneys, congestion and enlargement of the spleen, peripheral edema, and ascites. The causes of right-sided failure are mitral stenosis, myocardial infarction, diffuse myocarditis, primary diseases of the pulmonary vascular circulation, constrictive pericarditis, and, rarely, right-sided valvular lesions (stenosis of the tricuspid valve in rheumatic fever and congenital pulmonic stenosis).

Responses

Step 1: 1. hyperemia; 2. erythema
Step 2: hyperemia
Step 3: passive congestion or passive hyperemia
Step 4: 1. active hyperemia; 2. passive hyperemia or congestion; 3. active hyperemia or congestion; 4. passive hyperemia or congestion; 5. active hyperemia or congestion
Step 5: 1. local venous congestion; 2. local venous congestion
Step 6: 1. severe congestion and edema; 2. severe congestion and edema; 3. slight congestion; 4. severe congestion and edema
Step 7: 1. hemorrhage; 2. hyperemia
Step 8: hematoma
Step 9: 1. hemothorax; 2. hemoperitoneum; 3. hemopericardium; 4. petechiae; 5. ecchymoses
Step 10: 1. spontaneous; 2, traumatic
Step 11: 1. X; 3. X
Step 12: 1. threat to life; 2. iron-deficiency anemia; 3. threat to life; 4. iron-deficiency anemia
Step 13: 1. thrombus; 2. embolus
Step 14: 1. thrombotic embolus; 2. air; air embolism; 3. fat emboli
Step 15: 1. propagating thrombus; 2. mural thrombus
Step 16: 1. X; 2. X; 3. X; 4. X; 5. X; 8. X

REFERENCES

1. American Heart Association: Heart disease caused by coronary atherosclerosis, New York, 1962, The Association.

2. DeBartolo, Jr., H. M.: Ill. Med. J. **147**:158-160, 1975 (cause of hypertension).
3. Finnerty, Jr., F. A.: J.A.M.A. **231**:402-403, 1975 (hypertension).
4. Fishman, A. P.: In Beeson, P. B., and McDermott, W., editors: Cecil-Loeb textbook of medicine, ed. 13, Philadelphia, 1971, W. B. Saunders Co. (diseases of cardiovascular system, heart failure).
5. Gore, I.: In Anderson, W. A. D., editor: Pathology, ed. 6, St. Louis, 1971, The C. V. Mosby Co. (arteriosclerosis; aneurysms).
6. Gottlieb, L. H.: Hawaii Med. J. **24**:30, 1964, (fat embolism).
7. Haymaker, W., Johnston, A. D., and Downey, V. M.: J. Aviation Med. **27**:2, 1956 (decompression sickness in jet aircraft flight).
8. Hoak, J. C.: J. Iowa Med. Soc. **54**:331, 1964 (thrombocytopenia).
9. Johnson, R. L.: In Beeson, P. B., and McDermott, W., editors: Cecil-Loeb textbook of medicine, ed. 13, Philadelphia, 1971, W. B. Saunders Co. (alterations in atmospheric pressure).
10. Killip, T.: In Beeson, P. B., and McDermott, W., editors: Cecil-Loeb textbook of medicine, ed. 13, Philadelphia, 1971, W. B. Saunders Co. (ischemic heart disease).
11. Liban, E., and Rex, S.: Am. J. Clin. Pathol. **51**:477, 1969 (clinicopathology study of amniotic fluid embolism).
12. Lindheimer, M. D., and Katz, A. I.: In Conn, H. P., editor: Current therapy, ed. 26, Philadelphia, 1974, W. B. Saunders Co. (hypertensive disorders of pregnancy).
13. Marder, V. J., and Shulman, N. R.: Am. J. Med. **37**:182, 1964 (vitamin K deficiency and bleeding tendency).
14. Melby, J. C.: J.A.M.A. **231**:399-400, 1975 (hypertension).
15. Moolten, S. E., and others: Arch. Intern. Med. **84**:667, 1949 (thromboembolism).
16. Phibbs, B.: The human heart; the layman's guide to heart disease, ed. 3, St. Louis, 1975, The C. V. Mosby Co.
17. Quick, A. J.: Ann. Intern. Med. **55**:201, 1961 (blood factors).
18. Race, R. R., and Sanger, R.: Blood groups in man, ed. 4, Oxford, England, 1962, Blackwell Scientific Publications Ltd.
19. Ratnoff, O. D.: Arch. Intern. Med. **122**:93, 1963 (vitamin K deficiency and bleeding tendency).
20. Richter, M. N.: In Anderson, W. A. D., editor: Pathology, ed. 5, St. Louis, 1966, The C. V. Mosby Co. (blood and bone marrow).
21. Robbins, S. L.: Pathology, ed. 3, Philadelphia, 1967, W. B. Saunders Co. (circulatory diseases).
22. Scotti, T. M.: In Anderson, W. A. D., editor: Pathology, ed. 6, St. Louis, 1971, The C. V. Mosby Co. (disturbances in circulation of blood; heart).
23. Smith, F. R.: Dis. Chest **52**:15, 1967 (air embolism in scuba divers).
24. U.S. Department of Health, Education, and Welfare, Heart Information Center, National Heart Institute, Public Health Service Publication No. 154, Health Information Series 50, 1966 (varicose veins).
25. U.S. Department of Health, Education, and Welfare, Division of Biologic Standards, Public Health Service Publication No. 790, Health Information Series 98, revised 1966 (blood and Rh factors).
26. U.S. Department of Health, Education, and Welfare, Heart Information Center, National Heart Institute, Public Health Service Publication No. 146, Health Information Series 69, 1964 (high blood pressure).
27. Wintrobe, M. M.: Clinical hematology, ed. 5, Philadelphia, 1961, Lea & Febiger.
28. Wright, J.: Circulation **5**:161, 1952 (pathogenesis of thrombosis).
29. Young, L. E.: In Beeson, P. B., and McDermott, W., editors: Cecil-Loeb textbook of medicine, ed. 13, Philadelphia, W. B. Saunders Co. (hemolytic agents and mechanisms).

CHAPTER 10

Role of vitamins, minerals, and pigments in disease

Many organic and inorganic substances or nutrients are required in humans for maintenance of metabolic and reproductive activity, cell integrity, and tissue growth. The essential nutrients are protein, carbohydrates, fats, vitamins, and minerals. These nutrients are present in plants or animals eaten by humans. Simple deficiencies are those that exist when the source is inadequate and no predisposing factors, such as anorexia, are present. Simple deficiencies are rarely encountered in countries where living standards are reasonably high, but they are still common in many undeveloped countries. Conditioned deficiencies are those that exist because of some predisposing factor, such as a disease or condition that reduces intake, absorption, storage, or utilization of one or more of the essential nutrients. There may be interferences with intake, such as vomiting, loss of appetite, diseases of the mouth, or absence of the teeth, which modify the diet and may result in inadequate nutrition. Absence of teeth or ill-fitting dentures are often the reason for nutritional disorders in the elderly.

During absorption the end products of digestion must leave the lumen of the intestine, traverse the mucosal cells, and enter the terminal branches of the vascular and lymphatic vessels to gain entrance into the general circulation. This involves three mechanisms acting together or separately—active transport, facilitated transport, and passive diffusion. Impairment of these mechanisms interferes with the absorption of nutrients. In the gastrointestinal tract where the food is absorbed, enzymatic or biochemical dysfunctions may impair absorption of nutrients. Two common disorders that interfere with absorption and utilization of nutrients are diarrhea and diffuse inflammation of the bowels. The liver is a storage depot for nutrients, and if it is diseased, the buildup of adequate bodily reserves is reduced. The kidneys and bowels are excretory organisms. In disease states of these organisms, as well as of others such as the parathyroids and adrenals, interference with excretion may lead to selective losses of certain substances, for example, the inorganic elements.

Multiple deficiency states are common because a diet deficient in one component is usually deficient in others. Examples of this occur in such diseases as pellagra, beriberi, and kwashiorkor, which are discussed later. Malnutrition is a serious condition, particularly in children, since in many types of malnutrition, development of the brain is retarded and consequently the patterns of learning and behavior are very seriously affected.

An important function of food is the furnishing of energy. The energy value of food is called the caloric value, which in food chemistry is the large calorie. One gram of protein yields 4 calories; 1 gram of fat yields 9 calories; 1 gram of carbohydrate yields 4 calories. Adults require about 0.9 gram of protein per kilogram of weight daily for optimal nutrition.[10] This is coupled with enough carbohydrates and fats to maintain caloric balance. Although carbohydrates are necessary constituents of a balanced diet to supply energy, no fixed requirements have been established, since they can be completely replaced by protein and fats as energy sources. Proteins are essential for growth and repair. Fats contribute the most concentrated source of calories of all food nutrients. Although their chief function is to supply a source of energy, many fats also act as carriers of the fat-soluble vitamins—A, D, E, and K. They also furnish padding for vital organs, such as the kidneys, and as subcutaneous tissue they help to conserve heat.

National and international organizations have recommended daily dietary allowances for most of the nutrients for different age groups. These are available in many publications, notably those from FAO/WHO (Food and Agriculture Organization of the United Nations World Health Organization) and from the Food and Nutrition Board, National Research Council, National Academy of Sciences, Washington, D.C.

Tables of caloric values of foods are also available from many sources. These tables are of particular interest to those planning a diet for weight reduction. It must be stressed, however, that the existing recommended dietary allowance for nutrients does not cover the additional needs that arise from microbial disease, trauma, advanced malignancies, disorders of the gastrointestinal tract, or metabolic diseases and abnormalities. Persons consuming the recommended dietary allowance may not be adequately nourished, for they may have a disease that interferes with absorption or utilization of essential nutrients or accelerates their loss. When clinical examination by a physician raises the question of nutritional deficiency of a patient, medical history and dietary and biochemical data are required to confirm the diagnosis.[12]

Sodium, potassium, chloride, magnesium, fats, carbohydrates, protein, and water have been discussed in previous chapters. Other than a discussion of selected nutritional deficiency diseases in this chapter, information on these substances will not be repeated. This chapter will be devoted to vitamins, pigments, and minerals.

VITAMINS[4, 10-14]

When vitamins were first recognized as indispensable to health, it was believed that they belonged to the nitrogenous substances known as amines. Hence we have the name vitamin (from *vita*, meaning life, plus *amin*). Except for some vitamin K, they are not substances that human beings are capable of manufacturing, so that they must come from food or medications.

As a practical definition, vitamins have been defined as organic catalysts of external origin that are effective in small amounts but are essential for the maintenance of the normal structure and function of cells.[10] They are not utilized to furnish energy but act as essential components of the chemical mechanisms by means of which the food substances are metabolized. They do not enter significantly into cell structure, but act through the intracellular enzyme systems.

Most of the vitamins are available in animal or plant foods. The minimum daily requirements are well established, so a deficiency of any one of the vitamins can be remedied by improved diet, by parenteral injections in pure or concentrated forms, or by oral medications. Excesses over the minimum requirements of most of the vitamins are not harmful, but evidence exists that overdosage of either vitamin A or D may be detrimental to health. The effects of overdosage will be described under the specific vitamin in the following discussions.

Vitamins are usually designated by letters—A, B, C, D, E, and K—but the B complex embraces a number of substances, such as thiamin, riboflavin, folic acid, nicotinic acid (niacin), pyridoxine, and biotin. Some of these are better known by these names and are usually discussed in the literature accordingly.

Vitamin A[10-12]

Vitamin A is a fat-soluble, colorless primary alcohol (retinol). It is derived from certain yellow plant pigments known as carotenes. It is found preformed in animal tissue. It may enter the body as such from foods of animal origin (dairy products containing butter fat, liver, fish liver oils, and egg yolk) or through its precursors, the carotenes, which are primarily of vegetable origin. It is also present in fruits such as the papaya and mango. The known physiologic activities of vitamin A are (1) maintenance of the structure and function of certain specialized types of epithelium, (2) maintenance of normal skeletal growth, and (3) formation of aldehyde for vision, particularly in dim light. Skin and eye lesions and reduced resistance to infection occur with hypovitaminosis A.

Hypovitaminosis A is a deficiency of vitamin A. Low amounts of preformed vitamin A or an active carotene precursor in the diet are the most obvious and common cause of hypovitaminosis A. Any condition of the intestines that interferes with the absorption and conversion of carotene to vitamin A and its transport to the liver will contribute to hypovitaminosis A. Vitamin A deficiency is likely to occur in such diseases as sprue, fibrocystic disease of the pancreas, lymphomas, or lipodystrophy (Whipple's disease). The liver stores about 90% of the vitamin A in the body.[10] This is markedly reduced in cirrhosis and in other hepatic diseases where there is interference with intestinal absorption and conversion of carotene to vitamin A and its transport to the liver. In addition to the specific intestinal diseases mentioned here, operative procedures for removal of small bowel sections and excessive consumption of mineral oil are also contributing factors in hypovitaminosis A. Massive intestinal infections with *Giardia lamblia* (parasites inhabiting the duodenum and jejunum) and possibly ascariasis and hookworm infection (roundworms) are contributing factors to deficiency in vitamin A.[12] In kwashiorkor, a severe protein deficiency disease, inadequate amounts of vitamin A are stored in the liver, and the levels of vitamin A and carotene in the serum of children with this malnutrition disease are extremely low. It has been postulated that the transport of vitamin A to the liver is inadequate because of the lack of a protein carrier. It is believed that adequate vitamin A is a deterrent in infectious diseases, since it assists resistance to infection by maintenance of the integrity of mucosal surfaces.[10] Some bacterial infections, such as conjunctivitis, furunculosis, bronchopneumonia, and pyelonephritis are common in hypovitaminosis A; however, other mitigating factors are involved.

Xerophthalmia results from lack of vitamin A. In this condition, dry scaly lesions form on the scleral conjunctiva. Bitot's spots (triangular grayish areas in the scleral conjunctiva representing accumulations of keratinized epithelium) are seen in cases of prolonged mild deficiency. They may range from a few tiny air bubbles visible on the exposed conjunctiva between the corneal rim and limbus to white coatings overflowing onto the cornea. There is loss of light reflex, lack of luster, and decreased lacrimation. Keratomalacia (softening of the cornea) may develop, leading to ulceration, perforation, rupture, and destruction of the cornea. The final outcome is a scarred, opaque cornea and a sightless eye.

The loss of night vision or nyctalopia is generally the earliest physiologic effect of hypovitaminosis A.[10] In dim light, visual acuity is absent. Normal vision in partial darkness is dependent upon a pigment known as visual purple or rhodopsin in the retina. This pigment is formed by the combination of vitamin A aldehyde with protein. A continual source of vitamin A is essential for this combination. The most valuable test for vitamin A deficiency is to determine the speed with which vision adapts to feeble light.[10]

Xerosis or generalized dryness of the skin is characteristic of hypovitaminosis A. The follicular hyperkeratosis widely ascribed to a deficiency of vitamin A consists of a "goose flesh" appearance of the skin.[12] It is not altered by temperature or brisk rubbing, and it is most prominent on the skin of the outer forearm and thigh. The fully developed lesions are symmetrically distributed and consist of rough, horny papules projecting from hypertrophied hair follicles. The skin may look and feel like coarse sandpaper.

Massive doses of vitamin A lead to increased storage in the liver with resulting hepatomegaly. This condition is called *hypervitaminosis A*. The clinical picture in children is that of drowsiness, listlessness, irritability, headache, vomiting, and in severe cases, hydrocephalus with protruding fontanels, hepatosplenomegaly, hypoplastic anemia, leukopenia, precocious skeletal development, clubbing of fingers, and coarse, thin hair.[12] Some of the latter symptoms have been reported only in children who have been on prolonged overdosage of vitamin A. In adults, toxic symptoms appear only after prolonged overdosage (twenty to thirty times the recommended daily allowance).[10] The symptoms are hyperexcitability, bone pain, and headache. A history of excessive dosage of vitamin A and an increased cerebrospinal fluid pressure are diagnostic.

Vitamin A is not normally excreted in the urine. In some diseases such as those with liver and kidney disorders, advanced cancer, and febrile diseases, vitamin A is excreted in the urine, causing a depletion in the body. Appropriate laboratory analysis of the urine will give an estimation of the content of vitamin A.

Vitamins of the B group[5, 10-12]

A number of factors in concentrates from yeast, wheat germ, rice polishings, and other sources are known collectively as the vitamin B complex. The vitamin B complex comprises thiamin, niacin, riboflavin, pyridoxine (B_6), biotin, pantothenic acid, choline, folic acid, and vitamin B_{12}. All these are water-soluble. Not all produce diseases in humans when there is a deficiency, and most of the knowledge of their actions has come from animal experimentation. Deficiencies in several of these factors commonly exist together, but several disease entities are associated more or less specifically with deficiency of an individual factor. No known diseases in humans are recognized as caused by deficiency of the entire B complex.[10] Only those factors that produce disease in humans will be discussed. It is not clear at the present time what importance a deficiency of pyridoxide (B_6), biotin (vitamin H, or coenzyme R), pantothenic acid, or choline has in the production of specific diseases in humans. However, a combined deficiency of choline and methionine is believed to be the cause of fatty liver in alcoholism and kwashiorkor. Pantothenic acid level is below normal in pellagra, beriberi, and ariboflavinosis, but there is no conclusive evidence that a deficiency of it is a factor in the spontaneous occurrence of lesions in humans.[10] A pyridoxine deficiency in a commercial formula has been associated with hyperirritability and convulsions in infants when there was no other discoverable cause.[10]

Niacin. Niacin or nicotinic acid and its precursor, tryptophan, are believed to be responsible for pellagra when there is inadequate intake of either. The dietary sources are liver, lean meats, fish, whole grain cereals, enriched breads, dried peas, nuts, and peanut butter. Pellagra affects the skin, mucous membranes, gastrointestinal tract, and nervous system. The skin lesions occur particularly in the areas exposed to sunlight, but may occur in areas where there is irritation. The lesions are red, inflamed patches, resembling sunburn in the early stages, but they progress to roughened, keratotic, scaly, and pigmented lesions. The mucous membranes of the mouth and tongue are swollen and red, eventually progressing to ulceration. The digestive symptoms are dyspeptic disturbances and enteritis (inflammation of the intestines). The nervous system is affected late in the course of the disease, causing weakness, vertigo, and insomnia, and progressing to paresthesia.[5] Mental symptoms sometimes culminate in mania.[5] The victims are emaciated and may have macrocytic anemia.

Pellagra has traditionally been associated with corn diets because of their low tryptophan and niacin content. Also, it does not occur when the corn diet is supplemented with legume protein. Pellagra occurs in the corn-eating populations in several Middle Eastern and African countries. At one time it was common in the United States among low-income groups whose main diet consisted of pork fat and hominy grits made from degerminated corn.[12] The disease in the United States is now found mainly in alcoholics. Even when the niacin intake is low, if diets contain protein of animal origin or vegetable proteins of good quality, there may be sufficient tryptophan to prevent pellagra.

Thiamin.[5, 10-12] Thiamin is a water-soluble vitamin. It is widely distributed in foods but is rapidly destroyed in roasting and stewing of meat and cooking of vegetables, with as much as 30% to 50% being lost in cooking meat and 25% to 40% in cooking vegetables.[12] It is not stored in the body in significant amounts. The mechanism by which thiamin deficiency produces characteristic lesions in the nervous system is not clear, but it is believed that the degenerative changes in the peripheral nerves and central nervous system are perhaps the result of interrupted carbohydrate metabolism. The metabolism of the nervous system is believed to be dependent on carbohydrate oxidation.[10] Thiamin requirements are proportional to carbohydrate combustion, and a diet consisting largely of carbohydrate is an important contributing factor in the development of thiamin deficiency.

Three diseases are attributed to thiamin deficiency—beriberi, Wernicke's encephalopathy or Wernicke's disease, and Korsakoff's psychosis.[5] *Wernicke's disease* is associated with chronic alcoholism but is often found in individuals with a variety of debilitating diseases caused by diets consisting primarily of carbohydrates.[5] The disease is characterized by ataxia, disturbed ocular motility, mental dullness, impaired retentive memory, and at times disorientation. Polyneuropathy is occasionally a clinical manifestation. Eye disorders are diplopia, nystagmus, and occasionally ptosis and complete paralysis of eye movements and miosis. The symptoms and signs of alcohol withdrawal may be seen, such as delirium, confusion, agitation, hallucinosis, and tremulousness.[5] The principal lesions in the central nervous system are ganglion degeneration and focal demyelinating lesions in the nuclei surrounding the ventricles and aqueduct, particularly the floor and roof of the third and fourth ventricles.[10]

Korsakoff's psychosis is similar to Wernicke's disease, but the prominent feature is confabulations, that is, the tendency to invent fanciful replies to questions whose answers are not known to the patient.[5] Learning ability is defective, and there may be difficulty in forming visual and verbal abstractions. The most prominent and serious mental abnormality is disordered memory function, which may render the patient incapable of performing any but the simplest tasks. When this condition is combined with Wernicke's disease, it is referred to as the Wernicke-Korsakoff syndrome,[5] which may be complicated with other stigmas such as chronic malnutrition, cirrhosis of the liver, anemia, and mucocutaneous lesions. Ocular manifestations respond to therapy, but psychosis tends to be irreversible if well established.[12] In diagnosis the levels of blood transketolase (a coenzyme) activity are reduced prior to thiamin administration.[12]

Beriberi is the most common disease associated with thiamin deficiency. It occurs mainly in countries where polished rice is the diet staple. This diet is low in thiamin and high in carbohydrates. It is seen in rice-eating populations of Southeast Asia and the Indian subcontinent. Beriberi may also be associated with pathologic conditions that interfere with the ingestion or absorption of food, and it is found in alcoholism. Clinically the disease is manifested by multiple peripheral neuritis, emaciation, and disturbances of motion and sensation.[5] Involvement of the nerves may lead to paralysis of the limbs; muscular atrophy also occurs. The acute fulminating form is characterized by insufficiency of the heart and blood vessels.[10] Dyspnea, palpitation of the heart, and severe precordial pain occur. In older adults a chronic, dry, atrophic form is found in which there is wrist drop and foot drop. The beriberi of infants (particularly those 1 to 4 months of age) is associated with low thiamin in breast milk of mothers subsisting on rice diets.[12] The symptoms are vomiting, anorexia, cyanosis, dyspnea, edema, oliguria, constipation, and a cardiac crisis in fatal cases. These symptoms depend upon the stage of the disease—acute, subacute, or chronic. In cases of beriberi that have come to autopsy dilatation and edema of the heart are found.[10]

Riboflavin.[4, 10-12] Riboflavin was the first vitamin to be identified as a constituent of an enzyme system, which is important in cellular respiration.[10] It is water-soluble and is widely distributed in leafy vegetables, milk, and flesh of animals or fish. It may be destroyed in cooking or exposure of food to sunlight.[12] Deficiency of this vitamin produces lesions in the mucous membranes. Ariboflavinosis is caused by a diet deficient in riboflavin or by some conditioning factor that interferes with the absorption or utilization of the vitamin. The lesions occur on the skin, lips, tongue, and eyes, but may not occur until many months after the diet becomes deficient in riboflavin. Cheilosis and angular stomatitis are associated with riboflavin deficiency but are not pathognomonic,[12] since they occur in deficiences of niacin, iron, or pyridoxine. The early symptoms are burning and soreness of the lips, mouth, and tongue. The tongue is characteristically purple or magenta and is often deeply fissured. A seborrheic dermatitis may occur, as well as photophobia, lacrimation, and burning and itching of the eyes. Vascularization of the cornea by an ingrowth of capillaries into it is an early sign. The ocular lesions may progress to keratitis and ulceration of the cornea.[10, 11]

Ariboflavinosis may be associated with other deficiency diseases such as pellagra and kwashiorkor in low-income populations of developing countries. In the industrialized nations it is more likely to be associated with alcoholism and with long-standing infections, malignancies, and other chronic debilitating diseases.

Diagnostic bases are low urinary riboflavin excretion plus the clinical signs given above.

Vitamin B$_{12}$.[2, 5, 10-12] Vitamin B$_{12}$ is a water-soluble vitamin essential for normal function of all cells, but particularly those of the bone marrow, nervous system, and gastrointestinal tract. It has been called the antipernicious anemia factor or extrinsic factor of Castle. In a family of compounds with vitamin B$_{12}$ activity, cyanocobalamin (cyano group, or cobalt, or both, present in molecules) is the principal component. The chemical functions of vitamin B$_{12}$ are not known, but it is believed likely that it is involved in synthesis of DNA (deoxyribonucleic acid) and protein.[5] The principal source is foods of animal origin. Very little is present in vegetables. The diets in most countries, either industrialized or developing, as a rule contain enough vitamin B$_{12}$ to satisfy recommended dietary requirements. Deficiency states are not likely to occur except in the presence of malabsorption or lack of intrinsic factor. It is protein bound in food, and its absorption in the ileum depends on a gastric factor, called the intrinsic factor, which is a constituent of gastric mucoprotein and is secreted mainly in the fundus of the stomach. The B_{12} intrinsic factor is absorbed in the ileum and from there discharged into the bloodstream. It is transported to tissues from the plasma and stored in the liver. Deficiency of B_{12} results in development of megaloblastic anemia and subacute degeneration of the spinal cord, optic nerves, cerebral white matter, and peripheral nerves.[5, 10] Vitamin B_{12} is the extrinsic factor in pernicious anemia, but its absorption depends on the intrinsic factor in the gastric mucosa.

Pernicious anemia[8] is the most prevalent form of vitamin B_{12} deficiency. It is caused by failure of the gastric fundus to secrete amounts of intrinsic factor adequate to ensure intestinal absorption of vitamin B_{12}. The disease is characterized by chronic and progressive megaloblastic anemia, achylia gastrica (absence of hydrochloric acid and rennin from gastric juice), and neurologic and gastrointestinal damage, and it invariably benefits from parenteral administration of vitamin B_{12}.[8] The symptoms of the anemia are fatigability, weakness, faintness, pallor, and dyspnea. The neurologic complaints are paresthesias of the toes or fingers, progressing to impaired coordination of the lower extremities and fingers. These symptoms occur because of lack of oxygen being carried to tissue in the bloodstream. Cerebral symptoms are dullness, apathy, irritability, loss of concentration, and, possibly, frank psychoses, particularly in elderly patients.[8] Constipation or diarrhea is a common occurrence.

Pernicious anemia is uncommon in individuals under 35 years of age.[8, 10] Although no clear mode of inheritance is apparent, some patients have a family history of pernicious anemia.[10]

The association of clinical or laboratory evidence of vitamin B_{12} deficiency with gastric achlorhydria may suffice for diagnosis. A test for intrinsic factor is oral administration of radioactive B_{12} (for example, cyanocobalamin Co 57 or Co 60) along with a parenteral dose of nonradio-

active vitamin B_{12}—the Schilling test.[2] Very little of the radioactive vitamin is absorbed in pernicious anemia, as determined by subsequent measurement of radioactivity of the stool and urine. Several methods are being devised to assay gastric juice for intrinsic factor in vitro.[2]

Folic acid.[2, 7, 10, 12] Folic acid (pteroylglutamic acid) is synthesized by higher plants and also by microorganisms. It occurs richly in many vegetables as well as in liver. Several naturally occurring folates (substances with folic acid–like activity) are readily absorbed in the small intestine without the aid of intrinsic factor. Synthetic pteroylglutamic acid is absorbed readily, primarily in the jejunum. The principal effects of folic acid deficiency are in the blood and the gastrointestinal tract. The gastrointestinal manifestations may be similar to those of pernicious anemia but tend to be more widespread and severe, in part because of the greater likelihood of multiple vitamin deficiencies.[12] Cheilosis and glossitis commonly occur in severe cases. Diarrhea is often present. Blood findings include leukopenia and thrombocytopenia, as well as anemia. The marrow is richly cellular and megaloblastic with severe abnormalities of granulocyte precursors. Folic acid deficiency is much more common among the malnourished than is vitamin B_{12} deficiency, since body stores of folic acid and its derivatives in normally nourished individuals are relatively less extensive and stable than are those of vitamin B_{12}.[8] Because of its more rapid turnover, folic acid deficiency is more frequently found in intestinal malabsorption states than in vitamin B_{12} deficiency. It is a common complication of sprue, celiac disease, idiopathic steatorrhea, and intestinal short circuits (partial gastrectomy or other surgical procedures). The symptoms of folic acid deficiency may commence within several months of dietary deprivations. The overwhelming majority of patients with megaloblastic anemia have a deficiency of either vitamin B_{12} or folic acid. Diagnosis depends upon discriminating between these two disorders. Folic acid deficiency is suspected either after exclusion of vitamin B_{12} deficiency or by association of megaloblastic anemia with gross malnutrition, intestinal malabsorption, pregnancy, cirrhosis, chronic hemolysis, or anticonvulsant drug therapy.[8] In these conditions, folic acid deficiency is more common than vitamin B_{12} deficiency. The presence of severe oral or intestinal lesions supports a diagnosis of folic acid deficiency. Confirmation of diagnosis may be made by a therapeutic trial method with doses of vitamin B_{12}.[8] In folic acid deficiency, physiologic doses of vitamin B_{12} administered

parenterally daily are ineffective, whereas parenteral folic acid in daily doses is usually effective in producing full hematologic and clinical response.[12] Diagnosis may be established more quickly by microbiologic assay of the serum for folic acid activity. The urinary excretion of formiminoglutamic acid (FIGLU) during oral loading with histidine has been measured as a metabolic indication of folic acid deficiency.[2] Another method is determination of the blood level or urinary excretion of the vitamin after a test dose of tritium-labeled and nonlabeled folic acid.[2]

Vitamin C[4, 10-14]

Vitamin C is a water-soluble vitamin. It has been called the antiscorbutic vitamin, since its deficiency causes scurvy (Fig. 10-1). In vitamin C deficiency resistance to infection is reduced and healing of wounds is defective. It is particularly needed for the formation of normal connective tissue (collagen and ground substance). Humans are not able to synthesize ascorbic acid from glucose by way of glucuronic acid, since they lack the enzyme required for conversion of gluconate to ascorbate.[12] Therefore, if dietary intake of the vitamin ceases for several months, clinical scurvy develops. The ascorbic acid level in the blood falls rapidly in extensive wounds or burns. Vitamin C is available in fresh fruits, particularly citrus, and vegetables.

Scurvy or scorbutus is caused by a deficiency of vitamin C. The outstanding clinical symptoms are hemorrhages (cutaneous, mucous membrane, and muscular into joint spaces), lesions in the skeleton, and loosening of the teeth. The cutaneous hemorrhages range from petechial to massive extravasation, with the large hemorrhages corresponding to areas of trauma. Wherever there is mechanical stress, there may be hemorrhage into the muscles and fascia.

In infants, massive subperiosteal hemorrhage occurs, especially in the legs. The

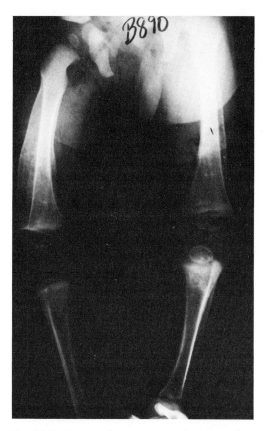

Fig. 10-1. Scurvy of extremities, showing white line of scurvy and ground glass demineralization, with thinned cortices, all of which are typical of radiographic findings of bone in scurvy. (From Young, C. G., and Likos, J. J.: Medical specialty terminology, x-ray and nuclear medicine, St. Louis, 1972, The C. V. Mosby Co.)

bleeding comes from capillaries whose endothelial lining cells have been damaged. In adults the gums become ulcerated, with loosening of the teeth and hemorrhage. In children the skeletal lesions, in addition to hemorrhages beneath the periosteum and into joints, are pathologic fractures through the rarefied bone at the metaphyseal ends of the long bones. Scurvy is most common in infants and young children during the stages when bone and connective tissues of all types are being formed. It is a disease in which the supporting tissues of the body are unable to produce or maintain intercellular substance. These intercellular substances include collagen, matrices of bone, dentin, and cartilage.

Early experiments traced this disease to a deficiency of ascorbic acid in the diet devoid of fresh fruits and vegetables. It still occurs in the United States, particularly in infants, in spite of knowledge of prevention.

The deficiency may be detected in laboratory procedures that measure the plasma or leukocyte concentration of ascorbic acid or the urinary excretion of the vitamin. Bone lesions are detected by x-ray examination. (See Fig. 10-1.)

Vitamin D[3, 10-12]

Vitamin D, a fat-soluble vitamin, has been called antirachitic vitamin. It is essential at all ages for the maintenance of calcium homeostasis and skeletal integrity. It is available in most foods of animal origin and in vitamin D–fortified milk. Vitamin D promotes absorption of calcium and phosphorus from the alimentary tract. Its deficiency causes rickets in children and osteomalacia in adults. Vitamin D is produced by ultraviolet rays upon the skin (vitamin D_3), but only the shorter rays are effective. Deficiency can occur only when the amount supplied in food or by sunshine is inadequate.

Rickets (Fig. 10-2) is often called infantile osteomalacia, since the bones lack hardening. It is a disease of young children in which the bones contain less than the normal amount of calcium and phosphorus. In the infantile form the osteoid tissue in growing bones is not calcified or hardened and deformities of the skeleton result. Sometimes bending deformities are present, such as the knock-knee in older children. Clinical symptoms are restlessness, irritability, and sweating. The children often have a potbelly, scoliosis, and delayed

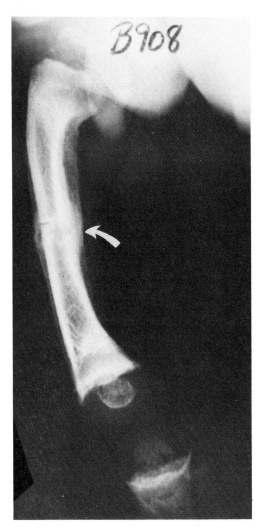

Fig. 10-2. Infantile rickets with healing pathologic fracture (arrow). There is bowing and demineralization of bone. (From Young, C. G., and Likos, J. J.: Medical specialty terminology, x-ray and nuclear medicine, St. Louis, 1972, The C. V. Mosby Co.)

dentition with defective enamel. In babies, fontanel closure is delayed. Because of lack of hardening of bones, fractures are likely to occur, as well as a pigeon breast and deformed joints.

Osteomalacia (softening of the bones) is an adult form of deficiency of vitamin D.[3] It is caused by a derangement of mineral metabolism, frequently associated with inadequate calcium or phosphorus or both in the diet, that leads to the osseous changes. In this disease, intestinal absorption of calcium may be decreased, and vitamin D may be deficient.[3]

Clinically it is expressed by pain in the bones, muscular weakness, loss of weight, and anorexia. Patients have a waddling gait and are subject to multiple, spontaneous pseudofractures. When fractures are multiple, healing is inadequate.

Diagnosis of rickets and osteomalacia from vitamin D deficiency rests on biopsy and roentgenographic (Fig. 10-2) and biochemical findings.[12]

Hypervitaminosis D (overdosage of vitamin D) is a syndrome characterized by hypercalcemia, hypercalciuria, and metastatic calcification.[10] Generalized calcinosis affects joints, synovial membranes, kidneys, myocardium, parathyroid glands, pancreas, pulmonary alveoli, lymph glands, arteries, acid-secreting portion of the stomach, and the conjunctivas and corneas of the eyes.[10,12] Demineralization of bones occurs in advanced stages. When calcium is mobilized from the bones, osteoporosis results. The symptoms include nausea, vomiting, and diarrhea.

Vitamin K[2,10,12]

Vitamin K, a fat-soluble vitamin, has been called the antihemorrhagic vitamin. It differs from other vitamins in that it can be synthesized in the intestine from bacteria, although it is available in the diet from leafy vegetables and other common foods. Vitamin K is necessary for the formation of vitamin K–dependent clotting factors by the liver (factors VII, IX, X, and prothrombin time).[2] It is absorbed from the intestines along with lipids with the aid of bile. It is not stored in appreciable amounts. If the parenchyma of the liver is severely damaged, it is not able to synthesize the vitamin K–dependent factors, even if adequate amounts are available. In newborn and premature infants the vitamin K–dependent coagulation factors are reduced, since the fetal liver is unable to produce adequate amounts of prothrombin from vitamin K. Several weeks are required for vitamin K to reach adult levels in the infant. Prophylactic treatment of premature infants and mothers at term with vitamin K has greatly reduced hemorrhagic disease of the newborn.

Other factors that interfere with the function of vitamin K are bishydroxycoumarin (Dicumarol) and other anticoagulants.[2] Conditioned deficiency of vitamin K occurs in biliary fistula, obstructive jaundice because of absence of bile from the intestinal tract, and in sprue and related diseases because of the failure of absorption of fat. Sterilization of the intestinal flora by antibiotics leads to diminished production or supply of vitamin K because of disappearance of normal flora.[2]

Diagnosis of vitamin K deficiency is made by laboratory determinations of prothrombin time, bleeding time, and clotting or coagulation time.[2]

MINERALS AND PIGMENTS[1,4,6,10-12,13]

Carbon, hydrogen, nitrogen, and oxygen are the basic constituents of all tissue cells, but in addition, a number of inorganic minerals are essential to human life. Some of these, such as calcium, phosphorus, magnesium, sodium, potassium, chlorine, and sulfur, occur in relatively large amounts in the body. Others are present in only trace amounts but are nevertheless vital to health in that they form essential components of certain enzyme systems. These include the metallic elements such as zinc, copper, manganese, selenium, and molybdenum. Deficiencies of these elements have been extensively studied in experimental animals, and some of the lesions produced are duplicated in humans in deficiency states. Manganese is an exception, since no lesions in the human being are known.[10] A sufficient amount of the minerals is ordinarily available in the diet. A deficiency of minerals is invariably caused by malabsorption in the gastrointestinal tract, usually as the result of disease, or particularly of renal diseases. An excess of these substances is usually the result of faulty excretion, increased mobilization, or an abnormally high level in the diet. The disturbances created by mineral deficiencies as a rule lead to metabolic and biochemical derangement associated with clinical disease.

Colored materials called pigments[10, 11] are deposited in the skin and internal organs in a number of conditions. Some of these pigments are formed within the body, and others are introduced into the body through the gastrointestinal tract, skin, or lungs. The main types produced within the body are melanin and the hemoglobin derivatives (hemosiderin and bilirubin formed from hemoglobin breakdown). Melanin is produced in the skin by melanoblasts (melanocytes), and it forms the normal coloring material of the skin and choroid coat of the eye. The degree of skin pigmentation varies in different races and in individuals. Pathologic increases of skin pigmentation occur in Addison's disease because of destruction of the adrenal cortices, in hemochromatosis (discussed under iron), and in localized pigmentation (cafe-au-lait spots) as seen in multiple neurofibromatosis and fibrous dysplasia of the bone. In leprosy, irregular patches of skin pigmentation form. Albinism, the absence of normal melanin pigmentation, is an inherited disorder. Pigmented nevi and malignant melanomas are tumors composed of melanoblasts. In the condition of melanosis coli, there is brown or black discoloration of the appendix or large intestine. Hemosiderin is discussed under iron, p. 129.

Bile pigment depositions in the tissues produce the condition known as jaundice or icterus.[1, 10, 11] The skin, scleras, and mucous membranes have a yellowish to orange or even greenish discoloration. It is caused by excessive bilirubin in the circulation. Some types are familial or hereditary. The inborn error in metabolism in the hereditary form is an inability of the liver to excrete bilirubin and its derivatives. Jaundice occurs in a number of diseases, notably erythroblastosis fetalis, icterus neonatorum, necrosis of liver cells from poisons, obstructions of the biliary tree by calculi, neoplasms, or strictures, and in organisms as in viral hepatitis.[1] It also occurs in a variety of hemolytic anemias.[9] Erythroblastosis fetalis is discussed in Chapter 9.

The most important exogenous pigments that gain entrance to the body through the lungs are coal dust, iron dust, and silica, which produce coal worker's pneumoconiosis (CWP), formerly called anthracosis, siderosis, and silicosis, respectively.[13] Other mineral dusts that present occupational hazards but to a lesser degree are beryllium, causing berylliosis; tin dust causing stannosis; and barium, producing baritosis. Occupational pneumoconioses can be caused by organic (vegetable) substances such as cotton dust (byssinosis), dust from sugar cane baled and stored for months (bagassosis), dust from moldy hay (farmer's lung), and dusts that cause an allergic reaction, irritating the lungs. Dust inhalation diseases, both environmental and occupational, have been grouped together under a common name—pneumoconiosis (from Greek *pneumo*, meaning lung, and *konis*, meaning dust).

A few years ago it was considered that only workers engaged in occupations where there was exposure to these dusts were in danger of developing lung diseases, but now it is recognized that the community at large may also be affected.[13]

Asbestos is used in thousands of ways as protection from fire and heat, for example, through insulation in buildings, fireproof clothing, and brake linings. Inhaled asbestos fibers cause the crippling disease known as asbestosis, which scars the lungs and interferes with the passage of oxygen into the blood. Asbestos fibers when inhaled become embedded in the lung and cannot be dislodged by the natural cleaning mechanism of the respiratory tract. Asbestos fibers often lead to development of certain cancers of the respiratory tract and digestive systems and are also the cause of pleural mesotheliomas.[13]

Silicosis was one of the first of the pneumoconioses to be recognized. It is a fibrosis of the lungs caused by breathing silica or quartz dust. All types of mining, such as gold, copper, lead, zinc, iron, anthracite and bituminous coal, produce silica, which is inhaled by workers. Silicosis may also occur from working in other industries such as foundries, sandblasting, concrete breaking, pottery and china manufacture, and granite cutting and polishing. The onset of silicosis is gradual, and it is often years before it is detected in the lungs. The condition is irreversible, and prolonged exposure increases vulnerability to tuberculosis, bronchitis, and emphysema.[13]

Black lung is now officially called coal worker's pneumoconiosis (CWP), since it occurs in workers in underground and surface coal mines where fine coal dust particles accumulate in the lungs over the years and darken the tissue to the color of coal itself.[13] A simple pneumoconiosis caused by coal dust may progress to massive fibrosis, often leading to severe disability and premature death.

Pigmentation of the skin and other tissues occurs when silver and lead are ingested or absorbed. The imporant diseases of these metallic poisons are argyria (silver poisoning) and lead poisoning. (See Fig. 12-1.)

Calcium and phosphorus[1, 10, 11]

The two minerals calcium and phosphorus are discussed together, since derangements of phosphorus metabolism are invariably associated with calcium and vitamin D levels (discussed under vitamins, p. 124). Both calcium and phosphorus are indispensable in bone formation and certain other physiologic activities. Both are normally maintained at certain concentrations in the blood by parathyroid function. The normal metabolism of calcium and phosphorus is dependent upon adequate dietary intake, vitamin D intake, and parathyroid function.

Calcium is the principal inorganic constituent of bone, dentin, and teeth enamel. It is mostly concentrated in the skeleton; therefore, an adequate intake is necessary for the proper composition of skeletal parts, particularly during the growing period. The demand for calcium and phosphorus is increased during pregnancy and lactation. Phosphorus is also present in large amounts in bone and teeth, but the ratio of calcium to phosphorus is about 2 to 1. When disturbances occur that result in excessive amounts of calcium being mobilized from the bone, phosphorus is also mobilized. Deficiencies in both can occur simultaneously. When calcium is absorbed from the gastrointestinal tract, the absorption of phosphorus is in part regulated by the same mechanism (intermediary metabolism of vitamin D) that applies to calcium. Phosphorus is abundant in ordinary foods, whereas calcium is dependent to a large extent on the amount of milk, milk products, and eggs that are ingested. A deficient intake of phosphorus is much less likely to occur than a deficient intake of calcium. Both are measured in the blood serum. Since the mechanisms of assimilation, excretion, and utilization are so closely related, both substances are considered in all pathologic disturbances affecting one or the other.

Calcium has four main functions: (1) formation of bone, (2) coagulation of blood, (3) maintenance of normal cell membrane permeability, and (4) maintenance of normal neuromuscular irritability. When an abnormal calcium metabolism causes low levels of body calcium, such as occur in hypoparathyroidism and vitamin D deficiency, tetany may result. Tetany is manifested by carpopedal spasm (flexion of wrist and ankle joints), muscular twitching and cramps, and sometimes by convulsions.

Derangements of calcium are referred to as hypocalcemia, a deficiency of calcium in the blood, and hypercalcemia, an excess of calcium in the blood. The most striking examples of these are hypoparathyroidism in the former and hyperparathyroidism in the latter. Other forms of hypercalcemia are caused by the demineralization of bone that occurs in some bone fractures, osteoporosis, and the immobilization of bone because of injury or paralysis. In the aged a physiologic atrophy of bone results from elevated serum calcium levels. Abnormal deposits of calcium also occur in the walls of blood vessels in arteriosclerosis. This is referred to as dystrophic calcification. Valvular function of the heart may be seriously impaired by calcific deposits in injured heart valves. Calcific deposits in the blood vessels or valves of the heart represent permanent deformity and scarring. Occasionally calcium salts are deposited in the skin and subcutaneous tissues and even in the deeper tissues, such as tendons and muscles. These are referred to as calcinosis. Calcium also enters into the formation of stones (lithiasis) in the collective system of the kidneys, biliary ducts, and salivary glands. In the late stages of chronic renal disease with renal failure, extensive mobilization of calcium may cause metastatic foci of calcium deposits in the kidneys. This type of bony disturbance is often called renal rickets or renal osteodystrophy.

Normally calcium salts are deposited only in bones and teeth. Any departure from this normal pattern is considered to be pathologic calcification, except in such instances as the calcium depositions in the pineal gland after puberty.

Iron[1, 9-11]

Iron is vital for health, although existing only in trace amounts in the body. Most of it is combined in complex pigments and enzymes (hemoglobin, myoglobin, and heme enzymes); the rest is protein bound. It is divided into red cell iron (hemoglobin), plasma iron, and tissue cell iron. As red cell iron we are familiar with it as hemoglobin (a combination of iron with proteins), the oxygen-carrying pigment necessary for the life of tissues and the organism as a whole. In the tissue cells it is present as a constituent of respiratory enzymes. Iron exists as an oxygen storage compound in muscle (myoglobin) and in many tissues in combination with protein. It is absorbed chiefly in the duodenum. It is stored in the liver normally and made available to tissues on demand. It is also stored in the reticuloendothelial cells of the spleen and bone marrow.

Iron is derived from diet and from breakdown of hemoglobin in red cells at their death. The red cells live about 120 days. The endogenous supply of iron results from the breakdown of hemoglobin into globin and hematin fractions and the further degradation of hematin into chemically active iron. This iron is either reconverted to hemoglobin in situ or carried through the blood serum to the storage depots (such as the liver) or tissue cells for aid in the formation of respiratory enzymes. When iron is lost for any reason, but through hemorrhage in particular, the serum iron is the first reserve called upon for synthesis of new red cells. Later the storage depots, liver, spleen, and bone marrow are utilized to replace the loss.

Iron deficiencies may occur from inadequate dietary intake. In women, however, the deficiency is often caused by excessive loss of menstrual blood and the depletion of iron stores. This depletion of iron stores occasionally occurs in pregnancy and lactation. Men seldom have iron deficiencies except through dietary deficiency or through loss of blood from hemorrhage or disease. Deficiencies also occur in the aged from their dietary habits. Any chronic blood loss will result in inadequate hemoglobin formation and eventually iron-deficiency anemias (hypochromic anemias). (See Fig. 18-29.)

When destruction of red blood cells is excessive, as in hemolytic anemias, large stores of iron accumulate in the body. Also in transfusions the red blood cells have a short life-span and are rapidly destroyed with resulting large deposits of iron. Decreased red cell formation may also cause excessive levels of iron. Prolonged excessive storage of iron causes hemosiderosis[6] (*hemo*, meaning blood, and *sidero*, meaning iron), a condition in which a pigment containing iron (hemosiderin) is deposited in the tissues. Hemochromatosis,[6] a systemic disease in which excessive deposits of iron are stored in the body tissues and organs over a number of years, is a disturbance of iron-pigment metabolism. It appears to be caused by excessive absorption of iron.

Iodine

Iodine is necessary for normal thyroid function, and deficiencies are related to thyroid lesions. These are discussed in Chapter 17.

Copper[6]

Copper is important in the formation and development of blood cells and is an essential constituent of several important enzymes. Copper toxicity is implicated in the heredofamilial aberrations of copper metabolism in Wilson's disease. In this disease copper is excreted in the urine instead of normally in the bile. The patients have cirrhosis of the liver and central nervous system damage, which is designated hepatolenticular degeneration.

Fluorine[10, 12]

Fluorine is incorporated into bone and teeth. To fight tooth decay it has been introduced into the water in those areas where it does not naturally occur. In communities where the water has been fluoridated, the incidence of tooth decay in children has been decreased up to 50%. Excessive amounts cause a mottling of the enamel. This may occur in children when enamel is being deposited in developing, unerupted teeth.

STEP-BY-STEP EXERCISES

Step 1. A number of organic and inorganic substances or nutrients are required in humans for maintenance of metabolic and reproductive activity, cell integrity, and tissue growth. Among these are the vitamins and minerals, which are accessory food nutrients present in plants and animals eaten by humans; vitamin K is the only vitamin manufactured in the body.

Mark the following statements *T* for true or *F* for false.

1. Vitamins and minerals are nutrients necessary for maintenance of a healthy body. ___
2. All the vitamins and minerals are present in foods. ___
3. Humans can exist without vitamins and minerals in foods because they are manufactured by the body. ___

Step 2. Deficiencies of minerals and vitamins exist because of an inadequate intake in food or failure of the body to absorb, utilize, or retain adequate amounts.

Mark the following statements *T* for true or *F* for false.

1. Diarrhea would interfere with the absorption of minerals and vitamins. ___
2. Food sources are always adequate and deficiencies exist only because of failure to utilize the vitamins and minerals. ___
3. Vomiting would interfere with absorption of the nutrients. ___
4. Absence of teeth or ill-fitting dentures would not interfere with adequate nutrition. ___
5. Many diseases might interfere with proper absorption and utilization of vitamins and minerals. ___

Step 3. The known vitamins useful to

humans are A, B complex (with certain exceptions of components), C, D, and K. Deficiency of A causes eye lesions, such as night blindness and xerophthalmia (dry eyes), which may lead to corneal ulcers, and also skin rashes. Deficiency of vitamin C causes scurvy, in which there are hemorrhages of the skin and mucous membranes and into the joints beneath the periosteum in children, also loosening of the teeth, usually in adults. Pathologic fractures may occur. Vitamin D is the antirachitic vitamin; a deficiency of it causes rickets. Symptoms are bony deformities and improper growth in children, and osteomalacia in adults. Vitamin K, the antihemorrhagic vitamin, may be made in the intestinal tract from bacteria. It is necessary for proper blood clotting.

Deficiency of which vitamin (A, C, D, or K) causes the conditions described?

1. Improper clotting of blood ___
2. Rickets ___
3. Scurvy ___
4. Osteomalacia ___
5. Night blindness ___
6. Bleeding gums ___
7. Corneal ulcers ___
8. Loosening of teeth ___
9. Bone deformities, particularly of the tibias ___
10. Hemorrhagic disease of neonate ___

Step 4. Vitamin B complex is made up of a number of substances, among which are thiamin or B_1, necessary for nutrition and function of the nervous system, riboflavin, and niacin. An example of a disease that results from thiamin deficiency is beriberi. Riboflavin deficiency results in severe abnormalities of the eyes with vascularization of the cornea by capillary ingrowth. Niacin or nicotinic acid deficiency may cause pellagra.

Deficiency of which components of the vitamin B complex can cause the following conditions?

1. Beriberi ___

2. Vascularization of cornea ___

3. Pellagra ___

Step 5. Many inorganic minerals, such as calcium, phosphorus, magnesium, sodium, potassium, chlorine, and sulfur, are present in the body in relatively large amounts and are necessary to human life. Others such as iron, iodine, copper, manganese, cobalt, and zinc are also essential to life, but they are present in smaller or trace amounts. Deficiencies of the minerals are invariably caused by malabsorption in the gastrointestinal tract, usually because of disease or excessive loss by vomiting, diarrhea, or in renal diseases. An excess of these substances is usually the result of faulty excretion, increased mobilization, or abnormally high levels in the diet.

Mark the following statements T for true or F for false.

1. Minerals, since they are present sometimes in only trace amounts, are not essential to life. ___
2. Deficiencies of minerals are always caused by inadequate amounts in the diet. ___
3. Minerals are lost in renal diseases and when vomiting and diarrhea are present. ___

Step 6. Two minerals indispensable in bone formation, particularly in growing children, are ___ and ___ .

Step 7

1. A deficiency of calcium in the blood is called ___ .
2. An excess of calcium in the blood is called ___ .

Step 8. In which of the following conditions would you expect to find a deficiency of calcium in the blood serum?

1. Demineralization of bone ___
2. Hypoparathyroidism ___
3. Hyperparathyroidism ___

Step 9. In which of the following would you expect to find deposits of calcium?

1. Arteriosclerosis ___

2. Calcinosis ___

3. Normal muscles ___

Step 10. Iron is essential, since it enters into the formation of hemoglobin, which is the oxygen-carrying property of the blood. Iron is lost in acute hemorrhages as well as in some chronic diseases, such as bleeding hemorrhoids and ulcers. It may also be lost excessively in abnormal menstrual flow. Iron is carried in red blood cells, and when they outlive their usefulness (120 days usually), they are not entirely lost to the body, since the iron they contained is reconverted for the use of tissues.

Mark the following statements *T* for true or *F* for false.

1. When a red cell dies at the end of its lifetime, the hemoglobin it contained is lost forever. ___

2. External free hemorrhages may result in an iron deficiency. ___

3. Repeated blood loss through bleeding ulcers might eventually result in iron-deficiency anemia. ___

Step 11. Which of the following conditions might be the result of excessive storage of iron?

1. Hemosiderosis ___

2. Hemochromatosis ___

3. Hemorrhoids ___

Step 12. Indicate whether iodine or copper contributes to the following functions.

1. Normal thyroid function _____

2. Formation of blood cells _____

SELECTED DISEASES CAUSED BY DEFICIENCY OF ESSENTIAL NUTRIENTS[12]

Diseases or conditions caused by deficiencies or derangements of vitamins and minerals were described in the previous discussions.

Marasmus[12]

Marasmus is a disease of protein-calorie malnutrition. The diets responsible for this disease are extremely low-calorie and are also deficient in proteins and other essential elements. Marasmus is characterized by growth failure in children and severe tissue wasting. The child is emaciated because of loss of subcutaneous fat. Atrophy of organs occurs, but the child is clinically alert and has a good appetite. Although growth stops or is impaired, since the child utilizes amino acids from skeletal muscles and other tissue and derives energy from fat deposits, no serious metabolic disturbances are seen.

Kwashiorkor[10, 12]

Kwashiorkor is caused by a deficiency in protein relative to calories. It is a common and sometimes fatal disease of infancy, occurring in tropical and semitropical areas of Africa, India, China, Philippines, and Central and South America among children who are not given sufficient protein. There may also be superimposed stress, usually of microbial origin.

It is characterized by edema, pellagroid skin lesions in the perineal region, on extremities, face, and trunk, dry brittle hair, anorexia, apathy, diarrhea, and fatty liver. Coexisting deficiencies of vitamin A, vitamin B complex, particularly riboflavin, and iron, may occur. There are profound biochemical changes, including a low total serum protein (a diagnostic characteristic), low levels of lipid fractions (neutral fat, fatty acids, phospholipids, and cholesterol), reduction in activity of a number of enzymes (lipase, trypsin, amylase, alkaline phosphatase), extremely low levels of vitamin A in the serum, potassium depletion, and other electrolyte changes secondary to diarrhea and vomiting.

Starvation[10, 12]

General atrophy of numerous tissues of the body occurs in starvation. Starvation may be caused by lesions of the digestive tract that interfere with assimilation of food, loss of appetite, or ability to relish food (anorexia nervosa), but profound degrees of wasting and emaciation of the body result from protein starvation. In individuals maintained on a low-calorie diet a negative nitrogen balance develops, and the changes are primarily those of protein starvation or deficiency. Loss of weight, hunger, edema, and atrophy of organs occur. Absence of spermatogenesis and ovogenesis results from atrophy of the testes and ovaries, respectively.[10] The cardiac and skeletal muscles become so small that they can be recognized only with difficulty in examination of tissues.[10] In children, growth of bones ceases. Severe malnutrition existed in concentration camps and prisons in World War II. It has also existed in numerous famines in many parts of the world. In correcting undernutrition or starvation, feeding must be gradual, similar to that of a newborn. Shock and death occurred in prison and concentration camp victims at the end of World War II when they were allowed to overeat.[12]

Responses

Step 1: 1. T; 2. T; 3. F
Step 2: 1. T; 2. F; 3. T; 4. F; 5. T
Step 3: 1. K; 2. D; 3. C; 4. D; 5. A; 6. C; 7. A;
          8. C; 9. D; 10. K
Step 4: 1. thiamin; 2. riboflavin; 3. niacin or
          nicotinic acid
Step 5: 1. F; 2. F; 3. T
Step 6: calcium; phosphorus
Step 7: 1. hypocalcemia; 2. hypercalcemia
Step 8: 2. X
Step 9: 1. X; 2. X
Step 10: 1. F; 2. T; 3. T
Step 11: 1. X; 2. X
Step 12: iodine; 2. copper

REFERENCES

1. Anderson, W. A. D.: In Anderson, W. A. D., editor: Pathology, ed. 6, St. Louis, 1971, The C. V. Mosby Co. (degenerative changes and disturbances of metabolism, minerals).
2. Bauer, J. D.: In Frankel, S., Reitman, S., and Sonnenwirth, A. C., editors: Gradwohl's clinical laboratory methods and diagnosis, ed. 7, St. Louis, 1970, The C. V. Mosby Co. (vitamin B_{12} and folic acid; vitamin K and coagulation factors).
3. Bennett, G. A.: In Anderson, W. A. D., editor: Pathology, ed. 6, St. Louis, 1971, The C. V. Mosby Co. (bones, rickets and osteomalacia).
4. Best, C. H., and Taylor, N. B.: The human body, ed. 3, New York, 1960, Holt, Rinehart and Winston (vitamins and minerals).
5. Dreyfuss, P.: In Beeson, P. B., and McDermott, W., editors: Cecil-Loeb textbook of medicine, ed. 13, Philadelphia, 1971, W. B. Saunders Co. (nutritional disorders of the nervous system).
6. Edmonson, H. A., and Peters, R. L.: In Anderson, W. A. D., editor: Pathology, ed. 6, St. Louis, 1971, The C. V. Mosby Co. (copper metabolism; hemosiderosis and hemochromatosis).
7. Godwin, H. A.: In Beeson, P. B., and McDermott, W., editors: Cecil-Loeb textbook of medicine, ed. 13, Philadelphia, 1971, W. B. Saunders Co. (folic acid deficiency).
8. Jandl, J. H.: In Beeson, P. B., and McDermott, W., editors: Cecil-Loeb textbook of medicine, ed. 13, Philadelphia, 1971, W. B. Saunders Co. (pernicious anemia).
9. Miale, J. B.: In Anderson, W. A. D., editor: Pathology, ed. 6, St. Louis, 1971, The C. V. Mosby Co. (hemopoietic system, blood).
10. Pinkerton, H.: In Anderson, W. A. D., editor: Pathology, ed. 6, St. Louis, 1971, The C. V. Mosby Co. (vitamin and mineral deficiencies).
11. Robbins, S. L.: Pathology, ed. 3, Philadelphia, 1967, W. B. Saunders Co. (deficiencies of vitamins and minerals).
12. Scrimshaw, N.: In Beeson, P. B., and McDermott, W., editors: Ceceil-Loeb textbook of medicine, ed. 13, Philadelphia, 1971, W. B. Saunders Co. (diseases of nutrition).
13. U.S. Department of Health, Education, and Welfare, Public Health Service (NIH), DHEW Publication No. (NIH) 74-188, 1974 (the dust inhalation diseases: pneumoconioses).
14. Wohl, M. G., and Goodhart, R. S.: Modern nutrition in health and disease, ed. 4, Philadelphia, 1968, Lea & Febiger.

CHAPTER 11

Diseases caused by physical agents or trauma

The physical agents that cause disease or injury are mechanical violence, such as automobile accidents, firearms, and home and industry accidents; changes in atmospheric pressure; changes in temperature; electrical injury; and radiation injury. All of these have one thing in common, the agent responsible for the injury came from outside the body. There was a collision of the body with some mass or object, as in a fall or in a moving vehicle accident, or with some object hurled or propelled by another, such as a bullet, missile, or knife. In almost all instances, kinetic energy or force was responsible for the injury. In all of them there is the implication that the normal state of rest or uniform motion of the body part was harmfully disturbed by an interference with its function or structure.

MECHANICAL VIOLENCE[15]

The most common manifestation of an injury to an organ or tissue is the wound. Any injury that causes a break in the skin or other body membranes or in the underlying tissues is known as a wound. Wounds are classified according to their size, location, manner in which the skin or tissue is broken, and the causing agent. In general, large wounds are much more serious than small ones because of the danger of severe bleeding, damage to underlying organs or tissue, and a greater degree of shock. Wounds are classified as abrasions, lacerations, contusions, incisions, penetrating injuries, crushing injuries, fractures, and bullet or gunshot wounds.

Abrasions represent a tearing away of the epidermal cells by friction. The corium may or may not be penetrated. Abrasions occur when the skin is rubbed off or scraped off, as in rope burns, floor burns, and skinned knees and elbows. They are potential sites of infection, since dirt and germs are usually ground into the tissues. Ordinarily, however, such a wound is of little significance and heals in a short time.

Lacerations are wounds in which the tissues are torn, rather than cut. These wounds have ragged, irregular edges and masses of torn tissue underneath. Lacerations are usually made by blunt, rather than sharp objects and are a common type of wound from machinery in industry. They often occur over the hands and skull where tissues are stretched thinner than at other sites in the body. External lacerations are frequently contaminated with dirt, grease, or other material that is ground into the tissues, and they also are likely to become infected. Lacerations often occur in abdominal organs (Fig. 11-1), particularly in a solid viscus (liver or spleen, for example), when the blunt trauma to the abdomen, back, or flank has been sudden and forceful. (See Fig. 18-2.)

Incisions are commonly called cuts. They are made by sharp cutting instruments, such as knives, razors, or broken glass. They tend to bleed very freely because blood vessels are severed. In this type of wound relatively little damage is done to the surrounding tissues since the edges of the wound are uniformly displaced to either side. They are not as likely to be-

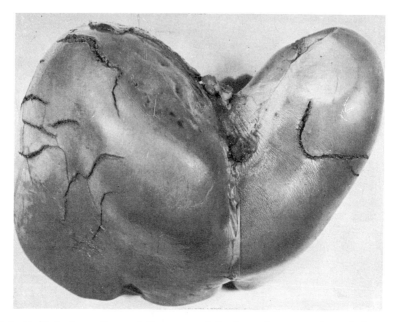

Fig. 11-1. Multiple lacerations of liver caused by lateral compression of thorax. (From Moritz, A. R., and Adelson, L.: In Anderson, W. A. D., editor: Pathology, ed. 6, St. Louis, 1971, The C. V. Mosby Co.)

come infected as abrasions or lacerations, because there is a free flow of blood, which washes out many of the microorganisms that might cause infection.

Contusions or *bruises* are injuries that produce the characteristic black and blue appearance at the site of injury. The underlying tissues are involved sufficiently for the walls of small blood vessels to be disrupted and cause interstitial bleeding, but there is no disruption of the epidermis. Usually the bruises appear on the surface soon after injury, but they may be deep, and hours may elapse before the extravasated blood is visible. Contusions can also occur in internal organs, particularly in those in which a viscus is crushed against the posterior wall of the abdomen. People with blood dyscrasias or who suffer from certain dietary deficiencies are prone to show extensive contusions from relatively mild injuries. Since the skin is unbroken in contusions, the probability of infection is practically nonexistent.

Penetrating or *puncture* wounds are caused by objects that penetrate some

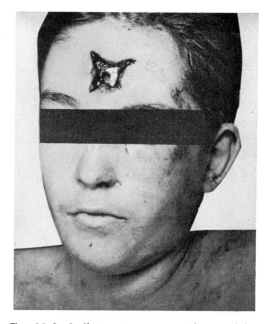

Fig. 11-2. Stellate entrance wound caused by propulsion of rapidly expanding gases into tissues. Muzzle of gun was in contact with skin at moment of firing. (From Moritz, A. R., and Adelson, L.: In Anderson, W. A. D., editor: Pathology, ed. 6, St. Louis, 1971, The C. V. Mosby Co.)

distance into the tissues, leaving only a relatively small surface opening. These wounds usually are made by nails, needles, wire, knives, or bullets (Fig. 11-2). As a rule, small puncture wounds do not bleed freely externally, but the large puncture wounds may cause severe internal bleeding. Broken ends of bones often cause puncture injuries, such as broken ribs penetrating into the lungs. There is always a danger of infection from penetrating wounds, since the object entering the tissues or organs may be contaminated with microorganisms.

About one half of the fatalities and injuries incurred in automobile accidents are from nonpenetrating abdominal wounds.[8] Add to the automobile accidents the number of internal wounds caused by forceful blows to the abdomen, back, and flank, and the rate of injury is appreciably increased. These types of wounds include rupture of an organ, lacerations, and contusions, with subsequent internal bleeding. The characteristics of blunt injury differ with the type and site, force of impact, strength of the abdominal wall, and condition of the viscera.[2] The solid viscera are more often involved with rupture or laceration from a sudden forceful blow. Turgid or distended viscera are also subject to severe damage, as in rupture of some fixed portion of the digestive tract or a distended urinary bladder. (See Fig. 18-2.) A strong tense abdominal wall is a deterrent in reducing the force of impact, but in elderly or inattentive people (asleep, comatose, or intoxicated) the protection afforded by a muscular barrier may be lacking.

Usually abdominal and extra-abdominal injuries are a part of multiple injuries to the body, such as those to the head, spine, chest, and pelvis.[10] The injury to internal organs may not be immediately evident but may be so severe that the patient dies from hemorrhage, shock, or suffocation. In abdominal trauma the spleen is often lacerated from the force of the blow or from associated fractured ribs.[16] Contusions of

the spleen may cause subcapsular hemorrhage. The characteristic symptoms or signs of splenic injury are pain, tenderness over the splenic area, muscle spasm, rigidity, or guarding.

Liver trauma with severe lacerations (Fig. 11-1) results in hemorrhagic shock and leakage of bile into the peritoneal cavity, causing bile peritonitis. The free bile exerts its effects on the venules and capillaries of the peritoneal cavity. These vessels lose their tone, and their walls become more permeable, permitting escape of large amounts of plasma into the abdominal cavity, precipitating shock.[7, 8]

The kidneys are in a relatively well-protected position, but nevertheless they are vulnerable to injury from forceful blows to the back and flanks. Severe contusions may result in serious posttraumatic sequelae, such as infection, hydronephrosis and impairment of function, hematuria, and hypertension.[16, 22] Hematuria is most often the characteristic symptom, but its absence does not preclude injury, for the tubules or ureters may be plugged, or the ureters may be transected singly or doubly, or there may be laceration of the renal pelvis with intraperitoneal bleeding.

When the bladder is ruptured (Fig. 18-2), extravasation of urine into the peritoneal cavity causes peritonitis. The main symptom is hematuria.

Pancreatic injury is rare, since this organ occupies a rather protected position in the abdomen, but it is serious when it does occur. There may be shock and traumatic peritonitis. Extensive retroperitoneal hemorrhage may be associated with pancreatic wounds and leakage of pancreatic secretion into the peritoneal cavity, producing fat necrosis.[16, 17]

In rupture of the bowel there may be abdominal distention, retrostalsis, and free air under the diaphragm, with increasing signs of peritonitis. Mesenteric vessels are often torn in conjunction with other abdominal injuries, and rupture of the diaphragm may occur.

Crushing wounds are particularly subject to infection because the microorganisms causing infection grow and multiply rapidly in the body cells injured by the wound. Crushing of tissues frequently accompanies lacerated wounds.

Nonpenetrating chest trauma includes the crushing injuries of the chest that interfere with respiration or systemic circulation. There may be tension pneumothorax (introduction of air into the thoracic cavity) or cardiac tamponade (acute compression of the heart from the effusion of fluid into the pericardium or collection of blood in the pericardium from rupture of the heart or a coronary vessel). In chest injuries, ribs may be broken and puncture the lung allowing blood to escape rapidly into the lower air passages. A foam composed of blood and air may be sufficiently obstructive to cause death by suffocation. Severe chest injuries are usually more critical than intra-abdominal trauma.[3, 10]

Concussion is a common type of injury to the brain. It is caused by a violent blow to the head or collision with a solid object. The symptoms are vertigo, loss of consciousness, nausea, weakness, and slow respiration. A concussion does not pose as serious a threat to life as a penetrating injury of the brain, which not only disrupts vital brain tissue but may also introduce infection. The neurons of the central nervous system are incapable of regeneration, and if damaged, they are lost forever. One of the serious consequences of mechanical injury to the head is the compression of brain tissue and the accumulation of intracranial blood. Secondary edema of brain tissues caused by a hematoma, for example, subdural, may give rise to fatal intracranial pressure. If the brainstem escapes damage, extensive and disruptive cerebral injury may be survived. (See Fig. 18-8.)

Peripheral nerve damage is common in injury. The nerves may be severed completely, and if so, their regeneration is slow and may not progress to complete restitution of all the nerve fibers.[18]

Fractures[4] are breaks in bones (Fig. 11-3); the two main types are simple and compound. The simple fracture is one in which the injury is internal; that is, the bone is broken but there is no break in the skin. The compound fracture is one in which there is an open wound in the soft tissues and skin through which the broken bone protrudes. A comminuted fracture is one in which the bone is splintered or crushed, with many disruptions in the continuity of its tissue. The compound fractures are more serious than simple ones, since there is always the danger of infection.

Fractures of the skull are particularly hazardous, since underlying brain tissue may be damaged. (See Fig. 18-18, *B*.) Sometimes the site of injury may show a depressed or caved-in appearance at the point of impact. At other times actual severance of bones can be seen, as in compound fractures or when foreign objects, such as glass or bullets, penetrate the skull. The symptoms of skull fracture vary. The victim may be conscious or unconscious, disoriented, confused, or restless. The pupils may be unequal in size and may not react normally to light. There may be bleeding from the ears, nose, or mouth. Paralysis or partial paralysis of parts of the body, such as the arms, legs, and face, may be present. Shock is a prominent symptom.

Fracture of the spine[11, 20] at any point may result in crushing or cutting of the spinal cord, causing paralysis or even death. (See Figs. 18-24 and 18-28.) The paralysis may be paraplegia—paralysis of both legs and the lowest part of the body, resulting from injury of the spinal cord at the level of the chest or lower back. It may cause quadriplegia or tetraplegia—paralysis of both legs and both arms, resulting from injury involving the spinal cord at the level of the neck.[11, 20] These paralyses may also occur from disease involving the spinal cord.

Symptoms of a spinal cord injury depend upon the level of the cord injury and not

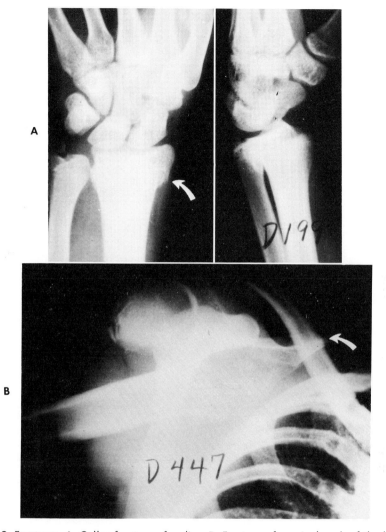

Fig. 11-3. Fractures. **A,** Colles fracture of radius. **B,** Fracture of surgical neck of the humerus (arrow). The surgical neck is the constricted part of the humerus below the tuberosities. (From Young, C. G., and Likos, J. J.: Medical specialty terminology, x-ray and nuclear medicine, St. Louis, 1972, The C. V. Mosby Co.)

the level of bone injury. Centrally the spinal cord is soft and easily squeezed and damaged by pressure from surrounding bones. Cord damage may occur above or below bone injury. A person may have a broken back without any cord injury, and thus he can escape paralysis. Complete severance of the cord most often results from a bullet or missile fragment, which might occur as combat injuries. Cord dam-

age might also occur from bruising and bleeding. Automobile accidents are the leading causes of spinal cord injury in the United States, but motorcycle and motor scooter accidents are increasing at an alarming rate. Young people often sustain injuries from falls from heights while mountain climbing and in sports such as football, diving (into a shallow pool of water), and skiing. Men sustain more traumatic spinal injuries than women, possibly because of their more dangerous sports and occupations.

An outstanding symptom of spinal cord injury at the neck level is the inability of a person to move the legs and arms. This type of injured person must be moved with the greatest of care to prevent further damage. His head and neck must be held steady while he is being moved. Four to six people are necessary for moving the body "all in one piece" without any bending or twisting. A person with injury at the chest or lower back level, who can move his arms but not his legs, is also lifted in the same manner without any bending or twisting of the body.[11, 20]

Fractures of the pelvic bones usually result from falls, heavy blows, or accidents that involve crushing. The danger in a pelvic fracture is that the organs enclosed and protected by the bones may be seriously damaged. Bladder rupture is partic-

ularly dangerous, as is severe internal bleeding because of tearing or cutting of large blood vessels by fragments of broken bone. Loss of ability to use the lower part of the body is a prominent symptom of pelvic injury.

Normally we think of fractures as occurring from accidents or blows from external origin, but in people who have diseased bones a relatively minor stress, such as twisting, may cause a break. Convulsive seizures may also result in broken bones. Violent muscular contractions in victims of electric shock from high voltage may also cause a bone fracture.

Other injuries to bones include dislocations, sprains, and strains. A *dislocation* is an injury in which a bone is forcibly displaced from its joint (Fig. 11-4). It is likely to bruise or tear the surrounding tissues. A *sprain* is an injury to a ligament of a joint with momentary dislocation of bones, causing tearing of the supporting ligaments and

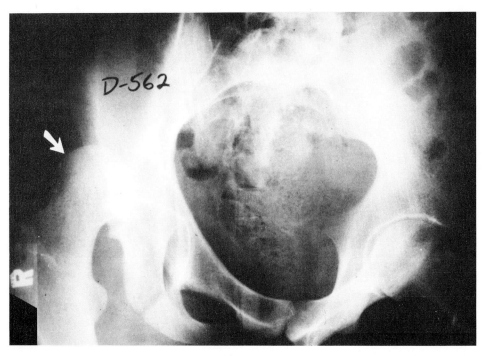

Fig. 11-4. Dislocation of hip, showing absence of head of femur in acetabulum. (From Young, C. G., and Likos, J. J.: Medical specialty terminology, x-ray and nuclear medicine, St. Louis, 1972, The C. V. Mosby Co.)

damage to the blood vessels and other soft tissues surrounding the joint. A *strain* is an injury caused by the forcible overstretching or tearing of a muscle or tendon. Blood may escape from the injured vessels in the immediate vicinity and cause discoloration of the tissues.

Bullet or *gunshot wounds*[15] (Fig. 11-2) may cause extensive and fatal damage. (See Fig. 18-8, *F*.) The extent of the injury is not governed by the size of the bullet entering the body, but rather by its speed and course of direction in the body and its point of entrance and exit. A bullet will continue to cause damage to all tissues in its path before it exits or becomes lodged in an organ or part of the body. When striking bone it may shatter fragments into adjoining tissues or organs, causing secondary damage. If the gun is in close contact with the skin, the expanding gases enter the tissues with explosive effects. The exit wound of a high velocity bullet is often larger than the entrance wound. Intracranial, intrathoracic, and intra-abdominal hemorrhages are invariably present in gunshot wounds, depending on entrance and course of the bullet. The primary effect of intracranial and intrathoracic injuries is interference with the respiration or systemic circulation through anoxia. Bullets in the head or heart may be almost immediately incapacitating to the point of death or may terminate fatally later.

Defense mechanisms in mechanical injury

The body is under stress to mobilize its defenses in any external injury. Hemorrhage is an immediate response to mechanical disruption of tissues. Blood will continue to flow from a wound until prevented from doing so by the body's own defenses of thrombosis, vasoconstriction, or the equalization of intravascular and extravascular pressures by a drop in the former or a rise in the latter. Outside interference with tourniquets, compression dressings and other therapeutic measures may be required to stop blood flow. When the small vessels (capillaries, arterioles, and venules) are damaged, vasoconstriction is an important defense mechanism in induction of hemostasis (stoppage of blood flow). This defense mechanism is also important in lacerations or crushing of vessels, large or small. When the disturbance is limited to the site of the defect in a vessel that has been incised, thrombosis is more effective in hemostasis.

The inflammatory response and repair of tissues in physical injuries follow the same principles given in Chapters 3 and 4.

INJURIES FROM EXTREMES IN TEMPERATURE[15, 18]

Exposures to extremes of heat and cold cause injury to the skin, tissues, blood vessels, vital organs, and in some instances the body as a whole. Above normal temperatures are generally more dangerous and more prone to cause injury than comparable degrees of lower temperature. The body can withstand a drop of 10° F in temperature with relatively few ill effects, but prolonged elevations of 6° or 7° F may cause serious injury.[18]

Hyperthermia is the term used to refer to heat injuries; these include high fevers, heatstroke, heat exhaustion, and burns and scalds. Heatstroke, heat exhaustion, and burns are discussed at the end of this chapter. Hyperthermia may be exogenous or endogenous in origin. Fever is an example of endogenous hyperthermia; it results from an imbalance in the amount of heat produced by the metabolic activity of the body and the dissipation of heat through skin radiation and respiration. High temperatures or fevers in infectious and inflammatory diseases may result in death from brain injury, presumably from damage to the vital centers in the medulla causing circulatory failure. An overall rise in the temperature of the circulating blood to a high level may lead to profound functional disturbances. These include generalized vasodilatation with resultant reduction in effective blood volume; rapid pulse and dilatation of the heart with impairment of cardiac efficiency; and stimulation of the respiratory centers first by rapid breathing, later by irregularity, and finally by suspension of respiratory activity. These systemic hyperthermic changes may occur with elevations of the body temperatures to injurious levels from inflow of heat or failure to eliminate heat developed by metabolic processes.

Exposure to excessive heat may result in either heatstroke or heat exhaustion. Both are classified as exogenous hyperthermia. The heat in these instances is absorbed through either the skin surface or inspired air.

Burns and scalds are caused by exposure to intense heat, either from fire, sunlight, hot solids or liquids, or contact with electric current.

Inspiration of overheated air, smoke, and combusted gases in burning buildings can cause damage to the respiratory passages and lungs. In mild cases, vesicles may form on the lips and mucous membranes of the mouth. Similar changes occur along the entire respiratory tract in severe exposure. If the exposure is intense, the mucosal surfaces of the tongue, oral cavity, and even the oropharynx and larynx may be charred. In the lungs there may be hyperemia and frank necrosis, with sloughing of the respiratory epithelium of the tracheobronchial tree associated with exudation of bloody serous fluid into the alveolar spaces.[18]

Injuries from low temperatures have both local and systemic effects on the body. The nonfreezing and freezing temperatures produce similar forms of local injury, different only in extent. Traditionally, cold injuries are categorized as chillblains, immersion foot, trench foot, and frostbite.[4] (See Figs. 18-7, *B*, and 18-13, *A*.)

Chilblains are a mild cold injury caused by repeated exposure for several hours to temperatures between 32° and 60° F. They are characterized by redness, itching, tingling, and skin inflammation.[4]

Immersion foot and trenchfoot are discussed at the end of the chapter.

INJURIES FROM CHANGES IN ATMOSPHERIC PRESSURE[9, 15]

Humans tolerate an increase in atmospheric pressure better than a decrease of equal magnitude. The effects of rapid increase in atmospheric pressure are far less injurious than those of decompression. The rate of change is an important factor in injury production. An injury called decompression sickness or caisson disease occurs when the atmospheric pressure is not lowered slowly, whether from a high to a normal pressure or from a normal to a low pressure. Decompression sickness is discussed in Chapter 9.

A rapid drop in atmospheric pressure may cause expansion of air in the paranasal sinuses and in the middle ears, with pain and an occasional eardrum rupture. In rapid increase in atmospheric pressure acute discomfort may be caused by inward displacement of the eardrums (aerotitis media).[1] This is seen sometimes in aviators or even passengers on aircraft, and a similar disturbance has been reported in submarine personnel.

Two conditions commonly affect unacclimatized individuals at altitudes over 9000 feet, and some at only 7000 feet.[9] One is *acute mountain sickness,* which may occur within a few hours after rapid exposure to high altitude. It is characterized by headache, exertional dyspnea, malaise, and weakness, which may be followed by insomnia, anorexia, nausea, vomiting, diarrhea, and abdominal pain. Cheyne-Stokes respiration, and tachycardia are usually present. The severe symptoms are unrelieved except by oxygen or descent to a lower altitude. An uncommon but sometimes fatal complication of rapid exposure to high altitudes is called *high-altitude pulmonary edema.* Persons engaged in severe physical exertion in an unaccustomed environment are most susceptible. Residents of high altitude areas who return to their mountain homes after living at sea level for a period of time are also susceptible. Symptoms are much like those of high-altitude sickness, but are progressive, with noisy breathing, rales, cyanosis, orthopnea, and hemoptysis.[9] Death may occur unless there is continuous oxygen therapy or descent to a lower altitude.

Blast injuries result from sudden changes in external atmospheric pressure that were initiated by an explosion. If the force of the explosion is transmitted through the air it is called an air blast; if through the water, an immersion blast; and if through more or less rigid structures, a solid blast.[15] The injuries differ with the type of blast. The walls or compartments of hollow viscera are particularly susceptible to blast injury. Multiple lacerations of the lungs are commonly sustained in air blast. However, with either air or immersion blast, diffuse injuries of both the thoracic and abdominal viscera may occur. Proximity to air or water explosions may result in virtual destruction of the body by the extreme turbulence of the air or water. Injuries to the feet are an expected hazard in a solid blast, such as might occur on a ship. Contact with solid walls is likely to result in crushing injuries or burial of the victim in the debris resulting in death.[15]

ELECTRICAL INJURIES[15]

The harmful effects from electrical injuries always depend upon the kind and amount of current, as well as the path of the current and its duration. The primary hazard in electrical injury is shock. Most of us have at one time or another suffered some degree of electric shock from defective wiring in home appliances. As a rule this type of shock is mild and only causes a tingling sensation in the hand, arm, or part of the body in contact with the appliance. Generally individuals are neutral, since usually they are grounded and at a zero potential. Electrical injury cannot occur unless some part of the body completes the circuit between two conductors. In major electrical equipment used in industry and in x-ray equipment in hospitals the operator is always at a lower potential than the equipment being used. This degree of difference of potential may be anywhere between 50 volts up to supervoltage.

Electric shock is discussed at the end of the chapter.

RADIATION INJURIES[5]

The sources of radiation danger are x rays, radium and its daughter product radon, radioactive isotopes, and other radioactive material. The danger of overexposure to radiation has been known for over 70 years, or almost since the discovery of x rays by Roentgen. Before the hazards were recognized, many pioneers in the field of roentgenology as well as some of their patients, suffered irreversible damage. Many of the side effects of radiation were discovered entirely by accident. Painful skin ulcers and epilation were among the first noticeable damaging effects. These side effects were resistant to all forms of treatment, and many eventually resulted in fatal cancer. Another harmful effect noted was the development of fatal aplastic anemia. These damaging injuries, of course, no longer occur unless through accident from overexposure. The methods of measuring the quantity of radiation being emitted at any given location have been worked out by physicists. They have established a tolerance dose by the estimation of the maximum total exposure to which any part of the body can safely be exposed continuously or intermittently over a given time. These standards are followed in the use of all radioactive materials, as well as with x rays.

Radiation absorption is manifested in different ways. Overexposure first produces an erythema of the skin, but the skin may later become dry and scaly and flake and peel. This may be followed by ulcerations or sores that will not heal. Hair is also affected and will fall out. The fingernails may become hardened and cracked, and the nail bed will show signs of ridging. The fingernail appearance may be the first sign of overexposure to x rays. Blood is sensitive to radiation, and those who work with radioactive substances in any form have repeated blood examinations to detect possible overexposure.[5]

We are all more or less exposed to environmental radioactive elements, since within the earth and on its surfaces are naturally occurring radioactive elements, such as uranium, radium, actinium, thorium, and many rarer substances. Even the houses we live in may contain radioactive stones! Our bodies and the food we eat contain components, such as potassium and carbon, that have naturally occurring radioactive isotopes. None of these pose a medical problem as far as hazards are concerned.

We are constantly reminded of the dangers of nuclear war. There has been a wealth of literature on protective measures in case of an enemy attack by atomic weapons. Much of what we now know about the effects of an atomic blast on human beings has been through studies of the victims of the atomic blasts in Hiroshima and Nagasaki, Japan, in 1945 at the end of World War II. The profound radiation changes found in these victims were largely confined to the highly radiosensitive tissues—the blood and blood-forming organs, the gastrointestinal mucosa, and the gonads. Extensive research has also been done with experimental animals.[5]

The systemic disorders of irradiation are radiation sickness, radiation cachexia, and radiation changes in the blood. Radiation sickness is characterized by nausea, vomiting, and psychic disorders, which appear promptly or within a few hours after exposure but usually terminate in about 48 hours. Radiation cachexia progresses slowly and is characterized by poor appetite, loss of weight, depression, and muscular weakness. It may appear months after massive exposure, and there is often an associated anemia and leukopenia. Some patients recover satisfactorily; others stabilize with a chronic ailment; and still others die. The injury to the blood and blood-forming organs is manifested by thrombocytopenia, leukopenia, and in severe cases, leukemia.[5]

The gonads are highly sensitive to ionizing radiation damage. A single dose of over 500 roentgens (r) to the ovaries produces sterility.[5] Cumulative effects of repeated small exposures can also produce sterility.

The nervous system of the embryo is highly sensitive to even small doses of radiation, but the mature nervous tissue is relatively radioresistant. The eyes develop cataracts after large doses.[5]

The skin is most frequently damaged, since it is the portal of entry for diagnostic or therapeutic purposes. Here it must be stressed that routine and special diagnostic x-ray examinations, as well as radiation therapy and radioisotope procedures, produce no serious or permanent damage to the body, since all are well controlled and the services are performed by personnel specially trained in the field of radiology.

STEP-BY-STEP EXERCISES

Step 1. Physical agents that cause injury or disease are classified as mechanical violence (automobile accidents, home and industrial accidents, and firearms), changes in atmospheric pressure, extremes in temperature, and electrical and radiation injuries.

Complete the blanks by identifying the type of injury.

1. Moving vehicle _____
2. Missile _____
3. Burns _____
4. Freezing _____
5. Sunburn _____
6. Overexposure to x rays _____
7. Shock from high tension wire _____
8. Gunshot blast _____
9. Atomic blast _____
10. Fall _____

Step 2. Mechanical injury involves some type of wound. Wounds are classified according to extent of tissue damage. Some are therefore much more serious than others, not only from the amount of hemorrhage involved, but also from the danger of introduction of infectious agents.

Identify the following types of wounds. (Refer to the text if necessary.)

1. Scraping of the skin by friction _____
2. Irregular tear by contact with a sharp instrument _____
3. Deep cut with edges uniformly displaced _____
4. Chest injury sustained from being buried under heavy debris _____
5. Violent blow to head with temporary loss of consciousness but no fracture _____
6. Breaking of long bone internally with no protrusion of bone through skin _____ _____
7. Breaking of long bone with protrusion of bone through skin _____ _____
8. Black and blue area of discoloration _____
9. Wound made by a nail entering deep into tissues _____

Step 3. In nonpenetrating thoracic or abdominal wounds the internal organs may be ruptured, lacerated, or severely bruised by the impact of a forceful blow to the body.

1. A blow to the body occurred over the spleen, but there was no internal hemorrhage. Would this be an abrasion ___, laceration ___, rupture ___, or contusion ___?
2. A sharp blow to the flank was followed by hematuria. Would this be a rupture of the kidney ___, bruise of the kidney ___, or rupture of the liver ___?
3. The thoracic cage has been injured and several ribs broken, and there is an accumulation of air in the thorax. Would this most likely have resulted

from a rib puncturing a lung ___, rupture of the diaphragm ___, or fracture of the sternum ___?

4. Several hours after an abdominal injury caused by a forceful blow to the intestines, there is distention of the abdomen with pain and retrostalsis. Would this most likely have resulted from the perforation of a segment of the bowel ___, laceration of the liver ___, or fracture of the pelvic bones ___?

Step 4. Bullet wounds may cause extensive and fatal damage. The extent of injury is not governed by the size of the bullet, but rather by its speed and course in the body and its point of entrance and exit. On the basis of this information and from what you have learned in the text mark the following statements *T* for true or *F* for false.

1. A bullet entering the brain would be more likely to cause instant death than one entering the lower abdomen. ___
2. A bullet entering the chest in the midline passes through the body and its point of exit is midback. The bullet would be likely to cause secondary damage by shattering bone into adjacent organs. ___
3. A bullet has entered the abdomen and come to rest in the liver. Probably no internal hemorrhage will result from this type of gunshot wound, since the bullet has lodged in an organ and has not gone completely through the body. ___
4. A bullet has caused intrathoracic injuries. These injuries would not be likely to interfere with respiration. ___

Step 5. Extremes of temperature may cause serious injury and even death. Temperatures above normal are referred to as hyperthermia; temperatures below normal are referred to as hypothermia. These terms are usually used to express extremes of temperature likely to result in disease or injury.

Indicate whether the following conditions would be classified as hypothermia or hyperthermia.

1. Temperature 105° F _____
2. Freezing of a portion of the body _____
3. Exposure to flames with burning of tissues _____
4. Heatstroke _____
5. Chilblains _____
6. Frostbite _____
7. Excessive exposure of skin to solar rays _____

Step 6. From the descriptions given, identify the following conditions.

1. A high temperature in infectious or inflammatory disease _____
2. Prostration from exposure to excessive heat _____ or _____
3. Mild cold injury to feet after repeated exposure for several hours to a temperature of 40° F _____
4. Severe cold injury following exposure to below zero (20° F) temperature _____
5. Exposure to solar rays with extreme redness of the skin _____
6. Charring of skin by a flame _____
7. Inspiration of overheated air and smoke in a burning building _____

Step 7. Rapid changes in atmospheric pressure may also be injurious to tissues, but the rate of change is an important factor.

Complete the blanks in the following statements.

1. When atmospheric pressure is not lowered slowly, whether from a high to a normal pressure or from a normal to a low pressure, a particular type of disease may develop that is called _____ _____.
2. Sudden changes in atmospheric pressure may also be initiated by an explosion, and the injuries are referred to as _____ injuries.

Step 8. The most hazardous effect of electrical injury is shock. The extent of injury will depend upon the kind and amount of current as well as the path of the current and its duration. Injuries range from superficial burns to deep burns and injury to vital organs, such as the respiratory center in the brain and the heart. Death may result from circulatory failure.

Mark the following statements *T* for true or *F* or false.

1. Electrical injury cannot occur unless you complete the circuit between two conductors. __
2. High voltage is much more likely to cause shock than low voltage. __
3. Electrical injury never causes severe burns. __
4. Electrical injury affecting the respiratory center in the brain may result in death. __
5. The heart is not involved in electric shock. __
6. If you are at a lower potential than the equipment you are operating, you are not likely to sustain a shock. __

Step 9. Sources of radiation danger are x rays, radium, radon, radioactive isotopes, and other radioactive material. Overexposure to any of these may cause tissues to die or be damaged. You are not likely to be injured by any of these if they are being used by skillful and specially trained personnel. Explosion by an atomic bomb however, is an exception, since injury from this source would be nonselective and would probably be from either a direct hit or radioactive fallout.

Mark the following statements *T* for true or *F* for false.

1. X rays are seldom harmful if being

used by radiologists or trained radiology personnel. ___

2. Radioisotopes are used in diagnostic and therapeutic procedures, but they are extremely dangerous because of the tissue damage they always inflict. ___

3. Nuclear fallout is not dangerous when you are not in the direct path of the explosion. ___

4. Radium or its daughter product radon are not dangerous therapeutic measures in the treatment of cancer. ___

5. All radiation materials or procedures are a source of danger. since all can inflict irreversible damage. ___

SELECTED TYPES OF INJURY
Heatstroke and heat exhaustion[4]

Exposure to excessive heat may result in either a heatstroke or heat exhaustion. In both the heat is absorbed through either the skin surface or inspired air. The two are very much alike as far as symptoms are concerned, with one notable exception. Sweating occurs in heat exhaustion but not in heatstroke.

In heatstroke the heat-regulating mechanism of the body fails. The body becomes overheated, with temperatures rising to between 105° and 110° F, with no perspiration so there is no cooling of the body. The skin is hot, dry, and red. The preliminary symptoms may be nausea, dizziness, headache, and weakness. Often the first symptoms, however, are collapse and loss of consciousness. Heatstroke may cause death or permanent disability.

In heat exhaustion the heat-regulating mechanism also fails, but in addition, blood flow is seriously disturbed, similar to the circulatory disturbance of shock. The body loses large quantities of salt and water through prolonged sweating. Heat exhaustion is sometimes accompanied by heat cramps in the muscles of the abdomen, legs, and arms. These cramps have been attributed to the loss of salt in profuse amounts. The preliminary symptoms, as in

heatstroke, are headache, nausea, dizziness, and weakness.

Burns[14, 19, 23]

Burns and scalds are caused by exposure to intense heat from fire, sunlight, hot solids or hot liquids, or contact with electric current. The type of heat producing the burn is called either dry heat, which causes desiccation and charring of tissues, or wet heat, which essentially boils the tissues, causing an opaque coagulation. The epidermis suffers the most intense effects, but burns may extend to affect deeper structures.

In a recent study of the epidemiology of burn injuries, about 50% of a consecutive series of 155 hospitalized burned adult patients showed a predisposition to becoming a victim of a burn injury.[12] Alcoholism led the list of predisposing factors because the burned patient had sustained the injury while under the influence of alcohol when he fell asleep in a chair or in bed and dropped a smoking cigarette. Other predisposing factors were senility, psychiatric disorders, and neurologic disease, respectively. The nursing home or hospital ranked second to the patient's own home as the characteristic site of the fire. Large fires in public buildings and aircraft accidents were infrequent sources of medically treatable burned people, since the most common outcome of these disasters was immediate death of the victims. Other causes of burns in hospitalized patients were attempted suicides and homicides, epileptic seizures, and attempts to start a fire by use of highly flammable substances.[12]

Burns are usually classified according to depth and extent of tissue damage. They are designated first-degree, second-degree, and third-degree (Fig. 11-5). First-degree burns are usually caused by gas explosions, brief contact with hot liquid, or prolonged exposure to the sun. Second-degree burns are usually the result of short exposure to flash heat or contact with hot liquid. Third-degree burns are caused by contact with

DEPTH OF BURN

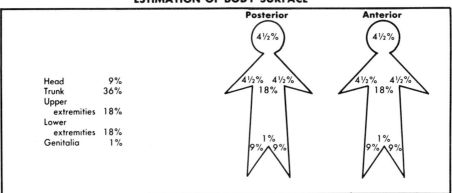

	Degree	Surface	Color	Pain
Epidermis	First degree	Dry No blisters	Erythematous	Painful, hyperesthetic
Corium	Second degree	Moist, blisters	Mottled red	Painful, hyperesthetic
Fat	Third degree	Dry	Pearly white or charred	Little pain, anesthetic

ESTIMATION OF BODY SURFACE

Head	9%
Trunk	36%
Upper extremities	18%
Lower extremities	18%
Genitalia	1%

Posterior

4½%

4½% 4½%
18%

1%
9% 9%

Anterior

4½%

4½% 4½%
18%

1%
9% 9%

SERIOUSNESS OF BURNS

Minor burn	Moderate burn	Critical burn
First degree	Second degree of 15 to 30 percent body surface	Second degree of over 30 percent body surface
Second degree of less than 15 percent body surface	Third degree of less than 10 percent body surface except hands, face, feet, or genitalia	Third degree of more than 10 percent of body surface or of hands, face, feet, or genitalia
Third degree of less than 2 percent body surface		

Fig. 11-5. Classification of burns. (From Therap. Notes **70:**236, Oct., 1963, Parke-Davis & Co.)

flames or hot objects. Burns that involve respiratory tract injury, major soft-tissue injury, or fracture are considered critical, as are electrical and deep acid burns. Severe burns produce physiologic, psychologic, and chemical injury and therefore affect the entire body. Shock always results if burns are extensive, and metabolic imbalance, toxemia, and possibility of infection are complications.[14, 19]

The first-degree burn heals rapidly, since no deep layers of the epidermis are involved. Second-degree burns usually heal in 10 to 14 days if there is no infection. If dermal burns are deep, however, healing is slow, usually taking 25 to 35 days, because the new epithelium is derived in part from the margin of the burned area and in part from the underlying hair follicles. Third-degree burns involve the full thickness of the skin and extend to the subcutaneous fat. The dermis is damaged to the extent that epithelial regeneration is interfered with. Skin appendages, hair shafts, sweat glands, and sebaceous glands are destroyed. The irreversibly injured dermis must be cleared away in the repair process before a new layer of epithelium can be generated. Before reepithelization can take place from skin margins, granulation tissue fills the defects, resulting in permanent scarring. Third-degree burns require skin grafting.[6, 23] A type of ulcer called Curling's sometimes develops in the duodenum following severe surface burns.

It is important to remember that the size of the burned area may be far more important than the depth of the burn. A first- or second-degree burn that covers a large area of the body is almost always more serious than a small third-degree burn.[18] A sunburn, which is usually a first-degree burn, can cause death if a very large area of the body is burned.

The extent of a burn usually is expressed as a percentage of total body surface. A rapid method of estimating extent of injury is the rule of nines, in which the body is divided into multiples of 9%. Because of differential growth rates, the percent of surface area of an infant's head is twice that of an adult; in a child up to 10 years of age it is about one and one-half times that of an adult. The trunk is only about two thirds that of adults.

Immersion foot and trench foot[4]

Immersion foot and trench foot are nonfreezing injuries. They are similar in symptoms, but the causes are different. Immersion foot is caused by exposure to cold water, 50° F and below for 12 or more hours, or to water approximately 70° F for several days.[4] Trench foot is caused by exposure to cold, damp weather for several hours to several days at 32° to 50° F.[4] Both immersion foot and trench foot are characterized by tingling, numbness, swelling of the legs and feet, and a bluish discoloration of the skin, with blisters and pain. The vascular alteration that takes place in immersion foot or trench foot causes partial or complete tissue ischemia. When the tissue is first chilled, vasoconstriction occurs and the tissue becomes pale, gray, waxen, or has a blotchy mottled bluish discoloration. When the tissue is warmed, the vascular damage may lead to marked dilatation of vessels, with hyperemia, severe swelling, and formation of large vesicles or bullae. If vascular damage is extensive, thrombosis and ischemia may occur, leading to infarction with gangrene of the injured part.[15]

Frostbite[4, 13, 21]

Frostbite consists of the cooling of tissues until ice crystals are formed. (See Figs. 18-7, *B*, and 18-13, *A*.) It is a freezing injury caused by brief exposure to extreme cold, 20° F or more below zero, or to near zero weather for several hours.[4] Superficial frostbite involves only the skin and perhaps the tissue immediately beneath it. Deep frostbite, however, involves all the tissues including the bone. The arms and legs are the parts of the body usually involved. Symptoms are first burning, stinging, and then numbness. Ice crystals in the skin give it a gray or white waxy color, but the skin can be moved over the bony ridges in the more superficial injury. A completely frozen part with ice crystals in its entire thickness has a pale yellow, waxy color. The skin in deep frostbite will not move over the bony ridges.

When a frozen part is thawed, it becomes red and swollen. Large blisters develop. The extent of injury is governed not only by the duration of exposure but also by the method of therapy in thawing the frozen parts. Dry heat may cause additional injury and possibly the development of gangrene.

When chilling reaches the freezing point, death of cells is almost inevitable. The ischemia leads to infarction necrosis, called dry or wet gangrene.[13] If the freezing is systemic, the skin becomes pale with marked vasoconstriction of vessels. As the hypothermia progresses, peripheral vasodilatation and hyperemia may develop secondary to injury of the vasomotor control of these vessels. Cooling of the peripheral blood soon causes depression of the temperature in vital organs, particularly the brain. Death may result from circulatory failure.

The fundamental factors involved in preventing frostbite are the production and conservation of body heat. If the body cannot produce sufficient heat, blood flow to the extremities is decreased, and insulation cannot prevent the occurrence of frostbite. In order for the body to maintain an adequate blood flow to the extremities, the individual must be healthy. For this reason people vary in their degree of susceptibility to frostbite. A person is much more likely to develop frostbite if exhausted for any reason, dehydrated, intoxicated, or subsisting on an inadequate diet.[13, 21]

Frostbite may also be caused by contact with certain chemicals that have a rapid freezing action. These are liquid oxygen, carbon dioxide, Freon, and other industrial gases. The injury is often referred to as a chemical burn, but actually the body tissue is frozen rather than burned.[4] Cold injuries of this type tend to be superficial as a rule, unless the chemical comes in contact with the eyes, in which case there is permanent impairment of vision because of damage to the eye tissues.

Electric shock[15]

The nervous system operates in an electrical manner, and any outside influence, if sufficiently strong, can affect it. Electric shock is most commonly caused by alternating current, usually because it is used more often than direct current, but direct current is more likely to be fatal than a high alternating current. A voltage of 110 A.C., or even less, may prove fatal if electric contacts are made on wet or moist skin. When the hands are wet or even moist, the current tends to go through the person to the ground instead of through the circuit, especially if the insulation is worn or there is a defective current. Dry skin offers about twenty times more resistance than moist skin to the passage of electric current.

The nervous system is involved in an electric shock, since it has control over the operation of the entire body. An electric shock can temporarily paralyze various organs under the nervous system control. An electric current flowing through the brainstem will cause death by inhibition of the respiratory centers. High velocity current can produce ventricular fibrillation of the heart, causing circulatory failure. This is the most serious consequence of electric shock. The heart itself may not be impaired physically, but since it operates like a tiny electrical system, its actions are disrupted and no blood is pumped to the body. Death follows quickly unless immediate measures such as cardiac massage are taken to start heart action. Breathing can be momentarily stopped in electric shock, because of paralysis of the respiratory center of the brain. Artificial respiration then becomes necessary to prevent death. The parts of the body in contact with a high tension current may be severely burned, for a high temperature is generated by the resistance of the body to burning of the tissue. When high voltage throws the body away from the contact, fractures may occur from the violent contraction of the muscles. Temporary deafness or blindness may also follow electric shock. After effects may consist of disorientation or even delirium, followed by a depressed mental state. In general the burns created by electricity follow the same pattern of inflammatory response and repair as hyperthermal injuries from all sources.

Responses

Step 1: 1. mechanical violence; 2. mechanical violence; 3. electric, radiation, or temperature; 4. temperature; 5. temperature; 6. radiation; 7. electric; 8. mechanical violence; 9. radiation; 10. mechanical violence

Step 2: 1. abrasion; 2. laceration; 3. incision; 4. crushing; 5. concussion; 6. simple fracture; 7. compound fracture; 8. bruising; 9. penetrating or puncture

Step 3: 1. contusion; 2. rupture of the kidney; 3. rib puncturing a lung; 4. perforation of a segment of the bowel

Step 4: 1. T; 2. T; 3. F; 4. F

Step 5: 1. hyperthermia; 2. hypothermia; 3. hyperthermia; 4. hyperthermia; 5. hypothermia; 6. hypothermia; 7. hyperthermia

Step 6: 1. fever; 2. heatstroke or heat prostration; heat exhaustion; 3. chilblains; 4. frostbite; 5. sunburn; 6. burn; 7. burn

Step 7: 1. decompression sickness; 2. blast

Step 8: 1. T; 2. T; 3. F; 4. T; 5. F; 6. F

Step 9: 1. T; 2. F; 3. F; 4. T; 5. T

REFERENCES

1. Ash, J. E.: In Anderson, W. A. D., editor: Pathology, ed. 6, St. Louis, 1971, The C. V. Mosby Co. (aerotitis media).
2. Baxter, C. F., and Williams, R. D.: J. Trauma 1:241, 1961 (penetrating injuries).
3. Burbank, C. B.: West. J. Surg. 69:277, 1961 (trauma).
4. Bureau of Naval Personnel, Training Publications Division: Standard first aid training course, Washington, D. C., 1965.
5. Dunlap, C. E.: In Anderson, W. A. D., editor: Pathology, ed. 6, St. Louis, 1971, The C. V. Mosby Co. (effects of radiation).
6. Garcia, F. A.: Surg. Clin. North Am. 43:507, 1963 (burns).
7. Glenn, F., and Thorbjarnarson, B.: Am. J. Surg. 101:176, 1961 (trauma).
8. Griswold, R. A., and Collier, H. S.: Int. Abstr. Surg. 112:309, 1961 (penetrating injuries).
9. Johnson, R. L.: In Beeson, P. B., and McDermott, W., editors: Cecil-Loeb textbook of medicine, ed. 13, Philadelphia, 1971, W. B. Saunders Co. (alterations in atmospheric pressure).
10. Kleinert, H. E., and Romero, J.: J. Trauma 1:226, 1961 (injuries).
11. Kruger, E. G.: N. Y. State J. Med. 63:682, 1963 (spinal injuries).
12. MacArthur, J. D., and Moore, F. D.: J.A.M.A. 231:259-263, 1975 (epidemiology of burns, the burn prone patient).
13. Mills, W. J., Jr.: Alaska Med. 3:28, 1961 (frostbite).
14. Morani, A. D.: J. Int. Coll. Surg. 39:36, 1963 (burns).
15. Mortiz, A. R., and Adelson, L.: In Anderson, W. A. D., editor: Pathology, ed. 6, St. Louis, 1971, The C. V. Mosby Co. (physical agents in causation of injury and disease).
16. Olinde, R. D. H.: South. Med. J. 53:1270, 1960 (injuries).
17. ReMine, W. H.: Surg. Clin. North Am. 37:1037, 1957 (trauma).
18. Robbins, S. L.: Pathology, ed. 3, Philadelphia, 1967, W. B. Saunders Co. (physical agents in injury).
19. Sako, Y.: Med. Clin. North Am. 46:383, 1962 (burns).
20. U.S. Department of Health, Education, and Welfare, National Institute of Neurological Diseases and Stroke, National Institute of Health, Public Health Service Publications No. 1745, Health Information Series No. 143, 1970 (spinal cord injury).
21. Washburn, B.: N. Engl. J. Med. 266:974, 1962 (frostbite).
22. Williams, R. D., and Zollinger, R. M.: Am. J. Surg. 97:575, 1959 (trauma).
23. Wynn, S. K.: Wis. Med. J. 60:469, 1961 (burns).

CHAPTER 12

Drug and chemical injury

Chemical injuries are generally referred to as poisonings. Poisons are substances that cause bodily disturbances, injury, or death by chemical means when introduced into the body by ingestion, injection, inhalation, or absorption. Poisonings occur in a variety of ways. They are often the result of suicidal attempts but are frequently accidental from an overdose or mistaken identity of a drug or substance. Poisons are also given with homicidal intent. Accidental poisonings rank as the most common cause of death in children under 5 years. Homicidal poisonings are less common than suicidal and accidental poisonings. Poisoning may also occur from the continuous use of a substance that is not normally dangerous if taken for a short time but that may have a cumulative effect if taken over a longer time.[3, 10]

Overexposure to a number of industrial chemicals is dangerous. These include ammonia, petroleum products, lead salts, mercury, carbon tetrachloride, and a variety of others. Some plants are poisonous when eaten or cause tissue damage when touched. Mushrooms (certain species) are a good example of foods that may be poisonous. Poison ivy is an example of a plant that causes injury on contact with the body. The venom of wasps, scorpions, spiders, bees, and snakes (certain species) are all potential dangers of poisoning. The venom of some snakes and scorpions may prove fatal when injected in a bite. The sting of bees and wasps may also be lethal if anaphylactic shock occurs in hypersensitive individuals.

The potential effect of a chemical agent is dependent upon several factors, such as the vulnerability of the individual tissues, mode of action of the agent, and its concentration. The action of poison is dependent upon the tolerance that the individual has for a particular substance. Some people seem to have a natural resistance to the action of certain poisons, whereas others are highly sensitive to them, and even a small amount might produce toxic effects, for example, the bee sting mentioned above. Drug addicts can tolerate doses of habit-forming drugs that might kill the average nonaddicted person. The age and general health of the individual also have a bearing on the action of the chemical. Infants, young children, and the elderly are more likely to be killed by small doses of poison than are young adults and middle-aged people. The action of the poison will be more severe, as a rule, if taken in large amounts, but the toxicity varies with the chemical. A few drops of one poison might be immediately fatal, whereas another poison might not be harmful unless taken in large amounts.[3]

The mode of entrance and the physical state of the poisonous substance also determine its effectiveness. Gases are absorbed more quickly than liquids and solids. In general the inhaled poisons are likely to be more effective than ingested poisons. Poisoning by skin absorption usually occurs quite slowly over a protracted period of time.[3]

Tissues and cells vary widely in their susceptibility to specific chemical injury.

Some chemicals are violently destructive to tissues; some act systemically and principally exert injuries on internal organs. Many poisons produce injury immediately upon contact with the tissue. The corrosive agents, which include both inorganic and organic acids and alkalis, damage tissue on contact. Acids when spilled or thrown on the skin cause extensive destruction of tissue manifested by necrosis, sloughing, and deep ulcerations. Corrosives taken orally cause violent damage to the intestinal tract, particularly the esophagus, paralleling the action of acids on the skin. The stomach rejects poison and reacts with violent nausea, vomiting, and hematemesis following ingestion. This regurgitation further adds to the initial damage to the esophagus. War gases damage the alveolar walls of the lungs on contact.[3, 10, 19]

Many poisons exert their effect only after absorption into the blood. They are then carried throughout the body, inflicting selective damage to various organs according to their susceptibility. The organs chiefly affected are the kidneys, liver, and those of the central nervous system and less commonly the heart, blood, and peripheral nerves. This is true of heavy metals, alcohols, barbiturates, ethyl ether, and opium alkaloids. Barbiturates and opium alkaloids do not injure the intestinal tract but when ingested in quantity, depress the central nervous system, with involvement of the cerebral cortex and then the vital centers of respiration and circulation. Death usually results from respiratory arrest. Alcohol when absorbed in lethal amounts acts as a central nervous system depressant or inhibitor, affecting the vital centers of respiration and circulation and causing respiratory arrest. Any drug or poison acting in a similar manner in depressing or inhibiting the respiratory center of the brain can cause death. Carbon monoxide inhalation has no effect on the lung tissues but acts as a systemic asphyxiant. Benzene damages principally the liver and marrow cells, although it is absorbed through the lungs and carried by the bloodstream to these tissues. Methyl alcohol affects principally the cells of the retina and optic nerve, leading to blindness, although these tissues cannot possibly be the portal of entry. The kidneys are particularly vulnerable to poisoning from mercury, bismuth, and the organic solvents because of their excretory functions, since all absorbed poisons leave the body mainly by this route. The proximal convoluted tubules are the most vulnerable. The colon is another organ involved in excretory functions and may suffer extensive damage because of the vast areas exposed to the large doses of poison. Since the liver is the detoxifying center of the body, it is commonly affected by poisoning, particularly from heavy metals, corrosives, and many organic solvents. The lesions are mostly hemorrhagic necroses. The blood change from poisoning is usually that of increased hemolysis, as occurs in lead poisoning. Another injury reflected in the hemopoietic system is aplastic or hypoplastic bone marrow.[10, 19]

The heart reacts to many poisons by swelling of the cardiac muscle fibers, particularly in cases of poisoning with heavy metals and those accompanied by anoxia. The peripheral nerves are affected by myelin (sheath surrounding the nerves) degeneration of the sensory or motor nerves or both, particularly with lead or bismuth poisoning.

All poisons exert their injurious effects only after their tolerance threshold is exceeded. This level varies with each specific agent. The pattern of tissue vulnerability and mode of action are relatively fixed constants for each chemical agent but vary with the toxic level. Concentration of even systemically absorbed agents varies within individual organs and may reach toxic levels in one organ without producing harmful effects in others. Some agents produce both local and systemic effects, whereas others are injurious only when absorbed. All these are variables that must be considered with each individual poison.[10, 19]

The symptoms of poisoning are variable and are not sufficiently uniform or characteristic in most instances to provide a sure means of identification.[3] Some symptoms mimic those of various diseases and cannot be readily distinguished. Symptoms also vary with the amount of poison taken and the length of time it has been in the system. Some agents produce fairly distinct degrees or stages of poisoning, with symptoms differing in each stage. There are, however, some general signs or symptoms that might indicate poisoning. Intense pain, nausea, vomiting, and hematemesis are symptoms of many chemicals taken orally. Caustic acids, alkalis, phenols, and metallic salts taken orally cause corrosion, swelling, and bleaching of the skin, mouth, and throat. Characteristic discoloration with black or brown stains on the skin or mucous membranes might indicate iodine poison, whereas yellow staining might be caused by picric or nitric acids. Some poisons also discolor the urine, either red, dark green, bright yellow, or black. In almost all cases of acute poisoning the victim has difficulty in breathing, and shock is almost always present. Paralysis or convulsions may be other signs of acute poisoning. The pupils of the eye may contract with some poisons and dilate with others.

If there is deep coma or mental derangement, the victim will, of course, be unable to relate the circumstances leading to his condition. In cases of attempted suicide the victim may suppress the details, even if physically and mentally able to identify the chemical agent. In cases of homicide the details will always be suppressed by the guilty party or parties. Some suicides and all homicides require investigations by both medical and legal authorities. Poison control centers are located at various medical establishments throughout the United States.[23] These act as clearinghouses for information about symptoms and treatment for all types of poisons. These centers are also able to identify the poisonous ingredients.

STEP-BY-STEP EXERCISES

Step 1. Poisons are chemical substances that when introduced into the body by ingestion, injection, inhalation, or absorption cause damage or injury to the cells. They interfere with the function or structure, or both, of an organ or organs and may affect the body as a whole.

Complete the blanks by indicating the route of the poison in gaining entrance to the body.

1. A chemical poison introduced into the stomach directly _____
2. A chemical poison introduced into the lungs _____
3. A chemical poison spilled on the skin _____
4. A chemical poison introduced by a hypodermic needle _____
5. Venom introduced into the body by snake bite _____

Step 2. Poisonous substances around the home include a wide variety of chemical agents. Many of these are drugs taken by a member of a family for a specific ailment, and dosage is controlled. Each household contains a variety of cleaning solvents that are particularly dangerous if taken orally in large amounts, or in some cases even in small amounts. A drug as harmless as aspirin if taken in excess can cause the death of small children. Most home accidents are caused by mistaken identity of a drug or substance or by small children taking drugs or household toxic substances left within easy reach. The following exercise is to test your general knowledge of poisons. This information is available on the labels of substances you may use around the house, and it is a constant subject of caution by public health officials. You may use any method you choose in responding. If you miss any of them, you will become wiser by learning the correct response. It might save your life or that of someone else.

Indicate which of the following substances might be lethal if ingested by a child or by an adult accidentally or with suicidal intent. Evaluate them on toxic qualities only. Some, ingested, might produce only gastrointestinal symptoms such as vomiting but would not be lethal.

1. Turpentine ___
2. Ammonia ___
3. Aspirin (ingested by small children in excess) ___
4. Barbiturates ___
5. Iodine ___
6. Kerosene ___
7. Benzene ointments ___
8. Gasoline ___
9. Spices ___
10. Table salt ___
11. Upholstery cleaners ___
12. Lye ___
13. Laundry bleaches ___
14. Soap flakes ___
15. Clogged drain solvents ___
16. Insecticides ___
17. DDT ___
18. Pesticides ___
19. Rodent killers ___
20. Vinegar ___
21. Paint removers ___
22. Cigarette lighter fluid ___
23. Varnish ___
24. Hand lotions ___
25. Quinine ___

Step 3. The cumulative effect of inhaling some poisons used in industry may cause serious damage; the accidental inhalation of poison in the home might also have serious effects or even cause death. This is another self-directed type of test. Some answers may be found in the discussion on selected chemical agents at the end of the chapter.

Indicate which of the following substances might cause damage if inhaled.

1. Ammonia ___
2. Carbon tetrachloride ___
3. Benzol ___
4. Ethyl alcohol ___
5. Morphine ___
6. Carbon monoxide ___
7. Air pollutants ___
8. Arsenic ___

Step 4. The following factors govern the ultimate effect on the victim of any chemical agent capable of toxic effects: (1) vulnerability of tissue, (2) tolerance of the individual, (3) age and health, (4) amount of dosage or exposure, (5) mode of entrance, (6) mode of action, (7) concentration, and (8) physical state (solid, liquid, or gas).

1. Two people are given the same dose of poison; one is in good health, and the other is chronically ill. Which one would tolerate the poison best: the healthy person ___ or the chronically ill person ___?
2. Would a 40-year-old man ___ or a 2-year-old child ___ tolerate a poison best?
3. Would an overdose of a habit-forming drug be tolerated best by a drug addict ___ or an infant ___?
4. Which one of the following might be most immediately fatal: a small dose of lethal poison ___ or a large dose of poison with low toxicity ___?
5. If swallowed, would an alkali ___ or ethyl alcohol ___ be more likely to produce immediate tissue damage?
6. If spilled on the skin, would a corrosive ___ or carbon tetrachloride ___ be more locally damaging?
7. Would a massive dose of barbiturates ___ or an ingested phenol ___ be more likely to produce coma?
8. Would a corrosive ___ or arsenic ___ be more likely to produce immediate vomiting with hematemesis?
9. Which of the following would produce tissue damage first: a poison absorbed through the skin ___ or an inhaled poison ___?
10. Are opium alkaloids ___ or organic solvents ___ more likely to cause intestinal damage?

SELECTED CHEMICAL AGENTS
Carbon monoxide[19, 20]

Carbon monoxide is a nonirritating gas, colorless, tasteless, and odorless, produced by imperfect oxidation of combustible carbon-containing material. It is extremely dangerous, since it gives no warning of its presence. It produces injury by inhalation, often from automobile exhausts, sewers, and manufactured gases used for heating or cooking in circumstances when ventilation is poor or practically nonexistent. It accounts for more deaths than does any other single chemical agent. The absorption of the gas is cumulative, and the toxic effects depend upon the duration of exposure and the concentration in the inspired air. It is a systemic asphyxiant. Its affinity for hemoglobin is many times greater than oxygen's.[20] It combines rapidly with red blood cells and interferes with the oxygen-carrying capacity of hemoglobin.

Because of a lack of oxygen or anoxia, the central nervous system is depressed. There is loss of consciousness, which may progress into deep coma and death. Chronic poisoning is caused by prolonged inhalation of relatively low levels of carbon monoxide. This type is characterized by changes in the central nervous system and anoxic changes in the kidneys, liver, and heart.

Chlorinated hydrocarbons[3, 10, 19]

Carbon tetrachloride is the best example of a chlorinated hydrocarbon that is poisonous if swallowed, inhaled, or allowed to contaminate the skin. The chlorinated hydrocarbons, such as chloroform, dichloromethane, and tetrachloroethane, as well as carbon tetrachloride, are used widely as solvents for cleaning.[3] They are commonly used for dry cleaning and the cleaning of electrical and electronic equipment. They are sold for home use under a variety of trade names.

Acute poisoning is most likely to occur from inhalation of vapor, which causes extreme irritation of the eyes, nose, throat, and lungs and when absorbed into the body damages the liver and kidneys. The symptoms of poisoning are often delayed, and the person may not realize his condition until he becomes dangerously ill some hours later. The general symptoms are headache, nausea, and mental confusion. An immediate fatal narcosis may result from acute poisoning.

Methyl alcohol[2, 10, 19]

Methyl alcohol is absorbed by ingestion or by inhalation of the fumes from liquid alcohol used in industry. When ingested, it causes patchy edema and hemorrhages in the stomach, which is the site of maximal exposure. Edema and hemorrhage also occur in the lungs when it is inhaled. The immediate effect is depression of the central nervous system and later profound intoxication. The prime toxic effect of methyl alcohol after absorption is its oxidation to formaldehyde and formic acid, both of which are extremely toxic. These substances attack the receptor cells of the retina. Brain tissues are swollen, and the cerebral vessels are congested. The clinical features point to central nervous system involvement and retinal damage with visual impairment or total blindness. Methyl alcohol was often substituted for ethyl alcohol in the making or selling of bootleg liquor during the era of prohibition, and this was responsible for a number of fatalities.

Ethyl alcohol[10, 12, 19, 24]

Ethanol or ethyl alcohol is the only one of several alcohols consumed by humans, and it is the only one that is known simply as "alcohol." The active ingredient, ethanol, is found in beer, distilled spirits, and wines. From earliest time humans have apparently been fascinated by the mood-changing effects produced by alcohol. In ancient times, alcohol in crude form was a valuable food and the nutrients of raw materials, including vitamins and minerals, were present. However, alcoholic beverages distilled by modern technology contain no minerals, vitamins, carbohydrates, proteins, or related essentials for well-being. One food value remains, however, and that is the rich source of calories usable for heat and energy but of no nutritive value. From a medical and physiological point of view, alcohol is an irritant, a sedative, anesthetic, antiseptic, drying agent, and a hypnotic agent. It acts as an analgesic, but unlike aspirin for instance, it reduces pain by putting the brain to sleep. Ethyl alcohol is also a habit-forming, potentially addictive, and poisonous narcotic drug. Because of the profound effects on the central nervous system it is considered a drug. In low doses alcohol stimulates, but in higher doses it becomes a brain depressant. The speed with which drunkenness and drunken behavior occur depends upon the rate of absorption into the bloodstream and also on the drinking history of the individual. Alcohol is not digested slowly before reaching the bloodstream, but is immediately absorbed into the blood after passing directly through the walls of the stomach and small intestine; thus, it is rapidly carried to the brain. Alcohol is metabolized in the body at a fairly constant rate, but if consumed faster than it can be broken down and burned, the alcohol accumulates in the body, resulting in higher and higher blood levels.

The following is a resumé of the blood alcohol levels responsible for certain behavior.[24] Thought, judgment, and release from tensions and inhibitions may be affected because there is depression of the cortex in the uppermost part of the brain. The blood level at this stage is .05%.* With increased drinking, the blood alcohol level at .10% causes depression of the motor areas of the brain and there is impairment of coordination of fine movements as well as ability to stand or walk steadily. A blood level of alcohol at .15% is the legal level of intoxication in many states, and a person with this blood level would be considered

to be under the influence of alcohol if apprehended while driving. At .20% there is depression of the midbrain. The person wants to lie down, and he has to be assisted in walking, dressing, or undressing. He is easily moved to tears or rage because of lack of control of emotions. At .30% blood level of alcohol, there is depression of the lower portion of the brain and the person becomes stuporous. At .40% to .50% blood alcohol level, there is depression of the entire area of perception in the base of the brain and the person is unconscious and may go into shock. At .60% level there is depression of the medulla in the lowermost portion of the brain, which controls the involuntary bodily processes—digestion, heartbeat, blood pressure, and breathing. At this blood alcohol level death rapidly ensues.[24]

Alcohol can frustrate sexual performance and impotence may result. This is usually reversible with return to sobriety. Because alcohol interferes with true sleep (REM—rapid eye movement or dreaming sleep), the person is irritable, tired, anxious, and has impaired concentration and memory.[24] If alcohol is consumed in conjunction with the taking of narcotics, tranquilizers, sedatives, pain relievers, motion sickness medications, or any drug that acts on the same brain areas as alcohol, this presents a hazard to health and safety and in some cases to life itself.[12]

There are a number of long-term effects of drinking alcohol in large doses over long periods of time. There may be damage to the heart, brain, liver, and other major organs. Prolonged drinking has long been associated with various types of muscle diseases and tremors. Recent research suggests that alcohol may be toxic to the heart and lungs. Liver damage may result from excessively heavy drinking. Cirrhosis of the liver occurs about eight times as often in alcoholics as among nonalcoholics.[24] Gastritis, ulcers, and pancreatitis occur frequently among alcoholics. Malnutrition of alcoholics is often blamed for the increased

---

*.05% indicates ½ drop of alcohol per 1000 drops of blood, .10% indicates 1 drop of alcohol per 1000 drops of blood, and so on.

occurrence of pneumonia and infectious diseases in alcoholics. Heavy drinking over a period of years may result in serious mental disorders, and also permanent, irreversible damage to the brain or peripheral nervous system. Wernicke's encephalopathy and Korsakoff's psychosis are associated with the protracted and abusive intake of alcohol and nutritional depletion. (See p. 120.) Delirium tremens is sometimes a fatal condition that occurs in alcoholism. The patient is confused, trembling, feverish, and has terrifying hallucinations. Delirium tremens is not simply a direct toxic effect of alcohol on the brain, but it is usually encountered after withdrawal in persons who have had a heavy intake for a prolonged period of time.

One of the devastating effects of alcohol is its influence on crime. Alcohol releases violent behavior in some. Half of all homicides and one third of all suicides are alcohol-related.[24] Drunkenness is frequently involved in child abuse and offenses against children. Alcohol is involved in about one half of the highway fatalities.[24] Economic losses are high, accounting for billions of dollars lost yearly from absenteeism because of alcoholism, and related losses are caused by costs for health and welfare services provided for alcoholic persons and their families.

About one out of twenty adult Americans suffers from alcoholism.[24] These individuals affect the lives of tens of millions of their family members, friends, and associates. Alcoholism usually takes from 5 to 10 years to develop.[24] Symptoms include drinking alone, drinking in the morning, or drinking before facing situations that bring on feelings of nervousness and unhappiness. "Blackouts" occur when a person cannot remember what happened while he was drinking. No one knows for certain what causes alcoholism, but it is considered a disease. In general, alcoholism appears to occur more frequently among individuals who have difficulty handling the normal everyday stresses of life, who are inwardly very dependent but outwardly put up a front. It also occurs frequently in those who want to escape from problems. There is probably no single cause for alcoholism, but rather a combination of reasons. Vitamin and hormone deficiencies have been suggested as causes of alcoholism, but if these are present in alcoholics, they appear to be the result rather than the cause of excessive drinking. To date, no chemicals in specific beverages nor any physiological, metabolic, nutritional, or genetic defects have been discovered through extensive research that would explain alcoholism. The prevention of problem drinking and alcoholism is so urgent that it has become a national health goal.

Phenols[10, 19]

The phenols include carbolic acid, cresol, and creosote. These are organic corrosives, which act locally as well as systemically. Poisoning may occur from ingestion, with absorption through the gastrointestinal tract, or from skin absorption. Contact with the skin produces an immediate necrosis of tissues and large chemical burns, which ultimately ulcerate and may become superficially infected. Swallowing of phenols produces immediate coagulation of the mucosa of the upper alimentary tract, followed by a sloughing necrosis of the tissues. Through either pathway, skin or gastrointestinal tract, the phenols cause central nervous system depression and vascular collapse. Profound coma may be followed by death within a few hours. If the victim survives for 48 hours or longer, there is necrosis of the renal and hepatic parenchymal (functioning) cells. The urine may have a brownish black discoloration and become smoky after standing in the light.

Alkalis and mineral acids[10, 26]

The alkalis include lye, lime, and ammonia; the mineral acids are hydrochloric, nitric, and sulfuric. All these are corrosive poisons that rapidly destroy or decompose the body tissues they contact. The general symptoms are burning pain in the mouth, with severe burning pain in the esophagus and stomach. This is followed by vomiting and retching. The contents vomited from the stomach contain shreds of tissue from the destroyed linings of the mouth, throat, esophagus, and stomach mixed with dark colored liquid. The inside of the mouth is eaten away. Swallowing, as would be anticipated, is very difficult, as is breathing. The abdomen is tender and distended. Body temperature is high. Death may be rapid from shock and circulatory collapse. In patients who survive, the permanent damage consists mainly of cicatricial stenosis of the esophagus and pylorus.

Arsenic[3, 10, 19]

Arsenic is a strong protoplasmic poison capable of causing death within 24 hours after ingestion of large amounts. It is a vascular poison, and the clinical manifestations are intense abdominal discomfort, vomiting, and later diarrhea, associated with peripheral vascular collapse. The progressive accumulation of small doses over a period of time gives rise to chronic poisoning, in which there is anorexia, weight loss, diarrhea, numbness and tingling of extremities, cutaneous pigmentation. and general debility. The absolute diagnosis of acute cases of arsenic poisoning consists in the examination of blood and soft tissues such as liver, brain, and spleen, which leads to recovery of arsenic. In chronic cases the increased amounts of arsenic in the urine constitute the best diagnostic approach. Concentration of arsenic in the hair and bone have been found months after death or cessation of exposure.

Lead[10, 19, 22]

Lead is a strong protoplasmic poison that may be accumulated in the body over a protracted period, eventually reaching toxic levels and causing tissue damage. Lead poisoning is particularly common in children who chew on furniture painted with a lead-base paint. It may also be absorbed through the respiratory tract; acute poisoning by inhalation is sometimes encountered in industry where large volumes of volatized compounds of lead are being used. Chronic poisoning with lead is more common in industry than acute poisoning, since the cumulative effect of small amounts of absorbed lead used in industrial processes is more likely to produce disease. Lead poisoning may also be caused by retention of lead from slightly acidic drinking water conveyed through lead pipes.

Lead is absorbed in the gastrointestinal tract and passed to the liver, then excreted back into the duodenum through the bile. Some is reabsorbed, but some is excreted in the feces. From the respiratory tract it rapidly enters the circulation, where it is carried to the bones and stored (Fig. 12-1), but some is excreted from the blood through the kidneys and feces at a fairly slow rate. The lesions are found in the gastrointestinal, nervous, and hemopoietic systems. A lead colic is produced in the intestines. The nervous system may be affected by a single massive dose or from cumulative effects. The outstanding manifestations of acute involvement of the nervous system are coma and convulsive seizures, particularly in children. A permanent complication in children who recover is residual nervous system injury with mental deficiency.

Mercury[17, 26]

Mercury is a metallic element. It is absorbed in the stomach, transiently stored in the liver, and thence excreted from the blood through the kidneys and colon. Acute mercury poisoning is almost always the result of accidental or suicidal ingestion; rarely is it from absorption of mercuric salts used therapeutically in injections, inunctions, or vaginal douches. The metallic mercury of the thermometer is highly insoluble and therefore is not dangerous if swallowed.

Bichloride of mercury is the compound usually involved in fatal poisoning. Its

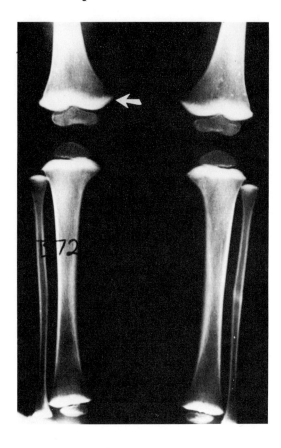

Fig. 12-1. Lead poisoning showing lead lines in metaphyseal ends of the long bones (arrow). This broad band of density is called the radiographic lead line. (From Young, C. G., and Likos, J. J.: Medical specialty terminology, x-ray and nuclear medicine, St. Louis, 1972, The C. V. Mosby Co.)

chief effects are in the gastrointestinal tract and the kidneys, which are the portals of entry and excretion, respectively. The mucosa of the stomach is destroyed by necrosis first, and later the colon is similarly affected. If survival is prolonged, ulcers develop. It is a nephrotoxic chemical, and within 24 hours after ingestion, oliguria develops, and later anuria followed by terminal uremia.[10]

In the condition called mercurialism the metallic mercury may produce chronic or acute manifestations, which differ from those produced by mercury chloride. The mercury may be inhaled, ingested, or injected. The symptoms of acute mercurialism are stomatitis and digestive disturbances and albuminuria and urinary casts. Chronic mercurialism involves primarily the central nervous system, with symptoms of tremors, exaggerated reflexes, and emotional instability.

Benzene (benzol)[8, 19, 26]

Benzol poisoning is usually the result of inhaling fumes produced in the manufacture of a wide variety of products, such as rubber, leather, paint, paint removers, fabric cleaning compounds, and cigarette lighter fluids. As in all inhaled poisons, the degree of poisoning is governed by the duration of exposure and the concentration of fumes. In the body benzene is converted into phenols and excreted from the kidneys. The toxicity depends on absorption of amounts in excess of the ability of the body to metabolize or excrete them, with the result that they accumulate in the body. There is first an irritative reaction in the respiratory passages, followed by flushing, cyanosis, dizziness, convulsions, and delirium in acute poisoning. Hemorrhages occur in the stomach and intestines. The brain becomes edematous and congested with subarachnoid hemorrhages. The chronic poisoning effects begin insidiously, characterized by peripheral blood findings of elevated red blood cell count and decreased white blood cells and platelets.

Salicylates[10, 15, 26]

Salicylates have become a leading cause of poisoning in the home in the past few years, particularly among children, because of the ready accessibility of aspirins in the household. They are also ingested for suicidal purposes. Salicylates taken in excess cause gastric irritation by the increase in free hydrochloric acid in the stomach. Other symptoms are dizziness, tinnitus, sweating, nausea, vomiting, fever, and hyperpnea. Sweating and vomiting lead to dehydration and water and electrolyte disturbance, particularly if there is also diarrhea. Acute intoxication in young children is often manifested by respiratory alkalosis followed by metabolic acidosis. This is caused by the drug sensitizing the respiratory center to carbon dioxide and results in the augmentation of a minute volume and a fall in carbon dioxide–combining power of the blood. The resultant respiratory alkalosis brings about compensatory renal loss of alkali with retention of chloride. If depletion of base continues, the urine becomes acid. Overdosage of salicylates also increases the metabolic rate and production of carbon dioxide that stimulates hyperpnea, with resultant further loss of carbon dioxide. The blood sugar level is raised, and there is formation of ketone bodies, with production of metabolic acidosis.[15] Clinically the symptoms resemble diabetic acidosis, and it is often difficult to distinguish between them.[3]

Barbiturates[10, 12]

The barbiturates are a sedative and hypnotic type of drug. Most of the cases of poisoning are the result of ingestion for suicidal purposes. Accidental deaths may occur in children from ingestion. Occasionally barbiturates are taken in conjunction with alcohol, and the central nervous system depression caused by the combination of the two may result in death.[12] Some of the barbiturates are slow acting, whereas others are fast acting, and ingestion above the minimal lethal dose causes death within an hour or less.[10] (See Table 3.)

The clinical manifestations are deep coma and depressed breathing. Inspissated mucus collects in the bronchial passages, obstructing the airways, and can cause death from suffocation. The systemic anoxia leads to vascular collapse, which has been attributed to either depression of the autonomic nerve centers or direct depressant effects exerted on the smooth muscle walls of blood vessels, causing vasodilatation and a drop in blood volume.[19] Death is usually the result of depression of the respiratory center of the brain. Barbiturates have no local effect at the portal of entry.

Morphine[25, 26]

Morphine is a hypnotic and sedative drug that produces coma, usually in less time than the barbiturates. The route of entry is usually by injection. The effect is an irregularly descending paralysis of the body. Death results from respiratory and circulatory failure. A drug addict can tolerate a dosage much higher than the usually lethal level. (See discussion on drug dependence, p. 161.)

Smog[10, 21]

The problem of air pollution is receiving increasing recognition in urban populations. The term "smog" implies smoke plus fog and originates from harmful atmospheric contamination. There are two recognized types. The first is the heavy, wet, murky atmosphere that occurs in areas where fog is prevalent. In fog of this type, sulfur dioxide is present, but there may be other substances such as soluble fluorides and chlorides plus unknown materials. Many deaths have been traced to this type of smog in London. The second type of smog occurs on windless sunny days. The formation of this type of smog depends upon pronounced accumulation of pollutants and strong sunlight. The sources of the pollutants are oxides of nitrogen from high-temperature combustion processes and hydrocarbons from vehicular exhausts. Although industry is involved and usually gets blamed for the pollution, vehicular exhaust is the greatest single pollutant. Added to this are open trash burning and sewage disposal by burning. The products formed by photochemical action may be more harmful than the primary action of the pollutants when encountered singly.

The effects of smog are not definitely known, but initial symptoms are eye irritations, chest pains, cough, and dyspnea. The effects are greatly increased in those with chronic respiratory diseases.

Poisonous plants[1, 13]

Many poisonous plants grow throughout the United States. Some of these contain toxic substances in the plant itself or in its seeds or grains. The common ones are chokeberry, jimson weed, stinkweed, and meadow saffron. Ergot sometimes grows as a fungus on various grains and is a source of potential poison.

The poisonous mushrooms are the *Amanita phalloides* and the *Amanita muscaria*. Both of these may cause death within a few days after ingestion. There is very little chance of poisoning from commercially grown mushrooms. The danger lies in the indiscriminate gathering of mushrooms for food by children or by those who are not able to recognize the difference between a poisonous and a nonpoisonous variety. *Amanita phalloides* has a white color and is often mistaken for the common mushroom *Agaricus campestris*, but no dependence should be placed upon color, size, shape, or general appearance. It often

takes the trained mycologist to distinguish the lethal types from the nonlethal. *Amanita phalloides* causes the greatest number of cases of mushroom poisoning. The symptoms often do not develop until 6 to 15 hours after ingestion, and the onset is marked by sudden, severe abdominal pain, intense thirst, nausea, vomiting, and sometimes blood and mucus in the vomitus. Collapse may soon follow, and the patient develops a peculiar yellow color. Confusion, delirium, and convulsions may occur Symptoms from *Amanita muscaria* often come on within 15 minutes after ingestion. They consist of salivation, excessive perspiration, nausea, vomiting, pain in the abdomen, and watery evacuations from the bowels. The pupils are contracted, and there is dyspnea.

The pathologic lesions of *Amanita phalloides* poisoning are hepatic necrosis and degeneration and necrosis of the proximal tubular epithelium of the kidneys. Fatty degeneration may also be found in the heart and brain, and there may be acute hemolysis. The principal effects of *Amanita muscaria* poisoning are stimulation of the myoneural junctions between the nerves and epithelial cells. Great muscular weakness occurs, and profound effects are in the peripheral organs.[1]

Venoms[3]

Spiders and scorpions are common in most parts of the world. Bites of tarantulas and black widows cause pain almost immediately, which spreads quickly from the region of the bite to the muscles of the back, shoulders, chest, abdomen, and ribs. Usually, severe abdominal muscle spasms are experienced. Bites from other poisonous spiders are not likely to be so immediately painful, but the victim may be affected with muscle cramps about half an hour afterward. The muscle cramps are first localized near the bite, but later they spread to other body muscles. Shock usually develops. The sting of a scorpion causes immediate intense pain, followed by numbness and paralysis of the area near the sting. Adults rarely die from either spider or scorpion bites.[3]

The poisonous snakes in the United States are the rattlesnake, copperhead, water moccasin, and the coral snake. The bites of rattlesnakes, copperheads, and water moccasins are hemotoxic (poisonous to the blood). The venom of the coral snake is a highly potent neurotoxin (poisonous to the nervous tissue). The symptoms of a bite from the rattlesnake, water moccasin, or copperhead are intense pain, severe headache, and thirst. The bite causes the escape of blood from the capillaries, which accumulates in the tissues. The bleeding from some of the internal organs into the intestines and excretory tracts may be detected by the presence of blood in the urine or feces.[3]

The bite of the coral snake causes an irregular heartbeat, followed by generalized weakness and exhaustion ending in shock. Severe headache, dizziness, and mental disturbances occur. Also, muscular incoordination and sometimes muscle spasms and twitching develop. Breathing may be difficult and labored. There may even be respiratory paralysis.[3]

DRUG DEPENDENCE, ADDICTION, AND INTOXICATION[10, 11, 25]

Although the word "addiction" is used in this text and in Table 3, the World Health Organization and Committee on Drug Addiction and Narcotics of the U.S. National Research Council have recommended substitution of the term "drug dependence" for "addiction." Drug dependence implies that the drug has been habitually misused until it poses a threat to physical health, psychologic functions, and ability of the user to adapt to the demands of society (authority and customs). At the present time the illegal use of drugs by young individuals (12 to 25 years of age) has almost reached epidemic proportions, particularly in the slums or ghetto areas of major cities. Illegal drug usage, however, is by no means con-

fined to these areas, for, in the United States it has spread to middle-class and upper-class suburbia, to colleges and universities, and to the armed forces. It is a subject of intense investigation by many local, state, and federal agencies, not only for suppression of illegal traffic but also for establishment of treatment centers for those who are drug dependent.

Drugs that produce psychic and physical dependence[11, 25, 27]

The drugs that produce psychic and physical dependence include opium types, barbiturates, amphetamines, opiate agonist-antagonist types, and ethyl alcohol. See Table 3 for further information on specific drugs. Only the opium derivatives, methadone, and amphetamines will be discussed here.

Opium derivatives. Opium is an alkaloid recovered from the seeds of the poppy (*Papaver somniferum*). The main derivatives of this poppy plant are opium, morphine, codeine, and heroin, collectively known as opiates. All of these are addictive narcotics. The symptoms of acute poisoning are unconsciousness, shallow respirations, and pinpoint pupils. The withdrawal symptoms are severe gastrointestinal cramps, sweating, tremor, and cardiovascular collapse.

Heroin.[4, 9, 11, 14, 18, 25] In the U.S. the chief drug in illicit traffic is heroin. It is particularly hazardous from a health standpoint, not only because of its drug-dependent influence, but also because it is often heavily contaminated with bacteria, fungi, yeast, spores, quinine, and diluting chemicals.[11] Heroin, as well as other drugs, is frequently adulterated with quinine, lactose, talc (magnesium trisilicate), baking soda, and mannitol. Sometimes an effort is made to purify the heroin by filtering it through cotton; thus, cotton fibers may gain entrance to the lungs and cause damage. Talc (magnesium trisilicate) is a common bulk filter, and when injected into a vein, lodges in distant arterioles, causing

Table 3. Up and down drugs*

Classes of legitimate drugs brand names	Description or slang names	Medical usage	Effects physical psychological	Dangers
SEDATIVES	Sleeping pills, Goof balls	Sedatives are used to induce sleep and relaxation. They are used to treat insomnia, anxiety, tension, high blood pressure, convulsions, epileptic seizures and mental disorders.	Sedatives depress the central nervous system. Other effects include muscle relaxation, impaired coordination, slowed reaction time, drowsiness, staggering, alterations of space perceptions. Loss of judgment and self-control, quick temper, incoherence, depression, and slurred speech may occur.	All barbiturates are addictive. Severe illness occurs if these drugs are withdrawn. Overdosage or rapid injection can cause blood pressure to drop, respiratory failure—coma or death. Combined with excessive alcohol they can cause coma or death. Seconal—caution advised if liver is impaired. Nembutal should not be used if liver is damaged since it is eliminated through the liver. If Nembutal is withdrawn abruptly, convulsions may occur.
Barbiturates Seconal (sodium secobarbital)	Red birds, Red devils			
Nembutal (sodium pentobarbital)	Yellow jackets			
Luminal (phenobarbital)	Purple hearts			
Amytal (sodium amobarbital)	Blue heavens, Blue devils			
Nonbarbiturates Doriden (glutethimide)	Goofers	(same as above)	(same as above)	Doriden poisoning is difficult to treat. Highly addictive.
Noludar				
Chloral hydrate	Knock-out drops, Mickey Finn (when mixed with alcohol)			
STIMULANTS *Amphetamines* Benzedrine (amphetamine sulfate)	Pep pills Bennies, Ups	Amphetamines depress appetite and are used in weight control as diet pills. They are used to combat fatigue and produce alertness; to alleviate depression by elevating moods; to treat narcolepsy, hyperkineticism, and other neurological diseases.	Amphetamines stimulate central nervous system. They produce insomnia, restlessness, euphoria, irritability, excitability, and tremors. Chronic use results in extreme weight loss, delusions, hallucinations, overconfidence.	After heavy prolonged use of amphetamines there is: tendency to be violent under delusions; susceptibility to severe exhaustion, malnutrition, pneumonia; possible development of high blood pressure, heart malfunction, brain damage; dependency; severe depressions if amphetamines are withdrawn. Methedrine, when injected in high doses, may cause hallucinations, heart attacks. Danger of infections from needles.
Dexedrine (dextroamphetamine sulfate)	Dexies, Dex			
Methedrine (methamphetamine)	Speed, Crystal, Meth			
Dexamyl	combination of amphetamines and a sedative	Dexamyl is used to treat mild depression.		

PAIN-RELIEVERS Opium derivatives		Use	Effects	Addiction / Notes
Morphine	Dope, M opium derivative	relieves severe pain	Opium derivatives depress the central nervous system; are known as narcotics. They impair intellectual function and coordination; can cause drowsiness, euphoria, nausea, itching, loss of appetite.	highly addictive narcotic, severe withdrawal pain; overdose can cause death.
Codeine	Schoolboy, Dope opium derivative	relieves minor pain and coughing		addictive
Paregoric	P.G., P.O. contains opium	counteracts diarrhea; used as a sedative		
Dilaudid	opium derivative	relieves pain		addictive: same dangers as morphine
Non-opiates Methadone	synthetic morphine-type drug	kills strong pain		addictive
Demerol	synthetic opiate	relieves pain, sometimes used in childbirth		addictive: more difficult to treat Demerol addiction than morphine
Meperidine	synthetic morphine-type drug	relieves pain	High doses cause excitement, tremors, convulsions.	
Percodan		relieves strong pain		addictive
Darvon	synthetic pain-killer	relieves minor pain, usually chronic or recurrent pains.		nonaddictive: some people develop dependencies, however
TRANQUILIZERS *Phenothiazine compounds* Thorazine Compazine Stelazine	major tranquilizers, chlorpromazine	used to treat severe psychiatric conditions; relieve minor anxiety; used as sedatives before surgery. Thorazine suppresses hallucinations caused by LSD.	Drowsiness, blurry vision, skin rash, and tremors may occur. Mental sluggishness, disturbed sleep, and depression may result after prolonged use.	Use of tranquilizers should not be discontinued abruptly. Non-addictive, but thorazine may be dangerous for liver and bone marrow. The combined effect of thorazine and the hallucinogen STP can be fatal–should not be used to tone down STP panic reactions.
Reserpine compounds Rauwolfia	major tranquilizers	(same as above)		

*Reprinted from the book "What everyone needs to know about drugs," published by U. S. News & World Report, Inc. Copyright 1970, U. S. News & World Report, Inc., Washington, D. C. 20037.

Continued.

Table 3. Up and down drugs—cont'd

Classes of legitimate drugs brand names	Description or slang names	Medical usage	Effects physical psychological		Dangers
TRANQUILIZERS—cont'd Equanil, Miltown (meprobamate) Librium (chlordiazepoxide)	minor tranquilizers	used to treat mild anxiety, tensions, minor emotional disorders; used to slow down over-active individuals; used to relax muscles			may be addictive
Valium (diazepam)		(same as above)	Valium does not usually cause drowsiness or loss of alertness.		may cause physical dependence resulting in severe withdrawal symptoms
ANTI-DEPRESSANTS *Dibenzapines* Tofranil Elavil		used to relieve moderate to severe depressions	elevation of moods stimulation		
Monoamine oxidase drugs Marplan Nardil Parnate Etonyl Niamid	MAO inhibitors; each has different chemical formula	used to alleviate depression—usually if no other drug is effective			Constant medical supervision required with MAO drugs; may have toxic effects on liver, brain, heart and blood vessels; should not be combined with strong pain relievers or taken after eating certain foods such as cheese.

arteritis and thrombosis, and eventually talc granulomatosis of the lungs[9] or liver.[16] Quinine used to dilute street heroin in low doses causes tachycardia and in high doses induces bradycardia. Paroxysmal atrial fibrillation may occur, and the arrhythmias may be lethal.

There are a number of cutaneous complications. Subcutaneous injections are called "skin pops," but later in order to achieve a quick "high," the veins are used. The needles may be contaminated with microorganisms, causing superficial abscesses, cellulitis, lymphangitis, lymphadenitis, and phlebitis. The users of needles are betrayed by the telltale track hyperpigmentation, cutaneous scarring, and venous thrombosis. There may also be a fairly characteristic necrotic punched out cutaneous ulcer. Some of the injection sites are exotic, such as veins of digits, ventral surface of the tongue, and even the dorsal vein of the penis.

Some of the other health hazards of the use of heroin are hepatitis caused by unsanitary needles used in injections; perforation of the anterior nasal septum with collapse and saddle deformity (rare) resulting from habitual sniffing of heroin; and myositis ossificans[4] caused by injury to the brachialis muscle by inept needle manipulation, called "drug abuse elbow." The neurologic disorders and complications of addiction to heroin[18] are numerous. These include coma, seizures, increased intracranial pressure, acute delirium, chronic organic brain damage, cerebral vascular accident, involuntary movement disorders, deafness, toxic amblyopia (may be secondary to quinine contamination), and acute and subacute polyneuropathy.[18] Infectious neurologic complications are bacterial meningitis, mycotic aneurysm, brain abscess, subdural and epidural abscesses, acute cerebral falciparum malaria, and complications of viral hepatitis and tetanus. All of these infectious neurologic complications are the result of using contaminated needles in injections.[18]

In heroin addicted pregnant mothers there are fetal effects, causing drug addiction of the newborn. In a mother who had tachypnea and respiratory alkalosis prior to giving birth the newborn had tremors, high-pitched cry, convulsions, and tachypnea.[14] The drug traverses the placenta easily, and withdrawal symptoms have been observed in about 70% of infants born of addicted women. If a maternal dose of heroin has been delayed, the withdrawal symptoms may develop in the fetus in utero. More commonly, symptoms occur 24 hours after birth but may be delayed several days. Many of the infants have withdrawal symptoms of sneezing, sweating, and yawning.

Respiratory arrest or convulsions, or both, may occur when pure heroin is injected. (See Table 3 for further information on specific opiates.)

Methadone.[11, 25] Methadone is an opiate type of drug now being used experimentally in treatment of individuals dependent on heroin or morphine. The patients are usually treated in special clinics or in hospitals and are gradually given up to 120 to 180 mg. of methadone in a single dose. Patients tolerant to this dosage will be cross-tolerant to as much as 30 mg. of heroin intravenously. The patient soon drops his dependence on heroin or morphine and will no longer seek it illicitly. The advantages of methadone maintenance are that the patient can return to school or work and can function in society, provided he is motivated and receives the maintenance dose of methadone. Patients become strongly dependent physically and psychically on methadone. The long-term effects of the drug are unknown at this time. Methadone is administered mainly in special clinics for treatment of addiction and is not ordinarily given by general practitioners.

Amphetamines.[6, 11, 25] The variants of amphetamine structure are known as pep pills, uppers, bennies, dexies, bombitas; methedrine is called meth, crank, splash, speed, or crystal. At the present time, however, there is a tendency to call all amphetamines "speed."

Amphetamines are taken occasionally to enhance alertness or to add impetus to one's performance. They have been used by students when studying for examinations, by drivers to stay alert on extended trips, by athletes to excel in competitive sports, and by military personnel while on prolonged marches or operations.[11] These are considered temporary uses, but prolonged use or overdosage impairs the judgment. Physicians have prescribed amphetamines to counteract fatigue in patients, as well as for depression and as a deterrent to obesity. The patients may continue to take them indefinitely because they have become addicted and cannot stop their usage without the resulting lethargic depression and the feeling that they cannot function without the stimulant. A tolerance develops for the drug, and dosage is increased to obtain a stimulating, exhilarating, or euphoric effect. The increase occurs sometimes over a period of a few days to months, but eventually the daily dose will be 50 to 150 mg.[6]

Users of amphetamines soon discover that oral consumption does not produce a "high" nearly as fast as snorting or injecting the substance intravenously and also that injection produces a more intense high. Some women may even inject the material into the vagina before intercourse. If a user is on a "speed run," he may inject up to 1000 mg. intravenously in a single dose and up to 5000 mg. in 24 hours.[6] This user is aptly described as a "speed freak." Some users combine amphetamines with barbiturates and even heroin, which is also used to come down from an amphetamine binge. If a user is on a "speed run," he is disinclined to eat, sleep, and he may ignore body care. Weight loss may reach as much as 10 pounds in a week.[6] During this experience the user is overactive, impulsive, and demonstrates defective reasoning and judgment, and eventually becomes paranoid. This combination causes him to engage in irrational behavior, which may lead him to hurt himself or others. Some bizarre accidents and homicides have been traced to amphetamine psychotics. A tragedy of amphetamine psychosis is that it may last long after the period of indulgence has ceased. Amphetamine intoxication causes compulsive behavior such as skin picking, bead stringing and unstringing, constant chattering, and pacing. If the dosage is raised too rapidly, the user though conscious may be unable to move or speak. The pulse is rapid, temperature elevated, and blood pressure increased. In intercourse, orgasm and ejaculation are delayed or impossible to achieve, and this may result in marathon sexual activity to the point of sheer exhaustion. In some users, however, there is a complete lack of interest in sexual activity. Other side effects of chronic high dosage are cerebral hemorrhage, cardiac arrhythmias, and a necrotizing angiitis in speed freaks. Dyskinesia includes jaw grinding. Hepatitis may develop from the use of unclean needles for injection.

When a speed user tries to "come down from a trip," after he has become exhausted and delusional, he suffers withdrawal symptoms of long periods of sleep, marked depression, apathy, numerous aches and pains, and a ravenous appetite. Depression may be so severe that it starts the user on another "speed run." Paranoid states are present sooner or later in all users of high dosages. Suicide may occur during or after the "speed run."[25] The user's experience can be terrifying or overwhelming because he suffers from delusions of persecution and is excessively suspicious of everyone. It is during the withdrawal phase that he may elect to commit suicide to relieve his symptoms.

Children are given amphetamines until adolescence to help them overcome hyperkinesia, but they do not tend to abuse the use of amphetamines as they grow older.

Drugs that produce psychic but not physical dependence[11, 25]

Drugs that produce psychic but not physical dependence include hallucinogens, cocaine types, cannabis types, and bromides. Of the hallucinogens the types most often used are lysergic acid diethylamide (LSD, LSD-25, and derivatives); mescaline (peyote, or mescal buttons); tryptamines (psilocybin, tryptomine, psilocin, including *Psilocybe mexicana*, a mushroom, and dimethyltryptamine, diethyltryptamine, and related compounds); hallucinogenic amphetamines (STP, DOM); cannabis types (marihuana, hashish, and tetrahydrocannabinols); bromides; and glue sniffing.

Hallucinogens. Hallucinogens cause changes in mood and sensory perception, hallucinations, chiefly optical, and moderate psychic dependence, but no physical dependence. They are used chiefly by young people who have rejected society and are in rebellion against their elders. A number of pseudoreligious cults have sprung up that use the drug to "expand their minds" to gain an insight into personal emotional problems. The harm in the use of these drugs is that the users withdraw from society, tend to use multiple drugs, and are victims of infections from unsanitary living habits. These drugs can trigger acute and chronic psychoses.

The clinical manifestations are changes in mood, mostly euphoric, with enhancement of sensations. People assume grotesque appearances; the user may feel that his body has altered, that his hands are like animal paws, and that he can see his blood and bones through his flesh. He may also feel that he is endowed with the power to fly through space. With heavy dosage he loses insight and may appear dazed. At such times he may attempt suicide or inflict psychotic attacks on others. Some users become permanently psychotic, and others experience "flashbacks" with return of symptoms. The flashbacks can occur months after drug action is terminated.

Such effects occur mainly in those who are marginally adjusted emotionally. On physical examination, the pupils are dilated but react to light; temperature and blood pressure are elevated; and sweating and gooseflesh occur. Deep tendon reflexes are hyperactive. LSD is the hallucinogen most often used. Most of the hallucinogens are taken orally or injected, but dimethyltryptamine and diethyltryptamine are smoked or injected.

Cocaine.[5, 11, 27] Cocaine was first used about 3000 years ago among the Incas. It came from coca leaves, and many Indian men and women of the Andean highlands are coca chewers. Scientific study began about 100 years ago, when cocaine was extracted from the coca leaves. Sigmund Freud, a great psychiatrist, believed that cocaine could cure morphine and alcohol addiction, but the enthusiasm subsided after a few unfortunate experiences. William Halstead, a great surgeon at Johns Hopkins, Baltimore, prescribed regional anesthesia with cocaine by blockage of peripheral sensory nerves.[5]

When cocaine is injected or inhaled, it produces a condition of hyperstimulation, overalertness, euphoria, and feeling of power. This "high" feeling, however, is short-lived, and to maintain euphoria, some users inject the cocaine intravenously every 10 minutes. The consequent restlessness and hypervigilance may progress to an unpleasant tension leading to paranoid thinking. When cocaine is discontinued, depression sometimes results. Like amphetamines, cocaine delays ejaculations and orgasm in sexual intercourse. Heavy use of cocaine causes weight loss, insomnia, anxiety, and paranoid thinking with hallucinations and delusions frequently occurring. A typical hallucination of cocaine psychosis is the belief that bugs are crawling over the skin. Violent behavior occurs, but the brief action of the drug prevents prolonged aggressive activities.

The local anesthetic action of cocaine is caused by blockage of transmission of pain.

It is a powerful constrictor of the small blood vessels. This accounts for ulceration of the nasal septum following the "snorting" of cocaine for long periods in high doses. Since tolerance and withdrawal symptoms do not occur, cocaine is not considered to be addictive. Craving to repeat the experience accounts for cocaine use.

There is dilation of the pupils, elevation of heart rate and blood pressure, and increased respirations after using cocaine. Overdosage produces tremors, convulsions of the temporal lobe seizure type, and delirium. Death may result from cardiovascular collapse or respiratory failure. Pure "cokeheads" as a rule comprise a small number of users. Those who use cocaine tend to use other drugs to supplement or modify its action, usually because high-grade cocaine is very expensive, selling for as much as $1,000 per ounce.[5] Street cocaine is usually adulterated with lactose, procaine, amphetamines, or strychnine. To maintain the cocaine state, as many as one hundred injections daily may be necessary. Cocaine has been called the "rich man's speed,"[5] and many who try it a few times cannot afford it and turn to other drugs or mind-altering substances they can afford. The classic "speedball" often simultaneously injects cocaine and heroin intravenously.[5] Some use cocaine while they are on a methadone maintenance program. Methadone can prevent the "high" when heroin is used but it does not interfere with the highs produced by cocaine, amphetamines, or sedatives.

To date the federal government has not restricted the manufacture of cocaine, but it is a controlled substance under law. Its topical use is widespread in medicine, particularly by otolaryngologists in the diagnosis and treatment of lesions of the tracheobronchial tree.

Cannabis (marihuana and hashish).[11, 25] Marihuana and hashish are products of the hemp plant, *Cannabis sativa*, which produces a resinous substance. The resinous substance is most abundant in the leaves and flowering tops of the plant. Dried leaves and tops are the marihuana (pot, grass, tea, reefers, muggles), which is smoked mainly in cigarettes. The compressed or concentrated resin is termed hashish. There is moderate psychic dependence, but no physical dependence. The chief arguments against its use in the United States are that it alters mood, judgment, and perception, and it may precipitate temporary psychotic states. In other parts of the world (India, Middle East, and North Africa), heavy abuse of extremely strong material has led to social deterioration and cannabis psychosis (mental deterioration). The clinical manifestations are silly behavior, euphoria, and mild sensory distortions, with the user believing that colors are brighter, music more beautiful, and touch more sensitive. These effects last about 2 to 4 hours after a dose of 7 mg. or less in one cigarette, and are followed by drowsiness and sleepiness. Doses exceeding this amount (14 to 20 mg.) produce anxiety, marked sensory distortions, and optical hallucinations. Tachycardia follows use of the drug in any amount. Conjunctivae are frequently red. The person under the influence of the drug has impaired memory for recent events and lacks the ability to concentrate, which are strong reasons why the drug should not be used. Occasionally marihuana or hashish has triggered panic and schizophreniform reactions in susceptible people.[11]

Bromides.[11] Bromides are sedatives. They accumulate in the blood, and the effects of poisoning appear slowly over a period of weeks. The symptoms are referable to the central nervous system and are manifested by irritability, impaired memory and cognition, emotional instability, and agitation. In severe poisoning, delusions, hallucinations, lethargy, and finally coma may occur. Tolerance and physical dependence do not occur.

Glue sniffing.[7] Juveniles are achieving an intoxicated state by sniffing or inhaling industrial solvents and aerosol sprays. The solvents include airplane glue (for model making), paint thinner, gasoline, and a variety of aerosols used in sprays as insecticides, furniture polish, disinfectants, hair sprays, antiperspirants, window cleaners, and other noxious material. Volatile solvents are properly classified as anesthetics, with an action like ether and alcohol, and like these they may produce a period of stimulation before depression of the central nervous system occurs.

The early symptoms are dizziness, slurred speech, unsteady gait, and drowsiness. Later excitement, irritability, and impulsive behavior develop, and injuries can occur during overactivity. Delirium, mental confusion, psychomotor clumsiness, a wide range of emotional responses and impairment of thinking are seen routinely. Illusions, delusions, and hallucinations may develop as the condition deepens. Ordinarily, a euphoric dreamy state is described, with sleep as the frequent endpoint. The intoxication lasts from a few minutes to an hour or two. Chronic and persistent cough may develop in habitual users. Also a rash has been described that developed around the nose and mouth in habitual users. No withdrawal symptoms have been described, but psychologic dependence is common.

Underprivileged children between the ages of 7 and 17 are more prone to sniff glue. Solvent sniffing is rare in adults, except among prison inmates and those engaged in its manufacture. By the late teens, the solvent sniffers have usually abandoned the practice. Unfortunately, many become chronic alcoholics, barbiturate users, or addicts.

The commercial solvents are poured into a balloon or plastic bag and then sniffed. Aerosol sprays may be sniffed directly from the can or sprayed into a container.

Many of the hazards associated with solvent sniffing are impaired judgment, irrational behavior, and injury of the brain, kidneys, liver, and bone marrow, probably representing a hypersensitivity to the solvents or a continued heavy dosage. Carbon tetrachloride can produce a hepatorenal syndrome. Death can result from respiratory arrest, and sudden death may be caused by cardiac arrhythmia. The fumes from the aerosols may occlude the airways by freezing the larynx, and although aerosols are not considered to be toxic chemically, it is believed that the adverse effects are the occluding of the pulmonary alveolar surface and the preventing of transfer of oxygen.

Responses

Step 1: 1. ingestion; 2. inhalation; 3. absorption; 4. injection; 5. injection

Step 2: 1. X; 2. X; 3. X; 4. X; 5. X; 6. X; 7. X; 8. X; 11. X; 12. X; 13. X; 15. X; 16. X; 17. X; 18. X; 19. X; 21. X; 22. X; 23. X; 25. X

Step 3: 1. X; 2. X; 3. X; 6. X; 7. X

Step 4: 1. healthy person; 2. 40-year-old man; 3. a drug addict; 4. small dose of lethal poison; 5. alkali; 6. corrosive; 7. barbiturates; 8. corrosive; 9. inhaled poison; 10. organic solvents

REFERENCES

1. Abul-Haj, S. K., Ewald, R. A., and Kazyak, L.: N. Engl. J. Med. **269**:223, 1963 (mushroom poisoning).
2. Bennett, I. L., Jr., and others: Medicine **32**:431, 1953 (methyl alcohol poisoning).
3. Bureau of Naval Personnel, Training Publications Division: Standard first aid training course, Washington, D. C., 1965.
4. Chung, B. S.: J.A.M.A. **227**:469-470, 1973 (drug-induced myositis ossificans circumscripta).
5. Cohen, S.: J.A.M.A. **231**:74-75, 1975 (cocaine).
6. Cohen, S.: J.A.M.A. **231**:414-415, 1975 (amphetamnie abuse).
7. Cohen, S.: J.A.M.A. **231**:653-654, 1975 (glue sniffing).
8. DeGowin, R. L.: J.A.M.A. **185**:748, 1963 (benzene).
9. Gottlieb, L. S., and Boylen, T. C.: West. J. Med. **1208**:16, 1974 (pulmonary complications of drug abuse).
10. Henningar, G. R.: In Anderson, W. A. D., editor: Pathology, ed. 6, St. Louis, 1971, The C. V. Mosby Co. (chemical injury).
11. Isbell, H.: In Beeson, P. B., and McDermott, W., editors: Cecil-Loeb textbook of medicine, ed. 13, Philadelphia, 1971, W. B.

Saunders Co. (drug dependence and intoxication).

12. Jetter, W. W., and McLean, R.: Arch. Pathol. **36**:112, 1943 (ethyl alcohol and barbiturates).

13. Kinsbury, J. M.: Extension publication of New York State College of Agriculture at Cornell University, Bulletin No. 538, Ithaca, N.Y., 1963 (common poisonous plants).

14. Klain, D. B., Krauss, A. N., and Auld, P. A. M.: N.Y. State J. Med. **72**:367-368, 1972 (tachypnea and alkalosis in infants of addicted mothers).

15. Lindsey, A., Jr.: J. Mississippi Med. Assoc. **2**: 486, 1961 (salicylate intoxication).

16. Min, K. W., and others: Arch. Pathol. **98**: 331-335, 1974 (talc granulomata in liver disease).

17. Noe, F. E.: N. Engl. J. Med. **261**:1002, 1959 (mercury poisoning).

18. Richter, R. W., and others: Bull. N.Y. Acad. Med. **49**:3-21, 1973 (neurological complications of addiction to heroin).

19. Robbins, S. L.: Pathology, ed. 3, Philadelphia, 1967, W. B. Saunders Co. (chemical agents).

20. Rowan, T., and Coleman, F. C.: J. Forensic Sci. **7**:103, 1962 (CO poisoning).

21. Sixth Annual Air Pollution Medical Research Conference: Arch. Environ. Health **8**:3, 1964.

22. Symposium on Lead: Arch. Environ. Health **8**:203, 1964.

23. U.S. Department of Health, Education, and Welfare, National Clearinghouse for Poison Control Centers, Public Health Service Bulletin, Sept.-Oct., 1962.

24. U.S. Department of Health, Education, and Welfare, Public Health Service, Alcohol, Drug Abuse, and Mental Health Administration. DHEW Publication 73-31, reprinted 1975 (alcohol and alcoholism).

25. What everyone needs to know about drugs, Washington, D.C., 1970, U.S. News and World Report, Inc.

26. von Hamm, E.: In Miller, S. E., editor: Textbook of clinical pathology, ed. 7, Baltimore, 1966, The Williams & Wilkins Co. (examinations for toxic substances).

27. Woods, J. H., and Down, D. A.: The psychopharmacology of cocaine. In Drug use in America: problems in perspective. The technical papers of the Second Report of the National Commission on Marihuana and Drug Abuse, Washington, D.C., 1973, U.S. Government Printing Office, vol. 1, 116-1939.

CHAPTER 13

Hypersensitivity and immunity

Hypersensitivity is the acquired capacity of the body to react in a heightenend and markedly intensified manner to a foreign agent or substance to which the body is exposed by parenteral, respiratory, oral, or other route. Hypersensitivity is useful when it protects the body from harmful effects of pathogenic bacteria and toxins. It is harmful, however, when it causes violent tissue reaction as in the host of allergic disorders. The hypersensitivity diseases are a complex group with varying pathogeneses, and in spite of the vast amount of research into the role and mechanisms of a number of these diseases, some areas are still not clearly defined.

To understand hypersensitivity diseases, you must have a knowledge of the meaning and application of the terminology involved, such as immunity, allergy, antigens, antibodies, and antigen-antibody reactions.

IMMUNITY[5, 12, 14]

With the discovery that infectious diseases were caused by living organisms, there followed investigations of the body's combative forces against bacteria and other poison-producing forms of life. The term "immunity" was applied to those combative forces and their mechanisms, and a new branch of medicine was established called immunology.[14] The early investigations were confined to the study of laboratory animals. Bacterial toxins were injected into these animals, and it was found that the animal mobilized specific substances that neutralized these toxins. These specific substances were called *antibodies*. It was further discovered that when diphtheria toxin was injected into an animal, it only developed antibodies specific to the diphtheria toxin; that is, these antibodies were ineffectual against other forms of bacteria. This process was called *active immunization,* since the body of the injected animal was forced by stimulation with the diphtheria toxin to produce antibodies to protect itself. Further investigations proved that if you took the serum of the immunized animal (containing specific antibodies) and injected it into another nonimmunized animal the latter would also gain a measure of protection against the same toxin. Proceeding a step further in the investigation, it was found that if the serum of the immunized animal were injected into an animal with a disease requiring the same specific antibodies of the immunized animal the latter animal would make a faster recovery. Since the serum used in these experiments contained antibodies to a specific disease that the injected animal had been forced to manufacture in its plasma, its transfer to another animal not active in producing its own protection gave only passive immunity. This process became known as *passive immunization.* In other words the latter animal borrowed its immunity from an animal that had built up protection with antibodies against the disease. This investigative work in immunizations has been the foundation of our present practice of immunizing people, particularly children, against a variety of infectious diseases that at one time exacted a high toll of life.[14]

Passive immunization is induced by injecting antitoxin. Its chief advantage is that it is prompt; the disadvantages are that it lasts a brief time, may produce serum reactions, and is economically unsound in group inoculations. However, if there is an epidemic, the immunizing dose of antitoxin will safeguard individuals until the danger has passed. Active immunity, on the other hand, is more lasting, but it takes longer to become effective. Active immunization is the type used against a variety of diseases such as poliomyelitis, typhoid (paratyphoid A and B), tetanus, cholera, typhus, plague, Rocky Mountain spotted fever, yellow fever, diphtheria, and influenza (some types). Vaccinations for smallpox also convey a measure of immunity. Immunization against measles may be passive for protection during epidemics. All active immunizations vary in length of time protection is afforded. For this reason, reinoculations are required from time to time for absolute protection. There are also a number of diseases in which one attack usually conveys a lasting immunity. These are plague, typhoid, smallpox, chickenpox, scarlet fever, measles, yellow fever, typhus, and mumps. Infections that do not confer lasting immunity are gonorrhea, pneumonia, influenza, glanders, dengue fever, relapsing fever, erysipelas, malaria, syphilis, tuberculosis, and occasionally diphtheria and scarlet fever, as well as those diseases caused by the pyogenic cocci.

Another type of immunity, infant immunity, is based on antibody inherited from the mother. The immune response at birth depends on the mother's immunologic history and her complement of gamma globulins (antibodies). This immunity is passive and usually wears off in 6 or more months.

Recent research has demonstrated the importance of the role of the thymus in immunity. The thymus functions to make possible immunity against certain micro-organisms and other forms of foreign proteins (for example, against tissue transplants from one individual to another).[6] Children with a thymic deficiency show increased susceptibility to certain infectious diseases.[6] In experiments on mice it has been demonstrated that mice thymectomized on the first day of life lost most or all of their capacity to produce antibodies. They lose weight and usually die within a few months.

ANTIGEN-ANTIBODY REACTION[6]

Antibody is formed by the host, and the antigen is the exogenous stimulating agent. The development of antibodies is one of the protective mechanisms activated when the body is invaded by disease-producing organisms. The other mechanism is the action of the white cells in engulfing and destroying the invaders. Antibodies start to protect the body as soon as the invaders are introduced. They accomplish this by causing the invaders to clump so that they cannot circulate freely in the blood, or in some instances they may simply inactivate the organisms so that the white cells can destroy them. Antibodies develop against each type of disease-producing invader to which the body is exposed. They may remain in the bloodstream for a long time after recovery from a specific disease, and during that time there will be immunity to that disease.

Although dissimilar, both allergic and immune responses are involved in the antigen-antibody reaction. The neutralization of the toxicity or infectivity of an invading antigen by its specific antibody is an *immune reaction,* which means that the body has an immunity to the offending antigen. If, on the other hand, an antigen enters the body and stimulates the antibody-producing cells to form antibody (reagin) so that when the same antigen again enters the body, it encounters antibody either in the bloodstream or in the sensitized cell, and the resultant antigen-antibody provokes a tissue cell reaction, this would be an *allergic response*.[14] Everyone has antibodies capable of producing an allergic or an immune response, since an antigen-antibody reaction occurs on contact with an antigen in both. A specific antibody elicited by a particular antigen will react with only that allergen. This is termed *specificity*. When a person is first exposed to a specific antigen (the sensitizing substance), he develops antibodies to that antigen, and this is called *sensitization*. For example, when you are first exposed to a pollen antigen, you acquire pollen antibodies. This is your sensitizing dose. If later you are exposed to the same pollen antigen and an antigen-antibody reaction is provoked with clinical manifestations of hypersensitivity or allergy, this means that you are sensitive to the pollen, and subsequent exposure will result in the same reaction. Antibodies form as a result of the sensitizing dose of antigen, but the antigen-antibody reaction occurs as a result of subsequent exposure. Certainly not everyone is sensitive to the introduction of foreign protein substances into the body. Some will have an immune response, whereas others will have an allergic response, depending upon the hypersensitivity of the individual.

HYPERSENSITIVITY REACTIONS[3, 6]

An antigen-antibody interaction is believed to be somehow responsible for all hypersensitivity responses.

Hypersensitivity reactions are divided into three categories—immediate type, intermediate type, and delayed type.[6]

The immediate type is the acute allergic or atopic type. It occurs in sensitized persons primarily after exposure to antigens encountered in the natural environment by inhalation, ingestion, or skin contact. The reactions begin about 5 to 10 minutes after the sensitized person comes in contact with the allergen, but this may be delayed when the antigen is topical or ingested. Immediate allergic reactions primarily involve smooth muscles, blood vessels, and

mucous glands, as occurs in hay fever, asthma, urticaria, and anaphylaxis. The term "anaphylaxis" is derived from Greek and means without protection.[14] It was adopted to distinguish it from prophylaxis, which means protection. Anaphylactic shock is caused by an antigen-antibody reaction, the severity of which depends upon the sensitivity of the person. In anaphylactic shock the foreign protein harmless on first injection proves dangerous or even fatal on reinjection in the same or even a smaller dosage. In the case of horse serum, death may follow the first injection, possibly because of a previous sensitivity acquired through food (horse meat) or contact with horses.

The symptoms of anaphylactic shock develop soon after injection of the foreign substance, for example, bee or wasp sting or injection of a medication such as penicillin. The characteristic symptoms are collapse, unconsciousness, cyanosis, and labored respiration, or there may be coughing, sneezing, choking, and urticaria. Not all these symptoms may occur, depending upon the severity of the shock, but death may result in a few minutes.

The intermediate type is between the immediate and delayed types. It can be readily produced in a variety of animals that have been injected with a variety of antigens, either intravenously or subcutaneously (Arthus reaction). This tissue reaction begins an hour or two after accumulation and disruption of polymorphonuclear leukocytes. The classic example is the Arthus reaction or phenomenon (local edema and necrosis following injection of the specific antigen in the sensitized animal, such as a rabbit). Serum sickness is another example of the intermediate type, but unlike the Arthus reaction, manifestations are diffuse and delayed. Serum sickness sometimes appears after an initial injection of a large dose of animal serum, such as horse tetanus antitoxin. The allergic reaction results from a single injection of the serum large enough to act as both a sensitizing and a challenging dose, but the reaction occurs after a latent period of 6 to 12 days in human beings. The symptoms are vomiting, fever, joint and muscle pains, edema, enlarged spleen and glands, widespread urticaria, and albuminuria.

The delayed type of hypersensitivity reaction is most often encountered as a consequence of natural infection by agents that usually produce chronic disease. Tuberculosis is a prime example. Other examples are brucellosis, tularemia, some fungal infections, and reactions to poison ivy, cosmetics, soaps, ointments, and so on —so-called contact dermatitis. The reaction does not begin for several hours and reaches a maximum after 2 or 3 days.

ALLERGY[4, 8, 10, 13, 14]

Allergy means altered reactivity of cells. The manifestations of allergy result from the combination of an antigen with an antibody formed by the host, which is generally in response to prior contact with antigen. The term "atopy" has been applied to the clinical allergies.[6] It is a disease in which heredity is believed generally to play an influencing role, except in contact dermatitis. Allergy cannot be inherited as a disease, since neither the substances that produce sensitivity nor the allergic manifestations themselves can be transmitted to offspring.[14] What is inherited is a predisposition to allergic manifestations. Clinical allergies, such as hay fever, asthma, urticaria, eczema, contact dermatitis, and those from food and drugs, are caused by noninfectious antigens of environmental origin. Allergen is the name applied to substances that may be protein or nonprotein but that are capable of inducing allergic responses or specific susceptibility. The pollen of ragweed is probably the most common allergen known. This type of allergen is an inhalant, but others include ingestants, injections, infections, and contact substances, such as chemicals and some plants.

The site of the allergic response or reaction is called the shock organ.[14] In humans these organs are usually the mucous membranes of the lungs (asthma), nose (hay fever or allergic rhinitis), stomach and intestines (gastroenteritis), as well as the skin (urticaria, rash, and erythema). All the characteristics of swelling of the mucous membrane or skin have been attributed to the union of the antigen with the cell-attached antibody causing injury to the cells. As a consequence of cell injury the minute blood vessels in the mucous membrane or skin dilate, and fluid from the blood seeps through their thin and expanded walls into the surrounding tissues. The blood cells, however, do not pass this barrier. Fluid in the tissues accounts for the swelling, which in turn provokes the symptoms. The symptoms vary with the organ under attack. The mucous membranes of the nose weep in hay fever; in asthma the small bronchioles swell, causing difficulty in breathing and the resultant wheezing; and in the skin, itchy wheals are formed.[14]

ALLERGY TESTS[7, 10, 11]

The spontaneous allergies of the wheal or erythematous type are frequently associated with circulating antibody in the blood. For this reason the antigen or antigens responsible can often be identified by skin testing with a battery of possible allergens, such as grasses, pollens, and extracts of other plants and substances. This identification is performed in two types of testing—the scratch test and the intracutaneous test. In the scratch skin test the allergenic substance for testing is gently rubbed into the skin after a small scratch has been made with a hypodermic needle. After a certain time the scratch will show inflammation if the person is susceptible to the allergen. In the other test a small amount of the allergen is injected into the skin (superficial layers) of the patient. After a period of 15 to 30 minutes, if the patient is susceptible, a wheal with surrounding edema will appear at the injected site.

An investigation for the cause of food and milk allergies requires the taking of a careful personal history with a complete list of the usual foods eaten by the patient. Since some of them, no doubt, will be implicated in causing allergies, a process of elimination of various suspected foods or drinks from the diet will often yield results in pinpointing the allergen.

AUTOIMMUNITY[6]

Autoimmunity[6] as a category of hypersensitivity reaction is now gaining widespread attention because of the increasing number of transplantations of organs, particularly the kidneys, and recently the heart. The mechanisms of rejection of foreign skin grafts and body organs on transplantation are also the basis of much animal experimentation. The immune mechanisms protect the body proteins, making a sharp distinction between self and nonself. The degeneration and rejection of homologous tissue and skin grafts are believed to be based on the formation of antibodies by the recipient to the grafted tissue.

In addition to the transplantation of organs or tissues, investigators are studying aspects of autoimmunity involving the proper conditions under which humans and animals will produce antibodies that will react with their own tissues in a group of diseases called the autoimmune diseases. Autoimmune diseases are believed by some to result from autoantibody formed in reaction to antigens in the individual's own tissues. Some believe that the autoimmunity is cell centered, and others that it is antigen centered. The group of diseases that may be considered autoimmune include the acquired hemolytic anemias, certain chronic leukopenias, allergic polyneuritis, some instances of thrombocytopenic purpura, some aspects of disseminated lupus erythematosus, and Hashimoto's disease (a type of thyroiditis). Other diseases believed by some authors to have an autoimmune basis are periarteritis nodosa, rheumatoid arthritis, glomerulo-

nephritis, rheumatic fever, and encephalomyelitis. Some of these are also members of a group called collagen diseases.

COLLAGEN DISEASES[3, 4, 6]

The collagen diseases have in common distinctive alterations of blood vessels and especially of the connective tissues. They are also believed to have a similar hypersensitivity pathogenesis. Collagen is the main supportive protein of connective tissue, as well as of skin, bone, cartilage, and tendon.

Each of the collagen or connective tissue diseases has distinct clinical patterns, but in general they are characterized by lesions in the joints, blood vessels, heart, skin, muscles, and serous membranes. The viewpoint varies as to which diseases might be considered as collagen diseases, but it is generally agreed that the following could be considered on this basis: serum sickness, disseminated lupus erythematosus, polyarteritis nodosa, rheumatic fever, rheumatoid arthritis, glomerulonephritis, dermatomyositis, and diffuse scleroderma. Representative collagen diseases with an implication of hypersensitivity are discussed on p. 178. Other diseases, such as rheumatic fever, glomerulonephritis, and rheumatoid arthritis, although considered by many as having a common pathogenesis of hypersensitivity reaction, are also sometimes involved in bacterial infections and other factors. Therefore these diseases are discussed elsewhere in the text.

STEP-BY-STEP EXERCISES

Step 1. Reaction in a heightened or intensified manner to a foreign agent or substance to which the body has been exposed by parenteral, respiratory, oral, or skin contact is called _____.

Step 2. Security against bacteria and other poison-producing forms of life is called _____.

Step 3. When a foreign material enters the bloodstream, a substance that is called _____develops in the plasma.

Step 4. The foreign substance that causes the substance referred to in *Step 3* to form is known as _____.

Step 5. Allergic signs and symptoms are a possible result of the combination of two substances referred to in *Steps 3* and *4,* and this would be called an _____ reaction.

Step 6. The process of rendering a person immune is called immunization. A person may have passive immunity, which means that there is transient immunization against a particular disease or foreign substance gained through the introduction into his system serum of animals already rendered immune. You might call this borrowed immunity, since the injected animal or person did not have to build up protection with antibodies against the disease but borrowed them from an animal that had the specific antibodies. In active immunization the acquired immunity is the result of the presence of antibody formed by the animal in response to the stimulating antigen.

Active immunization may be achieved by injecting antigen.

Passive immunization may be achieved by injecting antibodies (antiserum or antitoxin).

Complete the blanks in the following statements.

1. If antibodies or antiserum (antitoxin) are injected into a person, he acquires
_____ immunization.

2. If antigen is injected into a person and antibodies form, he acquires
_____ immunization.

Step 7. The immunity derived from active immunization and that from passive immunization differ. In passive immunization the antibodies disappear more rapidly from the bloodstream than they do in active immunization, indicating that the immunity conferred is of relatively short duration. The chief advantage of passive immunization is that it provides protection almost immediately, as might be necessary during epidemics of certain diseases. Active immunization, on the other hand, takes longer to be effective but is much more lasting than passive immunization.

Mark an *A* for active or a *P* for passive to indicate the immunizations most likely to be used for the following conditions.

1. Poliomyelitis __
2. Typhoid __
3. Cholera epidemic __
4. Tetanus following a major foot wound __
5. Diphtheria __
6. Recent bite of tick carrying Rocky Mountain spotted fever __
7. Influenza (certain types) __

Step 8. A number of diseases confer a lasting immunity once the individual has had an attack of a specific disease. These generally include most of the diseases of childhood, such as chickenpox, measles, whooping cough, and mumps, as well as the diseases of smallpox, yellow fever, typhoid, and scarlet fever. Other diseases, such as gonorrhea, influenza, malaria, syphilis, tuberculosis, relapsing fever, and pneumonia, do not confer lasting immunity from one attack.

Indicate from which of the following conditions one attack is likely to confer lasting immunity.

1. Measles __
2. Typhoid fever __
3. Syphilis __
4. Chickenpox __
5. Whooping cough __
6. Gonorrhea __
7. Mumps __
8. Pneumonia __

Step 9. Antibody is formed by the host after injection of antigen which is the exogenous stimulating agent. When the body is invaded by disease-producing organisms, two protective mechanisms are activated. One is the action of white cells; the other is the development of antibodies. Antibodies develop against each type of disease-producing invader to which the body is exposed. The combination of antigen (foreign invader) and antibody is called the antigen-antibody reaction. When antigen contacts its specific antibody and the reaction results in neutralization of the toxicity or infectivity of the antigen, this is an immune reaction. If allergic signs and symptoms result from the combination of the two substances, this is called an allergic reaction. Antigen-antibody reaction occurs on contact with an antigen in both allergic and immune responses.

Mark the following statements *T* for true or *F* for false.

1. Antibodies develop against each type of disease-producing invader. ___
2. The development of antibodies is one of the body's protective measures against disease. ___ ·
3. An antigen-antibody reaction resulting in neutralization of the toxicity of an invader is an immune response. ___
4. Allergic signs and symptoms are the result of an immune response. ___
5. Antigen-antibody reactions occur only in allergic responses. ___

Step 10. When a person is first exposed to a specific sensitizing substance (antigen) and develops antibodies to that antigen, this is called _____.

Step 11. Hypersensitivity reactions are divided into two types: the _____ type and _____ type.

Step 12. Complete the blanks with the type of hypersensitivity reaction, immediate or delayed, that is likely to occur within the specified time limits.

1. Ten minutes _____
2. One hour after ingested allergen _____
3. Twelve hours after exposure to poison ivy _____
4. Five minutes after playing with a pet dog _____

5. Twenty-four hours after taking a drug _____

Step 13. A severe type of immediate reaction following a second injection of penicillin in which the fatal outcome was prevented only with immediate therapeutic measures would be called _____ _____.

Step 14. Tetanus toxoid was administered to a patient, and several days later the patient had a fever, joint and muscle pains, widespread urticaria, and an enlarged spleen. This would be called _____ _____.

Step 15. The substances that give rise to allergic reactions are called _____.

Step 16. The site of the allergic response or reaction is called the shock organ. Identify the disease that would produce the allergic responses in the following:

1. Swelling of mucous membranes of nose with weeping _____ _____
2. Swelling of mucous membranes of bronchioles with coughing _____
3. Large irregular wheals on the skin _____
4. Irritation of mucous lining of stomach and intestines _____

Step 17. Experimentation has provided abundant evidence that under proper conditions humans and animals may produce antibodies that will react with their own tissues. This group of conditions is referred to as _____ diseases.

Step 18. A large number of diseases have a similar pathogenic hypersensitivity basis. These diseases involve the supportive protein of the connective tissue, as well as skin, bone, cartilage, and tendon. These diseases are called _____ diseases.

REPRESENTATIVE HYPERSENSITIVITY DISEASES

Systemic (disseminated) lupus erythematosus[1]

Before a discussion of the systemic manifestation of lupus erythematosus can be made, it must be mentioned that a discoid type involving mainly the skin is characterized by a butterfly lesion over the bridge of the nose and cheeks. Lesions, however, are not always confined to this area. This type may be a localized reaction to sunlight and without systemic complications.[1]

Disseminated or systemic lupus erythematosus is basically an inflammatory disease that affects the collagenous connective tissues in many organs and systems. It is believed by many to have a hypersensitivity etiology. Some believe it is caused by an external allergen, and others theorize that it represents autoimmune reactions developed by the patient to any number of antigens found within his own body.[1] It predominantly affects young females and is characterized by some or many of the following symptoms: photosensitivity of the skin to sunlight with skin rashes, joint and muscle pains, fever, malaise, anemia, lymphadenopathy, and splenomegaly. The glomeruli of the kidneys and the endocardium, myocardium, and valves of the heart may also be involved in later stages. The blood findings are leukopenia, thrombopenia, and excessive gamma globulinemia. When the kidneys are involved, there may be albuminuria, hematuria with casts in the urine, and an elevation of the blood urea nitrogen.[4,5]

This disease mimics many other systemic diseases, such as bacterial infections, rheumatoid arthritis, and rheumatic fever. The diagnosis therefore often depends on finding the classic L.E. cell in the peripheral blood or bone marrow aspirations or on finding antinuclear antibodies.

The disease may have an acute onset after excessive sunburn or exposure to sunlight, but usually the onset is insidious with a long protracted course. The death rate is high, usually occurring within 5 years of onset.[1] Because of the many systems involved, death may be the result of renal insufficiency, bacterial endocarditis, cardiac failure, sepsis, pneumonia, or pulmonary tuberculosis, or of any combination of these conditions.[1]

Polyarteritis nodosa[4,6]

The term "polyarteritis" means many vessels and is aptly applied to this disease, since it may involve any tissue of the body that contains arteries or veins. The arteries and veins have nodular swellings, which are beadlike and occur along the course of the vessels, thus justifying the use of the term "nodosa." It has also been called periarteritis nodosa. The disease is not confined to lesions around the vessels but affects the vascular coats of the vessels themselves.

There may be general systemic manifestations, as occur in disseminated lupus erythematosus, but in addition, polyarteritis nodosa has distinctive lesions of focal necrotizing inflammation of the walls of medium and small blood vessels, particularly the arterioles and small arteries. The vessel lumen may be swollen to the point of closure, with resultant thrombosis. This disease predominantly affects males, usually between the ages of 20 and 50 years. The disease may run an uninterrupted course leading to death, but on the other hand, there may be periods of remission. It is usually fatal, however, with death occurring as a rule in the first year. The characteristic symptoms are a low-grade fever, malaise, weakness, and leukocytosis. Disturbances in the kidneys, liver, and gastrointestinal tract are prominent. There is hematuria, albuminuria, abdominal pain and diarrhea or even melena, and muscular pain; the central nervous system may be involved as well.[4,6]

Many believe this disease is caused by hypersensitivity or allergy. A number of cases are associated with bronchial asthma and drug sensitivity on an allergic basis.[6]

Dermatomyositis and scleroderma[1, 6]

Dermatomyositis and scleroderma are systemic collagen diseases, but they have not been definitely linked to hypersensitivity reactions. These two diseases have much in common in clinical manifestations, with about the same age (30 to 50 years) and sex distribution (slightly more women affected than men).[6] The term "dermatomyositis" means involvement of the skin (*derma*) and muscles (*myo*); the term "scleroderma" literally defines itself, since *sclero* means hard and *derma* means skin. This disease is characterized by a tightly bound and nonelastic skin.

Dermatomyositis is associated with fever, joint pains, lymphadenopathy and splenomegaly, and edematous subcutaneous lesions of the skin. These symptoms are usually present in the acute stages. In the cases with insidious onset the symptoms are less marked, with low-grade fever and vague muscular and joint pains, malaise and weakness, and erythema of the skin. It is usually fatal within 3 years of onset.[6]

Diffuse scleroderma is mild in onset and runs a less rapid course than dermatomyositis. It is characterized by paresthesia, sensitivity to cold, stiffness of the joints and in the acute forms, nonpitting edema. The distinctive sign of this disease is the skin's loss of elasticity until it eventually becomes bound to the underlying tissues with no flexibility. When this occurs, there is decreased ability to move the body, and the muscles undergo atrophy from disuse and ischemia. The blood vessels in the muscles are constricted because of atrophy.[6]

Allergic disorders

Food allergy.[18] A specific food hypersensitivity or allergy can occur, characterized by recurrence of the same allergic symptoms whenever that food is eaten for as long as the person retains that specific allergy. Symptoms may involve the skin, respiratory or gastrointestinal tracts, or vital organs may be involved, leading to shock in rare cases. Both immediate and delayed forms of allergic response occur. The symptoms are affected by many factors, such as the quantity of food eaten, degree of change brought about by cooking food, and number of allergenic foods eaten in combination. Food does not have to be eaten, however, to cause symptoms, since inhaling the steam when the food is cooking provokes an allergic response. Insulin derived from beef or pork when used to treat human diabetes may cause an allergic reaction in a patient sensitive to these meats.

The most common symptoms of food allergy are urticaria, eczema, vomiting and diarrhea, but asthma, rhinitis, migraine headache, and serious shock may also occur. Some allergic reactions are confined solely to the gastrointestinal tract and may mimic other disorders of the digestive tract.

The most common food allergens are fish, seafood, berries (particularly strawberries), nuts, eggs, cereals, milk, beef, pork, chocolate, beans, peanuts, and fresh fruits of the peach family. Usually a food allergy develops after a number of exposures to the food, but the allergic individual may find that he reacts to foods that are members of the same biological family of plants. For example, if he reacts to brussel sprouts, he may also react to mustard, radishes, and cabbages, all members of the same family.

Drug allergy.[19] For thousands of years humans have been using various herbs and juices and saps from plants to treat their illnesses. Added to these medications are many sophisticated chemicals used in treatment of a myriad of diseases. With this exposure to drugs, it is only natural that adverse reactions would develop in some individuals.

In an allergic drug reaction there is at least one experience of previous exposure to the drug. Following this exposure there is a latent period during which the antibodies or cells sensitized to the drug are formed, usually a period of 1 to 2 weeks.[19]

When the drug is administered again, the sensitized cells lead to the symptons of allergy. The symptoms may be immediate or delayed. Most drug reactions are similar to those precipitated by pollens or food. Cutaneous reactions are common and include contact dermatitis and dermatitis medicamentosa. Allergic photosensitivity reactions may occur after any means of drug administration and consist of redness, skin lesions, scaling, and swelling on areas exposed to sunlight. Drugs are probably the most common cause of allergic urticaria, described later.

Systemic symptoms of drug allergy may affect any organ of the body. Anaphylaxis is a serious form of drug allergy but occurs less often than other reactions. Serum sickness is another generalized allergic drug reaction and was originally seen in response to injections of nonhuman blood protein. Today this reaction is seen less frequently because of the increased use of drugs and human sera. Animal serum, however, is still used to treat rabies, some snake and spider bites, gas gangrene, botulism, and diphtheria. Primary serum sickness begins 6 to 10 days after the medication is received. First symptoms are fever, rash, joint pains, itching, and inflammation of certain lymph glands. This usually lasts about a week.

Various blood cells may also be destroyed in drug allergy. Thrombocytopenia results if the platelets are affected. Red blood cell destruction causes hemolytic anemia, and injury to white blood cells results in agranulocytosis. If all three types of cells are affected in the bone marrow, an aplastic anemia develops. If circulating cells are injured, it is called pancytopenia.

Penicillin, sulfonamides, and aspirin are the three most common drugs involved in drug allergy, possibly up to 90%.[19] Penicillin is possibly the most common drug involved in allergic drug reaction, most often characterized by urticaria or other rashes, but serum sickness and anaphylaxis can occur.

The longer-acting sulfur drugs are a potential allergen. The reactions to sulfur drugs include urticaria, angioedema, rashes, blood disorders, and inflammation of blood vessels. Included in this category are medications such as sulfur antibiotics, diuretics, and oral hypoglycemics.

Other drugs causing allergic reactions are antituberculosis medications and antibiotics other than penicillin, barbiturates, local anesthetics, anticonvulsants, tranquilizers, vaccines, and antithyroid drugs, heavy metals, and organ extracts. Contrast media containing iodides used for certain x rays may also cause severe allergic reactions. There are also problems with skin testing for drug allergens. A detailed medical history is a must to discover what drugs the patient has taken. Too often laxatives, vitamins, birth control pills, pain relievers, nose drops, tonics, aspirin, ointments, douches, and suppositories are not considered to be drugs by the patient and are not mentioned, yet any one of these may cause a drug reaction.

Hay fever.[4, 6, 10, 11, 17] Hay fever is an allergic rhinitis. It is either seasonal caused by pollens or nonseasonal or perennial caused by antigens other than pollens. Dusts are common offenders.

Allergic rhinitis is characterized by edema, watering of the eyes, itching, and increased mucous secretions of the nasal mucosa, with sneezing. The term "vasomotor rhinitis" has been applied to both perennial allergic rhinitis and to the types with chronic edema of the nasal mucosa that are caused by nonantigenic irritants or that have a neurogenic or psychosomatic basis.

The mechanism of the triggering response to inhaled allergens can be explained on the following basis. The nose warms and purifies the inhaled air, removing dust particles, which are deposited on the mucosa. These are exposed to inhaled allergens. Hay fever is caused by sensitizing antibodies in the conjunctiva, nasal mucosa, skin, and blood plasma. When allergic pollens contact the sensitized mucosa, an antigen-antibody reaction is provoked. This causes the blood vessels to become engorged, which is followed by edema and increased mucous secretion, with itching and resultant sneezing. The physiologic effects are believed to be the result of release of histamine.

The allergic sensitization causing hay fever is the same type that occurs in infantile eczema, urticaria, bronchial asthma, and some forms of food allergy. Therefore, persons suffering from hay fever may also have manifestations of one of these forms of allergy. All the diseases of this group tend to occur in families, but none is inherited; as stated before, only the predisposition to become allergic to certain antigens is inherited.[6, 14]

The plants most often implicated in hay fever are ragweed and similar plants and grasses that are dependent upon wind dissemination of pollen for cross-pollination. These are seasonal for each type of plant, from early spring through late summer. In the United States ragweed grows abundantly, and hay fever is one of the most prevalent types of allergies in this country.[17]

Urticaria.[2, 15, 16] The term "urticaria" is derived from the Latin word *urere,* meaning to burn (Fig. 13-1). The pruritic erythematous or whitish swellings or wheals on the skin in this condition are characterized by burning or itching. Urticaria is commonly known as hives. The wheals occur most often in areas covered by constrictive clothing, but may occur anywhere on the body and are of various sizes and shapes. In giant urticaria or angioneurotic edema the wheals appear on the mucous membranes, especially the lips, the mouth, and in the throat, with laryngeal edema that may cause the patient to choke to death. The wheals are caused by the release of histamine in the skin from damaged mast cells. Mast cells are located along the finer cutaneous blood vessels and are a reservoir for histamine. As a result of the sudden release of histamine there is

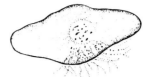

Damaged mast cell releases histamine

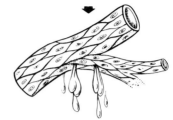

Increased permeability of blood vessels causes fluids and cells to pour into the dermis

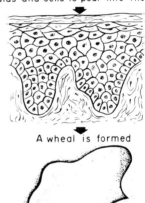

A wheal is formed

Fig. 13-1. Pathogenesis of urticaria.

a localized increase in capillary permeability that causes an outpouring of serum proteins and fluids into the tissues in the affected area, producing the characteristic wheal. The wheals may last from minutes to hours or even years, sometimes with inexplicable spontaneous remissions.[8, 16]

Urticaria may result from a variety of allergens; some are easily identified by skin testing, while others are identified only after extensive examination for the underlying cause. The precipitating factors may be ingestants, inhalants, contacts with fabrics or pets, therapeutic agents, infections, infestations with parasites, physical factors such as heat, cold, and light, or emotional stress or other psychologic factors. As can readily be seen, some of these factors are exogenous and others are endogenous. The acute or immediate type of urticaria is almost always provoked by exogenous substances, particularly food and inhalants such as danders and perfumes. Fresh berries, spices, chocolate, fish, and nuts are the foods most often implicated. A foci of infection is often a cause of chronic urticaria in children, with dental infections ranking high. The delayed type of response may become chronic because of the problems involved in identifying the proper allergen or inciting factor.[2, 15]

Although we commonly think of urticaria or hives as occurring mostly on the skin and other mucous membranes, it is believed they occur in the gastrointestinal tract and the meninges. The migraine type of headache may reflect urticarial processes in the meninges. Gastrointestinal upsets and headaches formerly believed to be the cause of cutaneous hives are now believed to occur as a result of wheals in internal organs.[13]

Asthma.[9, 10, 14, 20] Asthma is a noncontagious disease of the lungs. It affects nearly 9 million Americans, young and old. Symptoms of asthma are shortness of breath, choked breathing, wheezing, and a productive coughing of copious amounts of mucous secretions. Coughing is triggered by the body attempting to rid itself of the excess mucous in the lungs. During an attack, the victim struggles to breathe air into and out of his lungs through the bronchial airways, whose mucous linings have become swollen with fluid. During normal breathing there is no resistance in the airways, but during an asthmatic attack the spastic contractions of smooth muscles in the lung practically close the passageways of the bronchioli. When the bronchial tubes are closed, the stale air is trapped in the alveoli and fresh air is prevented from entering. Exhalation becomes increasingly difficult, and forced breathing results. If forced breathing occurs over a period of

time, there is danger of developing a concomitant emphysema. (See p. 314.) The wheezing sound is produced by air rushing through the narrow passageways during an asthmatic attack.

Asthmatics are generally categorized as extrinsic or intrinsic. Extrinsic asthma, as the name implies, is caused by outside factors. There is usually a history of allergies, which may also be common among other family members. Allergens include house dust, foods, animal danders and hairs, feathers, wool, cosmetics, pollen, molds, bermuda grass, fabrics, injections of bacterial origin, and fur. There is now growing evidence that air pollution may be implicated in causing asthma. Some people suffer asthmatic attacks from exposure to smog. Seasonal hay fever can also trigger asthmatic attacks.

The intrinsic category of asthmatics includes those in whom no external allergic factors can be identified, but who suffer from the same type of devastating attacks as extrinsic asthmatics. Most asthmatics fall in this category. Infection can be a significant factor in intrinsic asthma. In a network of asthma and allergic disease centers whose scientists are investigating the role of infection and related factors in asthma, it has been found that respiratory viruses, especially those responsible for the common cold, are a prominent cause of intrinsic asthma. The second most common cause is influenza virus. In a significant number of asthmatics aspirin has been found to be the cause of an attack, although the person might not have been allergic to it.

Emotional stresses are implicated as triggering attacks in many asthmatics, both children and adults, but these are considered more important as secondary factors than as primary causative ones.

When an asthmatic attack fails to respond to usual drug treatment, the individual is said to be in status asthmaticus. This is a sudden serious intense and continuous aggravation of asthmatic attack, which is marked by dyspnea to the point of exhaustion and collapse.

Asthma is not an inherited disease, but a strong predisposition to become sensitive to certain substances, such as foods and inhalants, is inherited.[14] Many asthmatics are members of families where the parents and siblings or close relatives have either asthma or hay fever.

Only recently have scientists begun to unravel some of the underlying complex mechanisms of allergy and asthma.[20] Recently it has been discovered that there is a unique kind of blood protein called immunoglobulin E (IgE), also called reagin, present in large amounts in patients with allergies and extrinsic asthma.[20] IgE is found only in small amounts in nonallergic individuals and intrinsic asthmatics. The IgE antibodies are formed in response to environmental allergens and attach themselves to specific cells, tissue mast cells in the mucous membranes and skin and basophils in the blood. According to the mast cell theory of asthma, the allergens are attached to the IgE antibody that is bound to the surface of these cells. The antigen-antibody reaction that results causes the mast cells to release their chemical contents—histamine and slow-reacting substance of anaphylaxis (SRS-A). These chemical mediators travel short distances to the affected respiratory tissue and cause secretion of fluid and mucus to increase and bronchial smooth muscle to constrict. Other released chemical factors cause the macrophages to accumulate with additional resultant inflammation. At the present time it is not known whether asthmatics have inherited an increased ability to make IgE or have an abnormality in mast cells.[20] Asthmatics may have an increased susceptibility to histamine or SRS-A release.

Contact dermatitis.[21] Contact dermatitis is a delayed type of response to allergens that results from contact of the skin surface with a variety of substances. Damaged skin is more susceptible to sensitization than normal skin. Circulating antibodies are not ordinarily demonstrated.

Almost anyone can develop contact dermatitis from repeated exposure to potent sensitizing agents, such as arsenicals, mercury compounds, sulfonamides, cosmetics, clothing dyes, paints, varnishes, plastics, topical medications, and plants. The contact may be limited to a specific area, but the symptoms of itching, redness, skin rash, or eruptions may be generalized.

The most notable example of contact dermatitis is the reaction to poison ivy, a plant. The lesions are often profuse and are characterized by edema, marked erythema, and vesicles and bullae. Dermatitis from contact with poison ivy does not occur immediately but is delayed for several hours or more, and then the lesions are more or less generalized.

Responses

Step 1: hypersensitivity
Step 2: immunity
Step 3: antibody
Step 4: antigen
Step 5: antigen-antibody
Step 6: 1. passive; 2. active
Step 7: 1. A; 2. A; 3. P; 4. P; 5. A; 6. P; 7. A
Step 8: 1. X; 2. X; 4. X; 5. X; 7. X
Step 9: 1. T; 2. T; 3. T; 4. F; 5. F
Step 10: sensitization
Step 11: immediate; delayed
Step 12: 1. immediate; 2. immediate; 3. delayed; 4. immediate; 5. delayed
Step 13: anaphylactic shock
Step 14: serum sickness
Step 15: allergens
Step 16: 1. hay fever; 2. asthma; 3. urticaria; 4. gastroenteritis (or equivalent response)
Step 17: autoimmune
Step 18: collagen

REFERENCES

1. Allen, A. C.: In Anderson, W. A. D., editor: Pathology, ed. 6, St. Louis, 1971, The C. V. Mosby Co. (hypersensitivity diseases).
2. Brodkey, M. H.: Nebr. State Med. J. 46:479, 1961 (urticaria).
3. Cluff, L. E.: In Harrison, T. R., and others, editors: Principles of internal medicine, ed. 4, New York, 1962, Blakiston Division, McGraw-Hill Book Co. (hypersensitivities).
4. Cooke, R. A.: In Prigal, S. J., editor: Fundamentals of modern allergy, New York, 1960,

Blakiston Division, McGraw-Hill Book Co. (allergies).

5. Hamilton, T. R., and Hamilton, B. W.: In Miller, S. E., editor: A textbook of clinical pathology, ed. 7, Baltimore, 1966, The Williams & Wilkins Co. (clinical immunology).

6. Hopps, H. C.: In Anderson, W. A. D., editor: Pathology, ed. 6, St. Louis, 1971, The C. V. Mosby Co. (hypersensitivity).

7. Kunkel, H. G.: In Beeson, P. B., and McDermott, W., editors: Cecil-Loeb textbook of medicine, ed. 13, Philadelphia, 1971, W. B. Saunders Co. (skin testing).

8. Robinson, H. M., Jr., and Robinson, R. C. V.: Clinical dermatology for students and practitioners, Baltimore, 1959, The Williams & Wilkins Co. (allergies).

9. Rubin, M. I.: In Nelson, W. E., editor: Textbook of pediatrics, ed. 7, Philadelphia, 1959, W. B. Saunders Co. (immunity, allergies).

10. Sherman, W. B.: In Prigal, S. J., editor: Fundamentals of modern allergy, New York, 1960, Blakiston Division, McGraw-Hill Book Co. (allergies).

11. Sherman, W.: In Beeson, P. B., and McDermott, W., editors: Cecil-Loeb textbook of medicine, ed. 13, Philadelphia, 1971, W. B. Saunders Co. (hayfever and allergy tests).

12. Sonnenwirth, A. C.: In Frankel, S., Reitman, S., and Sonnenwirth, A. C., editors: Gradwohl's clinical laboratory methods and diagnosis, ed. 7, St. Louis, 1970, The C. V. Mosby Co. (basic principles of immunology).

13. Sulzberger, M. B., and Wolf, J.: Dermatology: diagnosis and treatment, ed. 2, Chicago, 1961, Year Book Medical Publishers, Inc.

14. Swartz, H. Z.: Allergy, what it is and what to do about it, New York, 1966, Frederick Ungar Publishing Co., Inc.

15. Tudor, R. B.: Lancet **82:**273, 1962 (urticaria).

16. Unger, A. H.: Tex. Med. **56:**347, 1960 (urticaria).

17. U.S. Department of Health, Education, and Welfare, Public Health Service Publication No. 208, Health Information Series 17, 1967 (hay fever).

18. U.S. Department of Health, Education, and Welfare, Public Health Service, National Institutes of Health, DHEW Pub. No. (NIH) 74-533, 1974 (food allergy).

19. U.S. Department of Health, Education, and Welfare, Public Health Service, National Institutes of Health, DHEW Pub. No. (NIH) 75-703, 1975 (drug allergy).

20. U.S. Department of Health, Education, and Welfare, Public Health Service, National Institutes of Health, DHEW Pub. No. (NIH) 73-525, 1975 (asthma).

21. Wheeler, C. E.: In Beeson, P. B., and McDermott, W., editors: Cecil-Loeb textbook of medicine, ed. 13, Philadelphia, 1971, W. B. Saunders Co. (contact dermatitis).

CHAPTER 14

Infectious disease

An infection is an invasion of the body by microorganisms or biologic agents that cause tissue damage and disease. The microorganisms, regardless of whether they are bacteria, viruses, rickettsiae, fungi, protozoa, or helminths, cause disease only as an expression of their struggle for survival in the competitive biology of life. Bacteria and parasites, in particular, are dependent upon humans for life to a greater or lesser extent. Humans in turn prey on lower life for survival by consuming both plants and animals.

We survive in a crowded world of microorganisms, but only a relatively few of them are harmful. Many are incapable of producing disease; some coexist with us without injury to their host because of our mechanisms of natural resistance and immunity, evolved on a basis of live and let live with the world of microorganisms. Although we cannot deny the microorganism's existence in the biologic world, we have overcome their harmful effects in many instances through acquired immunity as a result of previous exposure. The ever-present flora of the skin, mouth, and body openings and surfaces do not gain entrance to our vital internal tissues because of the body's defense mechanisms and also through personal hygienic health measures that minimize their potential danger. Thus in this coexistence we have the ability to tip the balance in our favor through our knowledge of the harmful potentialities of certain microorganisms and by being on guard against them. Some microorganisms are beneficial such as the *Escherichia coli* flora of the intestinal tract, which produces vitamin K, an antihemorrhagic factor necessary for the maintenance of health.

Table 4 is included for reference on viruses, bacteria, rickettsiae, fungi, protozoa, and helminths that cause diseases, since it is not possible to describe in detail the many diseases attributed to these organisms in a discussion of limited scope. In addition to Table 4 a few representative diseases are discussed at the end of the chapter.

The infectious diseases have no doubt always plagued human beings, and some of them like leprosy were recognized in early Biblical history. Formerly many of them occurred in pandemics and epidemics of plague, cholera, smallpox, and typhus, taking a devastating toll of life. These have been largely eradicated from human existence through recognition of the causative agents and through methods of control or eradication. Some sporadic epidemics do, however, occur in thickly populated and poorly developed areas of the world. The last great pandemic was influenza following World War I (1914 to 1919), with an estimated 500 million cases and 15 million fatalities. Asian (type A) influenza occurred in pandemic form in 1957, but the loss of life and worldwide distribution was far less than occurred after World War I.[20] Most of the deaths that now occur in influenza epidemics are attributed to bacterial invaders—streptococcus, staphylococcus, pneumococcus, meningococcus, and

Text continued on p. 197.

185

Table 4. Infectious diseases

Disease	Infectious agent	Reservoir, source, mode of transmission	Principal organ or system affected; incubation period when known or applicable
Viral infections			
Chicken pox (varicella)	Varicella-zoster (V-Z) virus	Reservoir: infected person Source: nose and throat secretions Transmission: direct and indirect	Skin rash: systemic symptoms; incubation 2 to 3 weeks, 13 to 17 days
Cytomegalic inclusion disease	Herpes virus	Reservoir: man Transmission: possibly placental; other routes not exactly known	Salivary glands; inclusions found in other organs
Dengue fever	Arbovirus (group B)	Reservoir: man, mosquito Source: bite of infective mosquito	Skin rash, generalized aches and pains; incubation 3 to 15 days
Encephalitis, St. Louis	Arbovirus (group B)	Reservoir: infected mosquitoes Transmission: bite of infected mosquito	Brain
Encephalomyelitis eastern equine	Arbovirus (group A)	Reservoir: birds Transmission: mosquito infected by horse; man infected by bite of mosquito	Brain
Hepatitis, A and B	Virus types A and B	Reservoir: man Source: blood and feces of infected person Transmission: contaminated food, water and milk; possible intimate contact	Liver; gastrointestinal tract and kidney, when systemic; incubation variable 10 to 40 days
Herpes simplex (cold sore or fever blister)	Virus	Reservoir: man Transmission: direct contact as by kissing	Lips and buccal mocosa; may involve conjunctiva and facial skin
Herpes simplex, neonatorum	Virus	Reservoir: usually history of herpetic vulvovaginitis in mother	Necrosis in liver and adrenals; infant becomes ill fourth to fifth day after birth; may die in few days
Herpes zoster (shingles)	Varicella-zoster (V-Z) virus	Reservoir: man, usually known contact with chickenpox	Sensory nerve trunks; incubation 7 to 24 days
Influenza	Viruses A, B, and C have been identified	Reservoir: man Source: discharges from nose and throat of infected person; direct or indirect transmission	Respiratory symptoms, but may be generalized
Lymphogranuloma inguinale	Bedsonia (miyagawa-nella)	Reservoir: man Transmission: sexual intercourse	Primary lesion on genitalia (or cervix in women); inguinal lymph nodes incubation 7 to 12 days
Measles (rubeola)	Virus	Reservoir: man Source: secretions from nose and throat of infected person; intimate personal contact or by droplet spray or indirectly by fomites	Skin rash; disease becomes generalized; mucous membrane of respiratory tract; conjunctivae; incubation 14 to 21 days

Table 4. Infectious diseases—cont'd

Disease	Infectious agent	Reservoir, source, mode of transmission	Principal organ or system affected; incubation period when known or applicable
Viral infections—cont'd			
Measles, German (rubella)	Virus	Reservoir: man Source: nasopharyngeal discharges Transmission: direct contact, droplet spread, and fomites; may cross placental barrier and affect fetus	Skin rash; mild catarrhal symptoms; incubation 14 to 21 days
Mumps	Virus	Reservoir: man Source: saliva of infected person Transmission: direct contact, droplet spray, or fomites	Salivary glands, usually parotid; after puberty may affect testes or ovaries and may involve CNS; communicability as long as glands swollen
Poliomyelitis, acute anterior; spinal; and bulbar	Polioviruses types 1, 2, and 3	Reservoir: man Source: pharyngeal secretions and feces of infected persons Transmission: direct contact, droplet infection, milk (rare)	Voluntary muscles; anterior horns of spine; cranial and spinal nerves in bulbar type; incubation 2 to 14 days
Psittacosis (parrot fever)	Bedsonia (miyagawanella)	Reservoir and source: infected bird of parrot family or parrakeet; healthy bird may be carrier	Respiratory tract
Rabies (hydrophobia)	Neurotropic virus	Reservoir and source: infected dog, cat, wolf, skunk, vampire bat, and other animals, wild or domestic Transmission: bite of infected animal or saliva into wound	Central nervous system; incubation 10 days to 1 year or more
Smallpox (variola)	Virus	Reservoir: man Source: respiratory discharges of patient, lesions of skin and mucous membrane, or contamination with these Transmission: direct contact with infected patient; indirectly by contaminated articles or discharges	Cutaneous lesions, eruption generalized; systemic manifestations; incubation 7 to 16 days, commonly 12 days
Trachoma	Bedsonia (chlamydia)	Reservoir: man Source: ocular secretions of infected person Transmission: contact with ocular secretions	Conjunctiva, with later invasion of cornea, often leading to blindness
Yellow fever	Virus	Reservoir: man Source: man in urban areas; may be monkey or marmoset in forest areas; immediate source for man is infective mosquito Transmission: bite of *Aedes aegypti*	Liver; GI tract; kidney in systemic spread; incubation 2 to 5 days, maximum 6 days

Continued.

Table 4. Infectious diseases—cont'd

Disease	Infectious agent	Reservoir, source, mode of transmission	Principal organ or system affected; incubation period when known or applicable
Spirochetal infections			
Pinta	*Treponema carateum*	Reservoir: man Transmission: inoculation into skin, usually on exposed parts, from lesions; direct contact	Dermatoses; papular, macular lesions; in later stages there is depigmentation and severe atrophy of epidermis; incubation 7 to 20 days
Rat-bite fever	*Spirillum minus*	Reservoir: rat Transmission: bite of infected rat or mouse; reported from bite of dog, cat, pig, squirrel, ferret, and weasel	Inflammation or ulceration of bite lesion lymphadenopathy; rash; generalized spread; incubation 10 to 22 days
Relapsing fever	*Borrelia recurrentis*	Reservoir: man Source: infected louse Transmission: crushing of infected louse into bite wound or abrasion of skin	Petechial rashes; systemic febrile paroxysms alternating with afebrile periods; incubation up to 12 days, usually 7 days
Syphilis	*Treponema pallidum*	Reservoir: man Transmission: sexual intercourse; infected mother to fetus in utero; infected blood in blood transfusion (rare)	Chancre, primary stage; rash, secondary stage; systemic spread, tertiary stage (mainly cardiovascular, skeletal, and central nervous system); congenital, various deformities (saber shin, Hutchinson's teeth, deafness, blindness) and mental retardation in some; incubation period variable before chancre 10 to 90 days
Weil's disease	*Leptospira icterohaemorrhagiae*	Reservoir: rat or other wild animal, but also some domestic animals Transmission: contamination with urine or feces of infected animal	Liver with necrosis and liver cell degeneration; incubation 6 to 12 days
Yaws	*Treponema pertenue*	Reservoir: man Transmission: usually wound in contact with lesion of infected person; not a venereal disease	Primary yaw on exposed portion of body; secondary lesions are skin eruptions; tertiary lesions are ulcers and gummas of tibia and radius; other bone deformities; cardiovascular and CNS lesions; incubation 10 to 90 days
Bacterial infections			
Anthrax	*Bacillus anthracis*	Reservoir: animals, especially cow, but also sheep and horse Transmission: handling of infected wool, hides, and carcasses	Malignant pustule at site of entrance of spore; bloody mucinous edema in many tissues and serous cavities

Table 4. Infectious diseases—cont'd

Disease	Infectious agent	Reservoir, source, mode of transmission	Principal organ or system affected; incubation period when known or applicable
Bacterial infections—cont'd			
Botulism	*Clostridium botulinum*	Source: toxin produced outside body and introduced in food, usually home-canned vegetables	Symptoms start in gastrointestinal tract and spread to nervous system 3 to 4 hours after ingestion, but may start as long as 36 hours after eating infected food
Brucellosis (undulant fever)	*Brucella abortus* and *Brucella suis* in United States; *Brucella melitensis* in Malta fever (Mediterranean	Reservoir: usually cow, hog, goat Transmission: contact with infected animal; organism can pass through unbroken skin; ingestion of infected milk	Reticuloendothelial tissues; lymphatics; it is a septicemic disease with lesions in many organs
Chancroid	*Haemophilus ducreyi*	Reservoir: man Transmission: sexual intercourse	Chancroidal ulcers on and around genitalia
Cholera	*Vibrio cholerae*	Reservoir: infected person Source: feces and vomitus of infected person Transmission: contaminated water, food, hands, utensils, or flies	Acute intestinal infection; incubation 1 to 5 days
Diphtheria	*Corynebacterium diphtheriae* (Klebs-Löffler bacillus)	Source: direct contact and human carrier, although dust may contain virulent organisms for several days Transmission: contact with infected person and nasopharyngeal discharges	Mucous membranes of throat mainly; incubation 2 to 7 days: toxemia may be profound in this disease
Dysentery, bacillary	Various species of genus *Shigella*	Reservoir: man Source: feces of infected person Transmission: contaminated food and drink and asymptomatic carriers	Intestinal infection, mainly colon involved, but occasionally ileum; incubation 2 to 7 days
Escherichia coli infections	*Escherichia coli* (*Bacillus coli*)	Source: normally intestinal tract of man	Urinary infections; wound infection; intestinal infection as cause, or contributor
Erysipelas	*Streptococcus pyogenes* (group A)	Reservoir: man Source: respiratory discharges of same individual or exogenous origin Transmission: direct contact; indirect contact with fomites	Cellulitis lesion at portal of entry; incubation unknown but probably 2 days
Food poisoning	Usually *Salmonella* group; also *Staphylococcus*	Transmission: two types, ingestion of preformed toxin; ingestion of viable microorganisms; botulism is preformed type	Gastrointestinal infection; Salmonella incubation 12 to 24 hours; staphylococcic incubation 1 to 6 hours, with 3 hours average

Continued.

Table 4. Infectious diseases—cont'd

Disease	Infectious agent	Reservoir, source, mode of transmission	Principal organ or system affected; incubation period when known or applicable
Bacterial infections—cont'd			
Gas gangrene	*Clostridium welchii*	Source: exogenous, usually contaminated soil, etc. Transmission: wound or abrasion contaminated from soil (as in gunshot wound in battle)	Tissues in region of wound with spread through bloodstream throughout system; incubation 2 to 3 days
Glanders	*Malleomyces mallei* or *Actinobacillus*	Reservoir: animal, mainly horse, mule, goat Source: infected discharges from animal Transmission: through either skin or mucous membrane	Inflammatory nodules in mucous membrane of nose or skin, with ulcer formation; lungs, regional lymph nodes and many other organs affected by granulomas
Gonorrhea	*Neisseria gonorrhoeae*	Reservoir: man Source: sexual intercourse; infants may be infected by contaminated articles or by discharge from infected mother during birth process	Acute infection of reproductive organs—fallopian tubes in women and prostate and seminal vesicles in men, in addition to urethra; affects eyes in infants; incubation 2 to 10 days
Granuloma venereum	*Donovania granulomatis* (Donovan bodies)	Reservoir: man Source: organisms found free in discharge from lesion or intracellularly in cytoplasm of macrophages; venereal transmission is questioned; found mostly in lower economic strata where cleanliness is lacking	Vesicles, papules, and nodules may involve all of inguinal region from original papule on genitalia or in pubic region; incubation probably 1 to 4 weeks
Impetigo contagiosa	*Staphylococcus aureus* as a rule	Communicable disease limited mainly to children Transmission: direct contact; indirect contact with fomites	Initial lesions are vesicular and later crusted seropurulent plaques, usually on face and hands; incubation 2 to 5 days
Leprosy	*Mycobacterium leprae*	Reservoir: man Transmission: direct contact with infected individual; indirect contact with contaminated articles	Skin; nerves (peripheral); eyes; upper respiratory tract; can develop up to 20 years after exposure, but generally in 3 years.
Meningitis, meningococcal (fulminant type called Waterhouse-Friderichsen)	*Neisseria meningitidis*	Reservoir: man Source: nasopharyngeal discharges Transmission: direct contact from droplet spray; indirect contact from soiled linens or articles (rare); spread through healthy carrier or one recently recovered from infection	Rash on skin frequent, but main effects are on central nervous system, with involvement of meninges; incubation 2 to 10 days

Table 4. Infectious diseases—cont'd

Disease	Infectious agent	Reservoir, source, mode of transmission	Principal organ or system affected; incubation period when known or applicable
Bacterial infections—cont'd			
Paratyphoid fever	*Salmonella paratyphi; Salmonella schott-mülleri; Salmonella hirschfeldii*	Reservoir: man Source: feces and urine of infected person; carriers frequent during epidemics Transmission. direct and indirect; food and drink contaminated by hands of carrier (missed cases are common vehicles); milk, milk products, and shellfish frequently responsible	Generalized infection, involving lymphoid mesenteric tissues and intestines, with enlargement of spleen; disease is similar to typhoid only not so severe
Plague	*Pasteurella pestis*	Reservoir: wild rodent Transmission: bubonic plague (infective rat flea *Xenopsylla cheopis*); pneumonic plague (person-to-person contact); accidental infections in laboratory workers	Bubonic plague, buboes of lymph nodes and spread through bloodstream; both bubonic and pneumonic are septicemic diseases, with lungs and other organs involved; incubation bubonic 2 to 6 days; penumonic 3 to 4 days
Pneumonia, bacterial	*Streptococcus pyogenes* (group A hemolytic streptococci); *Staphylococcus aureus; Klebsiella pneumoniae* (Friedländer bacillus); *Haemophilus influenzae*	Reservoir: man Source: pulmonary discharges Transmission: direct contact with patient and carrier; indirect contact by droplet spread and fomites	Pulmonary involvement; incubation variable, usually short, 1 to 3 days
Pneumonia, pneumococcic	*Diplococcus pneumoniae*	Reservoir: man Source: respiratory secretions of infected persons Transmission: direct contact with patients and carriers: indirect contact with fomites	Pulmonary involvement; incubation believed to be 1 to 3 days
Pneumonia, primary atypical	PPLO—*Mycoplasma pneumoniae*	Reservoir: man Source: respiratory secretions of infected person Transmission: direct contact with patients or carriers, droplet spread, and fomites	Respiratory system, mainly lungs; incubation believed to be 7 to 21 days
Scarlet fever (scarlatina)	*Streptococcus pyogenes*	Reservoir: man Source: oral discharges of patient or contaminated articles, food, and water Transmission: direct or indirect contact (by droplet spray)	Erythematous fine rash and sore throat; hyperemia and marked red discoloration of skin; may become disseminated and involve many organs; incubation 2 to 5 days

Continued.

Table 4. Infectious diseases—cont'd

Disease	Infectious agent	Reservoir, source, mode of transmission	Principal organ or system affected; incubation period when known or applicable
Bacterial infections—cont'd			
Tetanus (lockjaw)	*Clostridium tetani* (tetanus bacillus)	Reservoir: man and domestic animals, particularly horse Source: soil, street dust, or animal or human feces Transmission: spores at sites of injury, burns, or wounds	Primary nervous system, peripheral nerves and anterior horn cells; incubation 4 days to 3 or more weeks
Tuberculosis (pulmonary)	*Mycobacterium tuberculosis* (tubercle bacilli)	Reservoir: man or infected cow Source: respiratory secretions or milk from tubercular cow (persons with extrapulmonary tuberculosis seldom transmit disease) Transmission: direct or indirect contact (droplet spray or fomites)	Pulmonary disorder but may be extrapulmonary; incubation from infection to primary lesion, 4 to 6 weeks; time of infection to progressive symptoms, may be years; first 6 to 12 months most hazardous
Tularemia (rabbit fever)	*Pasteurella tularensis*	Reservoir: wild animals, such as rabbit, hare, ground squirrel Transmission: direct contact with infected animal through unbroken skin, bite of insect (especially tick, horsefly, or deerfly), or eating poorly cooked infected meat; most dangerous infectious agent for laboratory worker	Suppurative or granulomatous lesions and septicemia; it begins as an ulcer, usually on hand or finger; incubation 3 to 5 days
Typhoid fever	*Salmonella typhosa*	Reservoir: man, patients and carriers Source: feces and urine of infected person Transmission: direct or indirect contact; food and water are principal vehicles	Gastrointestinal involvement becoming systemic; rose spots on trunk; lymphoid tissue involvement; incubation 10 to 14 days
Whooping cough (pertussis)	*Bordetella pertussis* (*Hemophilus pertussis*)	Reservoir: man; mainly a communicable disease of children Transmission: contact with droplet spray, fomites, or patients	Respiratory tract; incubation 4 to 16 days
Rickettsial infections			
Q fever	*Coxiella burnetii*	Transmission: probably tick among lower animals and occasionally man; probable inhalation of contaminated dust from skins of infected animals	Respiratory system mostly affected

Table 4. Infectious diseases—cont'd

Disease	Infectious agent	Reservoir, source, mode of transmission	Principal organ or system affected; incubation period when known or applicable
Rickettsial infections—cont'd			
Rocky Mt. spotted fever	*Rickettsia rickettsii*	Transmission: arthropod (tick) bite	Hemorrhagic lesions and rash; lesions occur in brain, myocardium and lungs. Rash occurs 2 to 5 days after onset of fever
Trench fever	*Rickettsia quintana*	Transmission: louse (bite or contact with feces of louse)	Macular rash; systemic spread; essentially a "war" disease; incubation is short
Tsutsugamushi fever or scrub typhus	*Rickettsia tsutsuga- mushi*	Reservoir: vole, mouse and probably other rodents (intermediate mammalian hosts) Transmission: bite of mite	Neurologic symptoms; systemic involvement with vascular lesions; ulcer at site of bite and regional lymph nodes enlarged; rash on palms and soles of feet
Typhus, epidemic murine or endemic	*Rickettsia prowazekii Rickettsia mooseri*	Reservoir: man Immediate source: louse Transmission: when infected body louse excretes rickettsiae in feces and man rubs feces or crushed lice into wounds or abrasions of skin; inhalation of dried infective louse feces as dust from dirty clothes	Central nervous system; may be systemic; incubation 5 to 20 days in epidemic type and 5 to 12 days in endemic type
Fungal infections			
Actinomycosis (actinomycetic infection)	*Actinomyces bovis*	Source: exogenous	Many forms—systemic; cervicofacial; abdominal; pulmonary; granulomas of brain
Aspergillosis	*Aspergillus fumigatus*	Source: exogenous; may be found in air; agent opportunistic, gains foothold in body with lowered resistance from preexisting disease or following therapeutic regimen Transmission: inhaled by farmers from infected hay or other materials	Lungs; may be disseminated including brain; cutaneous type may be found in ears
Blastomycosis, North American and South American types	*Blastomyces dermatitidis; Blastomyces brasiliensis*	Source: exogenous Transmission: North American type, inhalation of conidia (saprophytic source in nature unknown)	Pulmonary form with generalized bone and subcutaneous tissue involvement in N.A. lymph nodes and mucous type; lesions principally in membranes in S.A. type
Coccidioidomycosis, desert fever, valley fever, San Joaquin Valley fever	*Coccidioides immitis*	Transmission: inhalation of fungus usually from dust	Primarily pulmonary, but may be disseminated

Continued.

Table 4. Infectious diseases—cont'd

Disease	Infectious agent	Reservoir, source, mode of transmission	Principal organ or system affected; incubation period when known or applicable
Fungal infections—cont'd			
Cryptococcosis or torulosis	*Cryptococcus neoformans* or *Torula histolytica*	Source: exogenous	Granulomatous lesions in lungs; meninges may become involved
Histoplasmosis	*Histoplasma capsulatum*	Source: soil and dust where birds, bats, and chickens have left excreta Transmission: inhaled by man	Pulmonary infection; may become disseminated
Moniliasis or Candidiasis Thrush in infants	*Candida albicans* or other *Candida*	Source: buccal cavity in some people, also respiratory tract and feces of healthy people; opportunistic organism following prolonged antibiotic or steroid therapy	Cutaneous, vulvovaginal, gastric, intestinal, and endocardial infections
Sporotrichosis	*Sporotrichum schenckii*	Transmission: through wound by contaminated sharp object; florists and gardeners often victims	Nodular necrotic lesion at point of entrance; may become systemic and tends to be chronic
Protozoal infections			
Amebiasis	*Entamoeba histolytica*	Reservoir; infected person or asymptomatic carrier Transmission: ingestion of food and water containing cysts of *Entamoeba histolytica* or contaminated vegetables; food may be contaminated by flies or food handlers	Gastrointestinal tract as a dysentry and spread to liver or other parts of body; incubation 5 days in severe cases and several months in mild ones
Leishmaniasis or visceral leishmaniasis (kala-azar)	*Leishmania donovani*	Source: sand fly Transmission: bite	Reticuloendothelial system; incubation 2 weeks to 8 months; a cutaneous form is known as oriental sore
Malaria	*Plasmodium vivax* for vivax malaria; *Plasmodium malariae* for quartan type; *Plasmodium falciparum* for falciparum type; *Plasmodium ovale* for less common ovale type	Reservoir: man and mosquito Direct source: *Anopheles* mosquito Transmission. from man to mosquito and back to man	Reticuloendothelial system, liver, spleen, bone marrow; recurrent cyclic fever; incubation *P. falciparum* 12 days; *P. vivax* and *P. ovale* 13 days; *P. malariae* 30 days; *P. vivax* may have protracted incubation of 8 to 10 months

Table 4. Infectious diseases—cont'd

Disease	Infectious agent	Reservoir, source, mode of transmission	Principal organ or system affected; incubation period when known or applicable
Protozoal infections—cont'd			
Trypanosomiasis, American, or Chagas' disease	*Trypanosoma cruzi*	Reservoir: wild and domestic animals. Source: large biting bugs. Transmission: rubbing feces or crushed bug into abrasion or skin puncture, frequently mucous membranes	Conjunctivae from bites around eyes; lesions at point of entrance; lymphatic or hematogenous extension with edema; in acute Chagas' disease, heart and brain may be affected; may be chronic
Trypanosomiasis, African or sleeping sickness	*Trypanosoma gambiense* or *rhodesiense*	Reservoir: mainly man; also antelope, goat, and sheep. Source: tsetse flies. Transmission: bite of fly	Central nervous system with meningoencephalitis; lymph nodes enlarged and contain parasites; incubation 10 days to 3 weeks, but sometimes 2 or more years
Toxoplasmosis	*Toxoplasma gondii*	Reservoir: parasite in man and animals; possibly children acquire disease through sick pets; protozoon can cross placental barrier from infected mother; neonate may harbor disease	Congenital type, hydrocephalus; adult type, interstitial pneumonia and granulomas of cerebral tissues
Helminthic infections			
Ancylostomiasis or Hookworm disease	*Ancylostoma duodenale* or *americanum*	Reservoir: man. Source: contaminated soil. Transmission: organism penetrates skin, usually feet; worms grow in small intestine	Intestinal infection, with punctate hemorrhages of mucosa
Ascariasis	*Ascaris lumbricoides*	Reservoir: man. Source: contaminated soil. Transmission: ingestion of embryonated ova; worms grow to adulthood in intestines	Intestines, sometimes with obstruction; worms may migrate to biliary ducts, pancreatic ducts, appendix, and occasionally lungs
Distomiasis or fluke infection	*Fasciola hepatica* (sheep liver fluke); *Clonorchis sinensis* (Chinese liver fluke); *Paragonimus westermani* (lung fluke)	Reservoir: fascioliasis—man, sheep, and cow; clonorchiasis—parasitic in cat, dog, and man; paragonimiasis—ova need freshwater snail as first host, then man as intermediate host, as in all trematodes pathogenic to man. Transmission: eating raw fish in most instances	Fascioliasis — liver; clonorchiasis—liver and biliary ducts; paragonimiasis—lungs
Echinococcosis or hydatid disease	*Echinococcus granulosus*	Definitive reservoir: dog, wolf, or other carnivorous animals. Intermediate reservoir: sheep, cow, hog, and man. Transmission: usually infected dog; eggs or worm reach man directly or indirectly through	Hydatid cysts in liver or lungs

Continued.

Table 4. Infectious diseases—cont'd

Disease	Infectious agent	Reservoir, source, mode of transmission	Principal organ or system affected; incubation period when known or applicable
Helminthic infections—cont'd			
Echinococcosis or hydatid disease—cont'd		drinking water, soiled food, or soiled hands contaminated by dog feces	
Enterobiasis or oxyuriasis (pinworm or threadworm disease)	*Enterobius vermicularis; Oxyuris vermicularis*	Transmission: ingestion of ova deposited about anus and transferred by fecal contamination	Intense pruritus ani secondary to migration of adult female worms to perianal region; rarely, may migrate to uterus and fallopian tubes, and also to appendix
Filariasis or Bancroft's filariasis	*Wuchereria bancrofti*	Reservoir: man Source: bite of *Culex* mosquito, rarely *Aedes* and *Anopheles* Transmission: to man by mosquito and back to mosquito by man in life cycle	Elephantiasis; lymphatic vessels of lower extremities, retroperitoneal tissues, spermatic cord, epididymis and mammary gland
Onchocerciasis	*Onchocerca volvulus*	Reservoir: man Source: small flies (gnat or blackfly) Transmission: larvae introduce it into man with bite	Solitary or multiple cutaneous nodules; may involve eyes with eventual impairment of vision
Schistosomiasis or bilharziasis	*Schistosoma haematobium* (Africa); *Schistosoma japonicum* (Far East); *Schistosoma mansoni* Africa South America, Puerto Rico	Reservoir: principally man Source: fresh water contaminated by feces or urine, where *Schistosoma* penetrate snails Transmission: bathing or wading in infected water, with organisms entering skin	Regional lymph nodes; liver, spleen, intestines, and also lungs in some types; granulomas in body viscera in some types
Strongyloidiasis	*Strongyloides stercoralis*	Complicated life cycle of parasite: develops in intestine of man and is deposited in soil as ovum, where it further develops into filariform larva and is transferred back to man through skin or oral mucosa	Intestinal infection, mainly duodenum and jejunum; lungs may be affected by migratory phase of maturing larvae
Tapeworm disease	*Taenia saginata* (beef tapeworm); *Taenia solium* (pork tapeworm); *Diphyllobothrium latum* (fish tapeworm)	Reservoir: beef tapeworm—man definitive host Transmission: cattle ingest liberated eggs; man eats undercooked infected meat or drinks contaminated water containing larvae Reservoir: pork tapeworm—man definitive host	Gastrointestinal disorders and occasionally anemia or disease may be symptomless

Table 4. Infectious diseases—cont'd

Disease	Infectious agent	Reservoir, source, mode of transmission	Principal organ or system affected; incubation period when known or applicable
Helminthic infections—cont'd			
Tapeworm disease—cont'd		Transmission: man passes organism in feces; organism is ingested by hog; man eats infected pork Reservoir: fish tapeworm—man definitive host Transmission: man deposits organism in water; it is ingested by fish; man eats infected fish	
Trichiniasis or trichinosis	*Trichinella spiralis*	Transmission: hog becomes infected by eating uncooked garbage containing infected pork; man acquires disease by eating infected pork	Larvae become encysted only in striated muscles, although may reach heart, lungs, brain, and meninges
Trichuriasis or whipworm disease	*Trichuris trichiura*	Transmission: man deposits organism in soil and water and contracts disease through ingestion of food or water containing ova; ovum hatches in intestine of man	Habitat of worm usually ileocecal region; in massive infection there may be ulceration of intestinal mucosa and hemorrhagic diarrhea

Haemophilus influenzae. The acute respiratory viral infections, such as influenza, rarely cause death themselves; it is usually the result of these secondary or simultaneous invaders.[20] Through the use of the antibiotic miracle drugs even the dreaded bacterial infections and some of the viruses have to a great extent been brought under therapeutic control. However, the antibiotics cannot always be relied upon, since there is an increasing prevalence of organisms resistant to these drugs.

There are a number of reasons why infectious diseases, other than influenza and the common cold, are not prevalent or are practically nonexistent in our modern world. Extensive investigations in the discovery of the organisms responsible for disease have resulted in immunizations or vaccine for protection, as in diphtheria, smallpox, and measles. Discovery of the role of the insect in transmitting diseases has resulted in methods of eradication, as

in malaria and yellow fever. The control of the group of infections spread largely through human excreta is one of the most notable achievements in preventive medicine. The diseases in this category are the intestinal infections—typhoid fever, cholera, dysentery, and hookworm. The incidence of these diseases in any country today is an index of its sanitary conditions. Although the problem of influenza outbreaks remains, the use of influenza vaccine has at least served to forestall or weaken epidemics. It has been estimated that properly constituted influenza A and B vaccines can be expected to protect from 75% to 90% of vaccinated persons.[7] But the influenza virus has the ability to change antigenically, necessitating constant surveillance so that the vaccine may be altered if necessary.

Investigations of most of the biologic agents have resulted in positive identification of the organisms and the nature of their toxicity and invasiveness. Most investigative work on infectious diseases is now centered on the study of the viruses, since the common cold and respiratory infections are responsible for a morbidity rate that exceeds that of all other infections. Much of the investigative work has been prompted in the interest of controlling influenza and the common cold, but viruses as the cause of cancer are now the subject of intensive research. Animal experimentation in mice has proved that a particular virus produces leukemia in mice,[21] and the application of these findings to leukemia in humans is being intensively investigated. Studies of viruses by modern methods have resulted in many new and radical concepts being offered concerning the origin and nature of life. The implications of what these new concepts hold for the future in understanding the diseases caused by viruses can be found in modern textbooks of immunology, genetics, microbiology, and virology.

Since we hear so much about viruses in modern medicine, and since people are prone to blame the virus for almost all respiratory infections and a number of intestinal disorders, it is pertinent at this point to include a brief discussion of the virus. It should be pointed out that the virus is not responsible for a number of infections that are primarily confined to the respiratory tract. Initially there may have been a viral infection, but superimposed on this is the invasion of bacterial microorganisms in a number of cases of serious illness. These invaders, as pointed out previously, are the staphylococci, streptococci, pneumococci, and even the meningococci.

Viruses, unlike some of the other microorganisms, can exist for decades, like an inert chemical, without losing any of their virulence. Viruses remain quite lifeless outside a living organism, but once introduced into the body through respiratory or digestive tracts or through a cut or wound, they spring to life suddenly and can cause devastating damage to tissues. Once inside a cell the virus is capable of taking over the work of the cell and disrupting its normal activity. Viruses consist of information-laden nucleic acids surrounded by corresponding protein molecules This information has been obtained from the study of DNA and RNA, the basic materials of all life. Fortunately most viral diseases in humans confer lasting immunity, the exceptions being the common cold, influenza, and herpes simplex[39] infection.

SOURCES OF INFECTION[23, 29]

Most of the communicable diseases are specific for human beings and they are their own greatest foe in this regard. The communicable, or so-called contagious diseases, can be transferred by contact between an infected individual and a healthy person through various modes of transference, which are discussed below. Bacteria and viruses are the notable examples of microorganisms communicable person to person. Fortunately most of the microorganisms that cause communicable diseases are frail and soon die in the human environment, that is, in air, soil, or water. They cannot grow and multiply under adverse circumstances, which is why personal hygiene and sanitation play a major role in preventive medicine. Humans also harbor parasites, for example, helminths, which are transmitted through fecal discharges in the soil.[23]

Humans, however, are not the only source of reservoir of infectious diseases. One may contract infection from the lower animals, particularly through close association with domesticated animals. From domestic animals humans may contract a variety of diseases, such as rabies and echinococcus cysts from dogs; glanders from horses; trichinosis from hogs; undulant fever, anthrax, and tuberculosis, in part, from cattle; malta fever from goats; ringworm from cats; and psittacosis from parrots. In human environment also are rats, mice, and vermin capable of causing serious diseases such as plague, endemic typhus, rat-bite fever, and food infections. For example, humans may contract flukes from fresh-water snails, crabs, and fish; tapeworms and other animal parasites from meat; and intestinal disorders from food contaminated by insects such as cockroaches and flies. Through wild game they may contract tularemia from rabbits and Rocky Mountain spotted fever from a number of wild animals.[23]

PORTAL OF ENTRY[23, 29]

Before any of the biologic agents can cause anatomic or functional damage to the body, they must have a portal of entry. In general the gateways are the skin surfaces and respiratory, gastrointestinal, and genitourinary tracts. Through these channels microorganisms are conveyed in air, water, food, and soil. Most infections are taken in through the mouth in food and water, on the fingers and innumerable objects that are placed in the mouth, and through kissing. Others enter the nose through the air we breathe, which may be contaminated with pollutants or droplet infection. Examples of infections that may be transferred through the air we breathe are whooping cough, influenza, the common cold, and tuberculosis. Both the mouth and nose are gateways to the digestive and respiratory tracts and are closely related anatomically to the sinuses (air), central nervous system, blood vessels, lymphatics, and peripheral nerves. The genitourinary tract is a portal of entry for microorganisms of venereal diseases; also for trichomoniasis, moniliasis, and puerperal sepsis in women. The skin is a common portal of entry because of the enormity of the integument exposed daily to a large number of pathogens. If the skin is intact, however, most biologic agents cannot cross this barrier.

MODES OF TRANSFER[23, 29]

Biologic agents must have a means of transfer to a new host to maintain continuity of life. This is the only way there

can be a continuing source of nutrients available for their survival. If organisms could not spread from person to person or from animal to human, they would inevitably die when their host did. To spread to new hosts, they must have a method of leaving the body and a vector or vehicle of conveyance. These various methods of transference are generally the routes of direct contact, indirect contact, intermediate host, and by carriers.

Direct transference implies close contact with an infected individual. Infection spreads directly by microorganisms leaving the body through discharges from the nose, mouth, intestines, urinary tract, and from skin ulcers or sores. Direct infection can also be through sexual acts as in venereal diseases. It can be by kissing or contact with contaminated articles of clothing, utensils, or by almost any article handled by an infected person. Examples of infections contracted by direct transference are tuberculosis, diphtheria, scarlet fever, measles, influenza, common colds, cerebrospinal meningitis, whooping cough, mumps, and poliomyelitis. Contact with the feces or urine of a person suffering from typhoid, cholera, or dysentery may also directly transfer the organisms.

A large group of diseases are transmitted by indirect contact through the media of water, food, soil, and fomites. Infections may be conveyed long distances through food and water, whereas conveyance through the air as in droplet infection confines the organisms to the immediate vicinity. In the majority of infections conveyed indirectly, the microorganism is taken into the system through the mouth by food or water and discharged from the body in the feces. Infected feces and urine pollute drinking water when there are no sewage disposal plants and sewage from urban areas is dumped into open streams and rivers. This also happens in rural communities through the use of outhouses instead of modern sewage disposal methods. Contamination of water is a real danger during floods and acts of war when water purification breaks down.

Examples of infectious diseases contracted through water or food transference of microorganisms are typhoid, cholera, and dysentery. Water may also be connected indirectly with an infection as in ringworm of the feet contracted from contaminated floors and walks of locker rooms or swimming pools. Swimming pools are also instrumental in the spread of a few upper respiratory tract, conjunctival, ear, skin, and intestinal infections.

Upon recovery from an infectious process, such as typhoid fever, the body usually rids itself completely of the infecting agent. But in many instances the virulent microorganisms continue to live in the body. The person harboring the pathogenic organism is called a carrier. A carrier will show no signs or symptoms of the disease but will disseminate it through the handling of food or other articles, for example, clothing, bedding, towels, and eating utensils. The continued existence of many infectious diseases depends to a large degree on the dissemination of pathogenic organisms by apparently healthy and often immune carriers.

There are two types of carriers, the shedding carrier and the silent carrier.[11, 25] The shedding carrier poses the most danger, since he has the continuing capacity to infect others. The direct spread of staphylococcus from the shedding carrier is by droplets expelled from the nose that contaminate the skin and clothing. Anyone who touches the carrier or the contaminated bedding and towels may become infected. Hospital staphylococcal infections are often from healthy carriers among the personnel who have the organisms in their nasopharynx or on their hands and who contaminate food, hospital equipment, clothing, bedding, towels, and so on. Shigellae and salmonellae, the common causes of bacterial enteritis, are two other examples of bacteria spread through shedding carriers, mainly by food handlers.

Carriers of typhoid fever are continually shedding organisms. Viral hepatitis may be spread by asymptomatic carriers, the pathway of infection usually being the oral route after contact with articles or food contaminated by persons passing the virus in their feces. Diphtheria is a classic example of a carrier disease. Diphtheria organisms may be retained for months in convalescent carriers.[11, 25]

The silent carrier is able to spread infection only when he experiences renewed activity of his disease. Two notable examples of diseases in which the silent carrier plays a part are tuberculosis and syphilis. *Mycobacterium tuberculosis* infections may exist in the body for years, decades, or a lifetime and become active after long quiescence. Syphilis also may remain latent for years after a mild and sometimes unrecognizable onset. Typhus may be carried for many years in an asymptomatic, noninfective state. During a recrudescence the carrier of typhus may become infective, and the disease can be transmitted to a new victim through the intermediate carrier, the body louse. Recurrent herpes simplex[39] is a common viral disease in which the silent carrier harbors the latent virus, which becomes reactivated by sunlight, heat, or metabolic alterations and becomes a source of infection for others. Other diseases spread by silent carriers are brucellosis and malaria.

An animal in which a parasite passes its larval or nonsexual existence is called an intermediate host. A number of diseases require an intermediate host before they can be transmitted to humans. The intermediate host plays a significant role in the transmission of insect-borne diseases. This may be biologic or mechanical. Biologic transmission of parasites requires an incubation period in the insect, and the parasite passes part of its life cycle within the insect. Notable examples of this type of transmission are malaria and yellow fever by mosquitoes; Rocky Mountain spotted fever, relapsing fever, and tularemia by ticks; trypanosomiasis or sleeping sickness by the tsetse fly; typhus and trench fever by lice; and plague by fleas. In mechanical transmission of disease by insects the parasite is on the insect's proboscis at the time of injection, that is, when the individual is bitten. The body, mouthparts, legs, or outer surfaces of the insect may also be smeared with the virus, which is transmitted to humans through food or fingers. The excreta of insects may contaminate open wounds or scratches.[23]

The intermediate host also plays a major role in transmitting the tapeworm in cattle and hogs; flukes in fish, crabs, and snails; hydatid disease in dogs; and trichinosis in swine. In each of these the parasite spends some part of its life in the intermediate host.[23]

The soil is associated with the spread of such diseases as hookworm, whipworm, and tapeworm infestations. These are intestinal parasites, and the soil can be polluted by infected feces. After a stage of their cycle of development, sometimes through an intermediate host, the animal parasites reinfest humans. In the case of *Taenia solium,* which causes tapeworm infestation, the soil is contaminated by feces containing the eggs. Hogs devour the infection and return the disease to humans through infected meat. In similar soil pollution the eggs of other animal parasites deposited in feces continue their existence in humans through transfer from soil to humans through the skin. Some parasitic protozoa have resistant stages and may remain in the soil for long periods of time after fecal deposition. Anthrax is an example of a disease spread by spores found in pastures where there were once infected animals. The natural habitat and the great reservoir of tetanus are the intestines of herbivora. Spores of tetanus are contained in the intestinal discharges of humans and animals. Humans can be reinfected with both tetanus and anthrax from these sources.

CHARACTERISTICS OF INVASION AND TOXIGENICITY

Certain biologic agents characteristically invade a particular tissue of the body. Thus meningococci invade the meninges, and gonococci attack the urogenital tract. The rabies virus invades the central nervous system. In general the helminths invade the large and small intestines, and the *Salmonella* group invades both stomach and intestines. Some fungi, like those producing coccidioidomycosis and histoplasmosis, characteristically invade the lungs, although these may become disseminated later. The viruses that produce influenza and the common cold are more prone to invade the respiratory tract. Biologic agents like staphylococci and streptococci are able to find a suitable environment in virtually any site or tissue in the body.

The tissue selected extends down to include the individual cells. Bacteria survive outside cells and can multiply and grow on necrotic tissue debris. Rickettsiae, on the other hand, spend a large part of their life cycle within the cells. Viruses are able to survive only within living cells. Survival of biologic agents also depends on finding suitable nourishment and oxygen tensions. The biologic agent of tetanus, *Clostridium,* cannot gain a foothold in living healthy tissue but requires preexistent tissue damage or other bacterial agents to provide its nourishment until it can multiply and grow. *Clostridium* also can survive only in low oxygen tension. This is the reason superficial injuries well exposed to air provide an unsuitable environment for its survival. Deep penetrating injuries, on the other hand, that are sealed off from air at their surfaces offer an ideal environment.[22]

There are many variables in the ability of biologic agents to invade and multiply within the body. These differ with each class of pathogens, viral, rickettsial, protozoal, bacterial, and fungal. If they are highly invasive, they may permeate the vascular and lymphatic channels and become disseminated throughout the body.

They may cause bacteremias, toxemias, pyemias, or viremias and produce systemic manifestations. They do not necessarily remain confined to the organ of first attack or the portal of entry. For example, syphilis becomes disseminated shortly after development of the initial lesion (the chancre) by entering the bloodstream and later causing damage to the central nervous system, the aorta, and other viscera. In insect-borne diseases, such as malaria and yellow fever, the initial bite is not the site of the infection, but rather it is introduced into the bloodstream and is carried throughout the body and thus becomes a systemic disease.[23]

REACTIONS OF THE HOST TO BIOLOGIC AGENTS[22, 23, 29]

Whether an infectious disease develops depends on the ability of the defensive mechanisms of the host to prevent the invading agent from gaining a portal of entry or from surviving once it has entered the body. Some of the body's defense mechanisms against invading injurious agents were discussed in Chapter 3, and others were discussed under hypersensitivity diseases in Chapter 13. Since the defense mechanisms are of such tremendous importance in preventing and controlling infection, despite repetition the principles are stressed here.

The inflammatory response to any injury is the mobilization of defensive forces against infection. It has long been known that the body developed a different type of antibody against each germ or alien pathogenic invader. These invaders, named antigens, had a molecular construction sometimes called molecular warts that stimulated antibody production when introduced into the body. When viruses or bacteria enter the body and begin to damage the cells and tissues, a dynamic chain of events is put into motion. First, histamine and other chemicals are released that dilate the blood vessels. This is the body's first defense against injury. The body's

store of scavenger cells or phagocytic cells, localized principally in the spleen, liver, lymph nodes, and bone marrow, are dispatched to the scene of injury. These may be joined by isolated cells in the lungs, skin, blood vessels, and connective tissue. These phagocytic cells working themselves into the tissue surrounding the injury begin to engulf and dissolve the bacteria.[22] This would be an ideal defense if it were effective against all microorganisms, but it is unfortunately ineffective against certain stubbornly resistant pathogens. The body is not helpless, however, for it calls into action its second defense, antibodies and complement (a lytic substance in blood serum aiding in the breakdown of antigen in an intact cell). The antibodies neutralize a toxin or coat a bacterium so that the phagocytic cells can attack it, or they may cause the bacteria or viruses to clump together, preventing their entry into the cells. Subsequently the bacteria may be decomposed by this action. However, a certain number of parasites or bacteria resistant to all phagocytic action may gain an intracellular base, and from this survival they are able to spread infections being carried by the phagocytic cells themselves to various sites in the body by way of the lymphatics.

In addition to these mechanisms of defense, endogenous or exogenous, the body has a number of other remarkable, native resistance mechanisms. These include the intact skin and mucosal linings of the body that erect important barriers against invasion of pathogens. There are also other inherent physiologic mechanisms. These include the power of the saliva to dissolve some bacteria and of the gastric acidity to destroy most organisms when swallowed. The nose has hairs or cilia that trap dust and injurious particles before they have a chance to enter the pharynx and the lungs. Should these injurious particles find their way into the lungs, they are trapped in the mucous secretions, and a cough reflex expels many of them. Unfortunately this works to the disadvantage of others, since the microorganisms expelled in the cough are a potential source of spreading infection.

All these mechanisms may work effectively in the healthy individual to protect him against many pathogenic invaders, but if the body is debilitated or otherwise diseased, the barriers may break down and render it liable to invasion by microorganisms. This is particularly true in the very old whose vascular supply and adaptive mechanisms may be depressed because of the physiologic processes of aging. Malnutrition in any individual is a factor detrimental to his defense against disease. War and famine in the history of the world are notable examples of the effect of lack of food and proper nutrition in the development of epidemics of bacterial diseases. Chronic alcoholism and some metabolic disorders also interfere with nutrition, rendering the individuals more susceptible to infection. Very young people are susceptible to infections because of insufficient exposure that would normally build up immunity. Evidence of this is the preponderance of what are termed the childhood diseases of whooping cough, measles, mumps, scarlet fever, and so on.

Fortunately many infections confer a more or less lasting immunity, for example, the childhood diseases just mentioned. This acquired immunity is one of the most important mechanisms responsible for safeguarding against infection. Immunity may also be borrowed for a reasonable length of time against certain infections like smallpox, diphtheria, some influenzal viruses, tetanus, sleeping sickness, cholera, and typhoid. Infants up to the age of 6 months may have immunity inherited from their mothers, which ensures protection until such time as they have developed antibodies of their own.

CLINICAL FEATURES OF INFECTIOUS DISEASES[9, 12, 20, 22, 29]

Most infectious diseases have an incubation period (Table 4), which is the time lag between invasion and development of signs and symptoms of a pathogenic process. This varies with the different organisms responsible for the disease and may range from a few minutes to hours in botulism, a deadly toxemia from food poisoning, to years in leprosy. It may be numbered in days or weeks in many communicable diseases such as influenza, smallpox, measles, diphtheria, typhoid, and cholera. The same is also true of the incubation period of hookworm and other helminthic infestations, of the diseases carried by insects such as the mosquito, and of those transmitted by animals from ingestion of infected foods, as in trichinosis.

Many of the infections have generalized, clinical symptomatic manifestations, such as weakness, fever, chills, increased pulse and respirations, sweating, aches and pains, fatigue, and initial oliguria followed by polyuria, and may progress to prostration. These symptoms are caused by the disseminated systemic manifestations of an infection in most cases. As mentioned previously, the portal of entry does not manifest the sole clinical sign of a disease; the organisms may gain entrance to the blood or lymphatics and be carried throughout the body. Many biologic agents have a tendency to spread throughout the body if defensive mechanisms fail to curb or destroy them.

TISSUE AND ORGAN RESPONSES TO BIOLOGIC AGENTS[20, 22]

The portal of entry may show local manifestation of injury in some conditions. This is exemplified by the running nose in the common cold caused by hypersecretion of the mucosal lining, with invasion of viral agents. The pharyngeal or oropharyngeal tissues may also show varying degrees of inflammation in a number of bacterial or viral infections. In the venereal diseases the spirochete of syphilis causes a chancre at the portal of entry, either on the lips or genital organs. Gonorrhea causes a copious purulent discharge after settling in the genital organs. The gastrointestinal tract responds with diarrhea in a number of infestations with parasites and with food poisoning. Invasion of the lungs with biologic agents is characterized by coughing and increased expectoration. As mentioned earlier, many of the organisms have a predilection for certain tissues, such as meningococci for the meninges. The lymph nodes may respond by edema or lymphadenitis in the areas of drainage near foci of infection. This response is governed by the invasiveness and toxigenicity of the organism, which may spread from regional lymph nodes to a generalized lymphadenitis involving many nodes. Leukocytosis may be present with acute infections and with pathogenic cocci, but, on the other hand, leukopenia may occur in such infections as typhoid fever, miliary tuberculosis, malaria, and infestation with certain parasites.

The pattern of tissue response with inflammation and frank exudation varies with the specific biologic agents. In general, however, bacterial invasions usually evoke focal, suppurative, or necrotizing infections, which may progress to abscess formation or diffuse cellulitis.[9, 22] The suppurative purulent exudates, and in some cases pyogenic abscesses in solid tissue, may occur with invasion of gonococci, meningococci, pneumonococci, staphylococci, alpha hemolytic streptococci, coliforms, *Salmonella* group, *Haemophilus* group, and *Vibrio proteus*.[9, 22]

• • •

For a list of infectious diseases and their biologic agents, see Table 4.

A number of more or less common infections are described after the exercises.

STEP-BY-STEP EXERCISES

Step 1. Invasion of the body by microorganisms or biologic agents that cause tissue damage and disease is called

_____ .

Step 2. A disease that can be transferred by direct contact from one person to another through various means is called a

_____ disease.

Step 3. Not all infections are transmitted from person to person. Some infectious diseases are transmitted from animals to humans, particularly through close association with domestic animals. Infectious diseases are also transmitted to humans through food that came from animals or was contaminated by insects.

Mark the following statements *T* for true or *F* for false.

1. Humans are the only source or reservoir of infectious diseases. ___
2. Humans may contract infection from the lower animals. ___
3. Humans can contract infections from the lower animals only through association with them as pets. ___
4. Humans can contract infections through eating food that came from animals. ___
5. Insects cannot be considered vehicles for transference of disease. ___

Step 4. No biologic agent, whether it is bacterium, virus, fungus, protozoon, or helminth, can damage tissue and produce disease unless it has a portal of entry to the body. The portals of entry are the respiratory, gastrointestinal, and genitourinary tracts and the skin. This means that microorganisms can gain entrance to the body through the nose, mouth, broken skin, or through the openings of the genital organs and the rectum. The rectum is a portal of entry for the pinworm (seatworm) in children. Microorganisms can be present on the skin, in the air we breathe, in the food and water we consume, and in the genitourinary tract.

Complete the blanks with the portal of entry for the following diseases by designating whether respiratory, gastrointestinal, skin, or sexual contact.

1. Tuberculosis _____

2. Gonorrhea _____

3. Amebiasis _____

4. Hookworm infestation _____

5. Trichinosis _____

6. Syphilis (usual route) _____

7. Whooping cough _____

8. Common cold _____

9. Dysentery _____

10. Measles _____

11. *Salmonella* infection _____

12. Chickenpox _____

13. Rabies _____

14. Malaria _____

15. Streptococcal pharyngitis _____

16. Mumps _____

Step 5. Biologic agents must have a means of transfer to a new host to maintain a continuity of life. To spread to new hosts, they must have a method of leaving the body and a vector or vehicle of conveyance. These methods of transference are generally the routes of direct contact, indirect contact, intermediate host, and carrier.

Name the four methods of transference of biologic agents:

1. _____   3. _____
2. _____   4. _____

Step 6. Complete the following blanks with one of the methods of transference given in *Step 5*. (You may have to refer to the text to make the correct response.)

1. A disease such as tuberculosis that is contracted from droplet discharge

    _____

2. Typhoid fever contracted from drinking polluted water   _____

3. Ringworm of the feet contracted from a contaminated swimming pool

    _____

4. Cerebrospinal meningitis from close association with an infected person

    _____

5. *Salmonella* infection contracted from eating food handled by an infected waitress _____

6. Viral hepatitis after contact with contaminated articles from a person who is passing the virus in his feces

    _____

7. Kissing a person with infectious mononucleosis (probably but not proved) _____

8. Hospital staphylococcal infection from contaminated food or equipment handled by personnel with the organism present in the nasopharynx

    _____

9. Diphtheria from a person who is harboring that germ in the nasopharynx

    _____

10. Malaria from a mosquito bite

    _____

11. Tularemia from handling infected hides _____

12. Tapeworm from cattle or hogs

    _____

Step 7. Certain biologic agents characteristically invade a particular tissue or tissues of the body. Complete the blanks with the tissue or system commonly attacked. (You may have to refer to the text to make the proper response.)

1. Meningococci invade the _____.
2. Gonococci invade the _____

    _____.

3. Helminths invade the _____

    _____.

4. Coccidioidomycosis is a fungal disease that invades the _____.

5. Viruses are most likely to invade the

    _____ _____.

6. Salmonellae invade the _____

and _____ .

7. The virus of rabies invades the

_____ _____ _____ .

8. The fungus causing histoplasmosis

invades the _____ .

Step 8. If biologic agents are highly invasive, they may permeate the vascular and lymphatic systems and thus disseminate throughout the body. They may cause bacteremias, toxemias, pyemias, or viremias and produce systemic manifestations. They do not remain confined to the portal of entry or to the organs they first invaded.

Which of the following conditions are the result of systemic spread of the invading biologic agent?

1. Syphilis of the central nervous system ___
2. Malaria ___
3. Viral pneumonia ___
4. Yellow fever ___
5. Leprosy ___
6. Oropharyngitis ___
7. Gonorrhea ___
8. Syphilic aortitis ___

Step 9. The body has two important protective mechanisms that are activated when it is invaded by disease-producing organisms. One is the action of the white cells (phagocytic cells), and the other is the development of antibodies. In addition, the body also has a number of remarkable native mechanisms for protecting itself against disease or injury from microorganisms.

Mark the following statements *T* for true or *F* for false.

1. Saliva is able to dissolve some bacteria. ___
2. Cilia of the nose may trap dust and injurious particles before they can invade the lungs. ___
3. An intact skin is never a barrier to the invasion of microorganisms. ___
4. Mucous secretions in the lungs trap microorganisms which are expelled in the cough reflex. ___

5. Intact skin is a barrier against tetanus. ___
6. The inflammatory response is a protective mechanism. ___

Step 10. In responding to the following you may refer to Table 4; however, try to complete as many of the blanks as possible before doing so.

Identify the type of microorganisms involved (virus, bacterium, fungus, protozoon, helminth, rickettsia).

1. Staphylococcic pneumonia _____
2. Streptococcic pharyngitis _____
3. Common cold _____
4. Histoplasmosis _____
5. Amebiasis _____
6. Smallpox _____
7. Tularemia _____
8. Syphilis _____
9. Bacillary dysentery _____
10. Undulant fever _____
11. Tuberculosis _____
12. Rabies _____
13. Typhus _____
14. Typhoid _____
15. Diphtheria _____
16. Gonorrhea _____
17. *Haemophilus influenzae* infection _____
18. Whooping cough _____
19. Tetanus _____
20. Cholera _____
21. Rocky Mt. spotted fever _____
22. Psittacosis _____
23. Mumps _____
24. Coccidioidomycosis _____

25. Malaria _____

26. Filariasis _____

27. Echinococcosis _____

28. Food poisoning _____

29. Trichinosis _____

30. German measles _____

31. Enterobiasis _____

32. Herpes simplex _____

33. Poliomyelitis _____

34. Trench fever _____

35. St. Louis encephalitis _____

36. Sporotrichosis _____

37. Granuloma venereum _____

38. Tsutsugamushi fever _____

39. Hookworm disease _____

40. Scarlet fever _____

REPRESENTATIVE INFECTIOUS DISEASES

Some of the more or less common infectious diseases have been selected for discussion following. Table 4 includes all the major infections. Some infectious diseases are also discussed in Chapter 18.

Staphylococcic infections[6, 9]

A number of dieases and lesions are the result of staphylococcic infection. These include the furuncle (boil), carbuncle, impetigo, acne, paronychia, felon, abscess, osteomyelitis, arthritis, tonsillitis, sinusitis, otitis media, bronchitis, bronchopneumonia, acute enteritis, food poisoning, antibiotic-resistant staphylococcic infections, bacteremia, septicemia, and pyemia. Staphylococci may also be involved in mixed infections and associated with other pathogenic organisms.

Staphylococcus aureus (pyogenes), a gram-positive coccus, is the most common cause of pyogenic infections, such as those of the skin, subcutaneous tissues, and wounds. The infections of the head are a danger by threatening to spread and involve the brain either in abscess formation or meningitis.

Staphylococcic bronchopneumonia is particularly serious in infants and young children and carries a relatively high rate of mortality. In pyelonephritis of hematogenous origin, staphylococcus is often the causative agent.[9]

The clinical types of staphylococcic infection seen most often are impetigo contagiosa, furuncle or boil, carbuncle, paronychia and felons, and in wounds. Impetigo is a contagious infection largely confined to children, involving the superficial layers of the skin with pustules, vesicles, crust, and bullae. The boil or furuncle occurs most often in adults. It is a typical abscess formation that is usually localized but may be multiple (furunculosis). The carbuncle is a more complex focal lesion extending deep into the tissue with suppurative pockets. It is commonly found on the back of the neck. Paronychia and felons are suppurative lesions around the nailbed and are usually secondary to a penetrating wound or a hangnail. Wounds are often the site of staphylococcic infection, since most of them are contaminated with bacteria. Wound infection can spread, resulting in septicemia. Staphylococci are present on the skin in a number of people, and the carrier rate for *Staphylococcus aureus* in adults is about 50%.[9]

The antibiotic-resistant staphylococci are a hospital problem, constantly threatening infection of surgical incisions and wounds, and causing bronchopneumonia or staphylococcic food poisoning from carriers. Staphylococcic food poisoning is probably the most common type of food poisoning.[9] The symptoms appear rapidly and are of relatively short duration, with recovery prompt as a rule. The incubation period lasts about 3 hours and rarely beyond 6 hours after one eats food contaminated by a strain of staphylococci that produce enterotoxin. The usual symptoms are nausea, vomiting, severe abdominal cramps, and diarrhea. Staphylococcic organisms can remain stable in stored refrigerated food for a very long period and are extremely heat resistant to destruction of the enterotoxin.

Streptococcic infections[9, 27]

About 90% of the streptococcic infections are caused by *Streptococcus pyogenes* (beta hemolytic streptococci).

The thick purulent discharge of staphylococcic infection is in contrast to the thin watery exudate of streptococcic infection. This, however, is not a hard and fast rule, for there is a wide diversity of reaction in streptococcic infections, and pyogenic reactions do occur.

The focal lesions produced by streptococcic pyogenic infection are otitis media, appendicitis, impetigo wound infections, tonsillitis, and pharyngitis. The more generalized diseases caused by streptococcic infection include puerperal sepsis, bronchopneumonia, meningitis, erysipelas, scarlet fever, and septicemia. Streptococcic infection may also be concerned in rheumatic fever and glomerulonephritis.

The frequency of streptococcic infection is the result of its wide distribution in nature. *Streptococcus pyogenes* is found in the throat of about 5% to 10% of adults.[9] It is often disseminated by nasal carriers who infect their hands and clothing. They are much more likely to spread infection than the oral carriers. *Streptococcus viridans* (alpha or nonhemolytic streptococcus) is found in the nose and throat of normal individuals and is a normal inhabitant of the small intestine.

The streptococcic sore throat or nasopharyngitis is caused by beta hemolytic streptococci. It may remain localized to the pharynx and tonsils. The pharyngeal tissues are swollen and red, and the tonsillar crypts contain purulent exudate. Symptoms are toxemia with malaise, headaches, fever, and peritonsillar abscesses. This infection can spread to the cervical lymph nodes. Otitis media and sinusitis are frequent complications. Streptococcic sore throat has occurred in epidemics as a result of ingestion of contaminated milk, from either infected cows or carriers of the organism. Streptococcic bronchopneumonia is almost always the result of a worsening of streptococcic pharyngitis or of an infection superimposed on whooping cough, influenza, measles, or other viral respiratory infection. The signs and symptoms of this type of pneumonia are generally severe and often are complicated by pleural empyema.[9]

Pneumococcic infections[9, 10]

Pneumococcic infection, as the name implies, is primarily an infection of the respiratory tract, which is the portal of entry for the organism. Many of the cases of bronchopneumonia and lobar pneumonia are caused by infection with *Diplococcus pneumoniae*. In addition to involvement of the lungs, the paranasal sinuses and middle ear are often the seat of the infection. Brain abscesses may also result from septic thrombosis of venous sinuses in the brain. Meningitis in both adults and children is often the result of pneumococcic infection. Other complications are pleural effusions, empyema, lung abscess, purulent pericarditis acute bacterial endocarditis, myocarditis, and mastoiditis.

Meningococcic infections[9, 29, 33]

Meningococcic meningitis, also called cerebrospinal meningitis, epidemic cerebrospinal meningitis, and spotted fever, may be sporadic, endemic, or epidemic, with children and young adults being most often affected. The usual etiologic agent is *Neisseria meningitidis*, but it may also be caused by a number of other bacteria, viruses, or other microscopic organisms. The most common form is bacterial meningitis. The bacteria may be present in the body with no effect, or they may cause serious illness. The source of infection is often a healthy carrier or someone who has recently recovered from the infection. Healthy carriers may harbor meningococci in the nasopharynx. Even with a large number of carriers, as occurs during an epidemic, the disease is not highly contagious.

Meningococci enter the body through the nose and mouth and are spread by droplets in the air after sneezing and coughing or by direct contact. The disease is spread more easily in crowded quarters as in military barracks or institutions.[33] It occurs more often in winter and spring and is more common in temperate climates.[33]

Meningitis usually begins with local nasopharygeal infection, sudden severe headache, and stiffness and pain in the neck, shoulders, and back. The fever is high, and there is often nausea and vomiting. The presence of spotted areas of erythema (a rash) that progress to petechial hemorrhages is common. In the fulminant forms, massive purpuric hemorrhages occur. Symptoms may progress to delirium, stupor, or even coma. Without modern treatment meningococcic meningitis is fatal in about one half of the cases, and those who survive may be deaf or paralyzed.

Fulminant meningococcemia (Fig. 14-1) runs a violent and rapid course, with death usually resulting within 24 hours after onset of incapacitating symptoms. Peripherovascular collapse, shock, cyanosis, and cutaneous hemorrhages occur. When the adrenal gland is involved and hemorrhage is present, the disease is called Waterhouse-Friderichsen syndrome.[9]

Amebiasis[30]

Amebiasis is an infection of the bowel caused by *Entamoeba histolytica*. When it occurs in a severe form, it is known as amebic dysentery. It occurs occasionally in

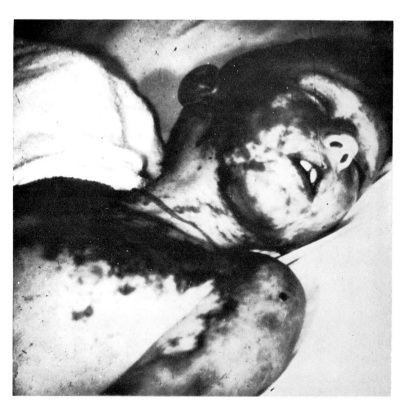

Fig. 14-1. Purpura in fulminating meningococcemia. (From Wehrle, P. F.: In Top, F. H., editor: Communicable and infectious diseases, ed. 7, St. Louis, 1972, The C. V. Mosby Co.)

the United States but is more common in the tropical climates. In its mild form, generally with no serious effects, the infection is believed to be carried by 3% to 5% of the population as a whole.

Amebiasis is contracted by swallowing parasites in polluted food and drinking water. The infective stage is the cyst, which contains the parasites. Once the cyst is inside the body, the parasites come out and develop into an active form called the trophozoites, which multiply and may invade tissues. In chronic amebiasis some trophozoites continue to multiply in the body, but others revert to cyst stage and are passed in the feces. In amebic dysentery the cysts are not formed, and only relatively fragile active stages are found in the stools.

Amebiasis is associated with poor sanitation. Not only can the infection be contracted from drinking water, but also from food contaminated by flies and other insects that have fed on human waste matter. Leafy vegetables also become carriers of the disease when they are grown with the use of human fertilizer or washed in polluted water. Careless food handlers may also be responsible for spread of the infection.

The symptoms are headache, fatigue, flatulence, nausea, tenderness of the abdomen, bowel irregularity, and a variety of symptoms associated with gastrointestinal disturbances. In amebic dysentery the abdominal pains may be severe, with diarrhea, blood-streaked feces, fever, and chills. If spontaneous recovery occurs, it may be followed by repeated attacks. Amebic abscess may develop in the liver whether or not the patient has had previous bowel infection. Colonic ulcers and sometimes skin ulcers are present in acute amebiasis.

Diagnosis is made by microscopic examination of the stools for the presence of amebas.

Ancylostomiasis[12, 23]

Ancylostomiasis (uncinariasis, hookworm disease) is one of the most prevalent diseases in the world. It is caused by *Ancylostoma duodenale* (old world hookworm) or *Necator americanus* (new world hookworm). The usual mode of transmission is through the skin. The mode of exit is through feces containing eggs of the parasite which are deposited in the soil, where larvae are hatched. In about five days the larvae reach the infective stage and can penetrate the skin, generally through the feet between and beneath the toes. As the larvae penetrate the skin, a dermatitis known as ground itch develops. Most of the people who acquire hookworm disease live in impoverished and unsanitary areas and usually wear no shoes. This is particularly true of children. After piercing the skin the larvae enter the subcutaneous tissue and proceed through the lymphatics or venules to finally reach the pulmonary circulation. From here they pass up the tracheobronchial tree and eventually enter the gastrointestinal tract. As they pass through the lungs, they produce petechial hemorrhages and areas of transient bronchopneumonia. When they reach the duodenum and first portion of the jejunum, the adult parasites attach themselves to the mucosa walls, producing punctate hemorrhages and at the same time feeding on the blood of their host. This results in severe hypochromic macrocytic anemia and iron deficiency. Anemia is one of the most characteristic symptoms of hookworm disease. The symptoms are proportional to the number of hookworms present and the nutrition and resistance of the host. When infestation of young children is severe, growth as well as sexual and mental development may be retarded. The prevention of soil pollution is the key to eradication as well as the wearing of shoes.

Appendicitis[26]

Appendicitis is a rather common disease, affecting all age groups, but is uncommon at the extremes of age and is most frequently seen in older children and young adults. The mortality rates are the highest

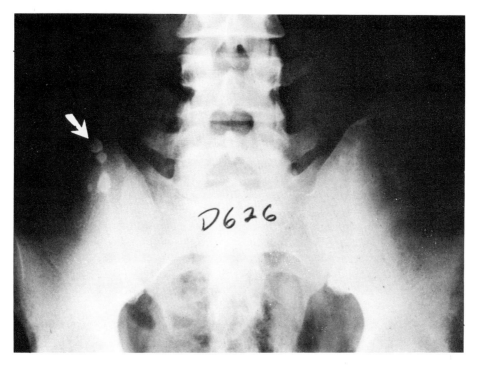

Fig. 14-2. Appendix showing fecalith (arrow). (From Young, C. G., and Likos, J. J.: Medical specialty terminology, x-ray and nuclear medicine, St. Louis, 1972, The C. V. Mosby Co.)

in patients between 5 and 14 years of age and over 55 years. It is the most common disease process requiring intra-abdominal surgery in infants and children. The high mortality rate in the older age group has been attributed to the presence of cerebral lesions that impair the ability of these patients to feel or express pain. Physical diagnosis may be handicapped by their weakened musculature and lack of response. Also, concomitant pulmonary, cardiac, or renal disease may exist, which lowers resistance to an attack of appendicitis and makes these patients a poor risk for surgical procedures.

The chief cause of acute appendicitis is infection. The inflammation begins as either a focal ulceration or as a diffuse phlegmon, which eventually involves all coats of the vermiform appendix. The appendiceal artery is an end artery, and its tributaries are prone to blockage by an obstructed appendix, such as a fecalith (Fig. 14-2). Stasis from partial or total obstruction can lead to infection. Infection leads to vascular thrombosis, local necrosis, and infarction, which can result in perforation, abscess formation, or peritonitis. The infection may be caused by *Escherichia coli*, which is a normal inhabitant of the intestinal tract. Streptococci may also be involved, which can invade the appendix from other sources, such as in patients with a history of frequent upper respiratory infections.

The initial symptom of acute appendicitis is abdominal pain. The pain may be severe or mild and is usually followed by anorexia, nausea, or vomiting. Pain is often localized in the epigastrium or periumbilical area, but frequently it will shift downward and to the right. It may be localized in the right flank, with maximum tenderness in this area if the appendix is retrocecal. In some patients, particularly young children, the pain may not localize but be diffuse over the entire abdomen.

Bronchitis[10, 17]

Bronchitis is an infection that often follows influenza or a cold or is part of a general acute upper respiratory infection. In the early stages it has to be differentiated from whooping cough, measles, diphtheria, and the primary atypical or virus pneumonias.

The normal bronchial tree is essentially free from bacteria, but external agents can disturb the epithelium lining the respiratory tract to the extent that its self-cleansing action is lost or impaired. The external agents include the chemical and physical irritants, allergens, and a number of infectious organisms. The industrial irritants are fumes or dusts from the manufacture of various products that pollute the air in urban areas. The average person inhales approximately 15 million milliliters of air per day, and this air is heavily laden with staphylococci, pneumococci, streptococci, *Haemophilus influenzae*, and a number of viruses, in addition to irritants from air pollution. The primary respiratory infections are usually viral, but bacterial invasion is frequently present in the mouth and nasal flora.

The factors that contribute to chronic bronchial disease are age, debility, previous respiratory infections or disorders, cardiac diseases, influenza, colds, and climate—weather and season.

In bronchitis involving the trachea, larynx, and bronchi, called laryngotracheobronchitis, the mucous membranes of the larynx, trachea, and bronchi are inflamed, swollen, boggy, and covered by mucinous or mucopurulent secretions. If this form is mild, it is usually self-limited and results in complete healing. The great danger is that of the infection extending into pneumonia.

In acute bronchitis the onset of pneumonia is more likely and more severe in infants, the elderly, and chronically ill or debilitated individuals. A prior infection with some influenza virus seems to predispose to development of bronchitis, and if it is acute, it may be followed by bronchopneumonia. Symptoms of acute bronchitis are high fever, rapid pulse and respiration, leukocytosis, dyspnea, cyanosis, profuse sweating, chills, headache, chest pains, and a viscid pinkish or rusty sputum. The complications are shock, severe dehydration, meningitis, and endocarditis.

In suppurative mucopurulent bronchitis the contact with irritants causes an increased blood flow and mucous secretions. Polymorphonuclear leukocytes emigrate into the walls of the bronchi. The cough reflex follows with further trauma to cilia and mucosa, and pus cells accumulate in the lumina. The exudate changes from clear and watery to a yellow, mucoid purulent type. This type can lead to chronic bronchial disease if the acute reaction persists.

A predisposing factor in ulcerative bronchitis is exposure to intensely irritating substances such as industrial fumes, chemicals, or dusts, with development of bacterial, fungal, or viral infection. This type is characterized by intense inflammatory reaction, with some localized necrosis of mucosa. It is not a different entity from the mucopurulent type but represents a degree of greater response. The continuing infection destroys large areas of surface epithelium, resulting in permanent damage to the underlying walls. If *Staphylococcus aureus* or *Streptococcus pyogenes* is involved, there is a tendency for the infection to spread rapidly, leading to early necrosis and expansion of abscesses. The inflammatory changes may spread into peribronchiolar tissues and adjacent alveoli and produce ulcerative bronchiolitis or bronchopneumonia.

In chronic bronchial disease the predisposing factor may be a complication of other chronic pulmonary disease. The causative agents may be pneumococcus and *Haemophilus influenzae*. The disease occurs oftener in men, with the onset usually in middle or old age. The disease is usually afebrile, with the main symptoms being a loose and constant or paroxysmal cough. (See Fig. 18-22, *C.*) Sputum may be scanty or abundant, mucoid or purulent, but if bloody or foul, it is usually indicative of other pulmonary disease.

Emphysema is considered to be the most predictable of the sequelae of chronic bronchial diseases. In addition to the features of bronchitis, emphysema also involves dilatation of the alveolar spaces, with compression, narrowing, and rupture of the alveolar walls. (See Fig. 18-12.)

Gonorrhea[29, 38]

The etiologic agent of gonorrhea is *Neisseria gonorrhoeae.* It is the most common and widespread of all the venereal diseases and is worldwide in distribution.

In the United States gonorrhea has reached the epidemic proportions in many states and communities. The national average of the occurrence of gonorrhea is 429 cases per 100,000 population, but this is probably not a completely accurate statistic, since there are many cases not reported to health authorities by physicians in private practice. The 15 through 25 age group is most often affected. The increase of male homosexuality has had an effect on the incidence of venereal disease.[18, 19] Recently there has been concern over gonococcal proctitis and pharyngeal gonorrhea in homosexuals and pregnant patients.[18, 19, 40]

The organism is transmitted usually by sexual intercourse, except for infants, who become infected by contact with an infectious discharge from the mother during birth or later from infected hands and articles. The incubation period varies with the virulence of the organisms, but as a rule it is 2 to 10 days after sexual contact.

In the male the symptoms are a burning sensation in the urethra and on urination a purulent exudate at the urethral orifice. The inflammation may extend to involve the prostate, seminal vesicles, vas deferens, and epididymis. Abscess formation may occur in the prostate and seminal vesicles.

Sterility may result from destruction of the epididymis by the inflammatory process. Scarring and stricture of the urethra may result.

In the female the first symptoms are an irritating discharge, burning on urination, and swelling of the Bartholin glands. (See Fig. 18-34, *E.*) Sometimes, however, the discomfort is minimal, so that she may be unaware that she is infected. During pregnancy or immediately after delivery, the infection may invade the endometrium and spread to the fallopian tubes, causing an acute purulent salpingitis and tubo-ovarian abscesses. This may be followed by pelvic or generalized peritonitis and be fatal. In chronic cases the pyosalpinx and tubo-ovarian abscesses (Fig. 14-3) may lead to pelvic involvement with adhesions and result in chronic pelvic inflammatory disease. There is severe pain, menstrual disturbances, cessation of ovarian function, and sterility.

In both acute and chronic stages of gonorrhea the bloodstream is invaded, and a frequent extragenital manifestation is gonorrheal arthritis. (See Fig. 18-23, *C.*) Other systemic manifestations that may occur are skin lesions, bacterial endocarditis, and general peritonitis.

Infants who have contracted the infection during the birth process have severe purulent conjunctivitis, which may lead to blindness if unattended.

Hepatitis[5, 15, 31]

Hepatitis is an inflammation of the liver. In the United States most cases of hepatitis are caused by viruses—hepatitis virus type A (formerly known as infectious hepatitis) and hepatitis virus type B (formerly known as serum hepatitis).

Hepatitis A is one of the most common communicable diseases, especially in children. The causative virus is present in the feces, blood, and urine of infected individuals and is communicated through close contact. It may also be spread by contaminated water and food, including raw or

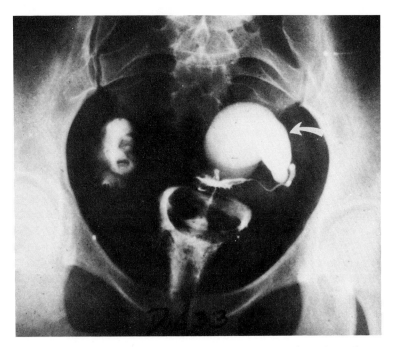

Fig. 14-3. Tubo-ovarian abscess. Arrow points to the immensely enlarged ovary. (From Young, C. G., and Likos, J. J.: Medical specialty terminology, x-ray and nuclear medicine, St. Louis, 1972, The C. V. Mosby Co.)

inadequately cooked clams and oysters gathered from polluted waters. It is also possible to contract hepatitis type A through blood transfusions or contaminated needles used for injections, but these occurrences are uncommon. In the case of blood transfusions the virus is transmitted by the parenteral route. The disease has a higher rate among donors of plasma and platelets as contrasted with whole blood donors.[15] It has been speculated that the virus may have been perpetuated in the equipment or water used to balance the centrifuge utensils and thus could have been easily transmitted to the original donor, since plasma and platelet donors become recipients when given back a portion of their own blood. Recently, an outbreak of hepatitis type A in a bone marrow transplant unit has been reported.[15]

Hepatitis A usually begins about 4 weeks after exposure, but it may occur as early as 2 weeks or as long as 6 weeks.[31] In the case of bone marrow transplants referred to previously, the overt disease developed within a period of 3 months.[15] The most common symptoms are loss of appetite, fatigue, anorexia, headache, nausea, mild fever, sore muscles, pain in the abdomen, and dark urine. The most characteristic sign is a yellowing of the white of the eyes or a yellowish or jaundiced appearance of the skin. Jaundice, however, may not be present in all affected persons. Hepatitis A is usually mild in children and lasts about 2 weeks; it is more severe in adults, lasting about 4 to 6 weeks. It may be severe in the elderly who may be suffering from other debilitating diseases.

Hepatitis type B can be acquired through transfusions of blood or blood products containing the virus and also through the use of contaminated needles, including tattoo needles and other instruments used to puncture the skin. The use of communal needles by drug addicts is a prevalent way of spreading the disease. Proper sterilization of a needle shared in the commune is not a common practice of drug addicts. The virus has also been associated with ear-piercing performed by nonmedical personnel. Children are less commonly infected than adults or young teenagers, which may be partly because of the prevalence of drug addiction in the latter group and use of contaminated needles for injections. Hepatitis B is also present in body secretions and may be transmitted through saliva or as a venereal disease by semen.

The incubation period may be long—2 to 6 months after exposure. Symptoms are similar to those of hepatitis type A, except they develop more slowly and are more apt to include skin rash and joint pains. It is frequently much more severe than hepatitis type A and recovery takes longer. The mortality rate is between 1% and 10% of the patients.[31]

There are no vaccines against either hepatitis A or hepatitis B. Immune serum globulin provides temporary protection against hepatitis A. The standard immune serum globulin does not appear to be effective in prevention of hepatitis B. However, the hepatitis B antigen test, or Australia antigen test, is a specific blood test for hepatitis B and is useful in making a correct diagnosis, and in screening out would-be donors whose blood is positive to hepatitis B antigen.[31] This screening should reduce the number of cases of hepatitis B resulting from blood transfusions. Once a person has had hepatitis A or hepatitis B, his immunity to the specific type is probably lifelong. However, immunity to one type does not confer immunity to the other.

Also other viruses such as cytomegalic viruses and Epstein-Barr viruses may cause hepatitis. There are other cases of probable viral hepatitis where the virus has not been definitely demonstrated. These have been postulated as being caused by hepatitis C.

Herpes zoster (shingles)[35]

Shingles is an acute inflammation of the nerve cells, characterized by pain and rash. Pain may be present as a nagging or burning in or under the skin, with no apparent reason. The pain in the abdomen has been mistaken for appendicitis or cholecystitis; pain in the chest has been mistaken for pleurisy and heart disease; pain on the face has been confused with neuralgia. Other symptoms may include headache and fever. With the appearance of the rash of closely grouped small watery blisters on reddened skin, the diagnosis of shingles is evident. Blisters are usually, but not always, limited to one side of the body and follow the course of a nerve that has been attacked by the shingles virus. The disease affects both sexes and all races, but it is usually a disease of adults. Children and even newborn, however, have been affected. A rash on the forehead, nose, or eyelid during an acute stage may affect the eye, resulting in scarring of the cornea, threatening vision if treatment is not prompt and effective. Shingles on the face may also affect the ear, which may lead to temporary or lasting loss of hearing. In the early weeks of pregnancy, shingles may injure the developing fetus. The damage reported is similar to that often found in babies whose mothers had German measles or rubella in early pregnancy.

Every year there are about 166,000 persons affected with shingles, but this may not be accurate since mild cases may not come to the attention of a physician.[35]

The finding that shingles and chickenpox (varicella) are caused by the same virus has been confirmed repeatedly; varicella-zoster (V-Z) virus is the cause of both diseases.[35] When shingles follows a known exposure to shingles or chickenpox, the incubation period is about 7 to 24 days, usually about 2 weeks. When there is no known exposure to shingles or chickenpox, the theory is that the chickenpox virus has been lying dormant in the body and then becomes active again as shingles.

Histoplasmosis[1]

Histoplasmosis (Fig. 14-4) is a fungus disease caused by *Histoplasma capsulatum*. It is usually a mild, transient, pulmonary infection that leaves residuals of calcified

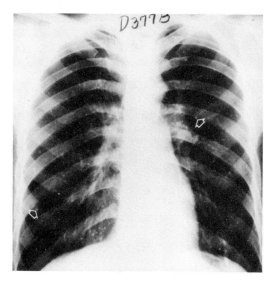

Fig. 14-4. Histoplasmosis. Arrow points to areas of infiltration. Healed histoplasmosis is seen as scattered small round calcifications. (From Young, C. G., and Likos, J. J.: Medical specialty terminology, x-ray and nuclear medicine, St. Louis, 1972, The C. V. Mosby Co.)

foci in the lungs and bronchial lymph nodes. The infection may spread from the lungs to other organs, often with fatal outcome within a year. Macrophages are involved in dissemination, which accounts for the fungi in the spleen, liver, lymph nodes, and bone marrow.

Histoplasmosis may be contracted from soil or dust containing excreta from birds, chickens, and bats. Endemic areas in the United States are in the upper Mississippi River and Ohio River regions, but sporadic cases occur in most of the states. Other endemic areas include Latin America, as well as other parts of the world. Histoplasmosis is also found in dogs and other animals. The histoplasmin skin test is positive after a patient recovers.

Symptoms of bone marrow involvement are anemia and leukopenia. In the initial form with pulmonary involvement an upper respiratory infection with cough and fever occurs a week or two after contact with excreta of the fowls previously mentioned.

Many nodules develop in the lungs, which later become calcified and inactive. (See Fig. 14-4.) Extrapulmonary involvement includes lesions such as nodules and ulcers in the skin, intestines, spleen, liver, meninges, heart valves, and adrenal glands. The adrenals are favored organs because of the abundance of steroids they contain. These patients may develop Addison's disease.[1]

Infectious mononucleosis[16]

Infectious mononucleosis is a viral disease. It occurs mainly in young adults and children. It is contagious and in several instances has occurred in epidemics. It has been called the kissing disease.

The symptoms are slight fever, malaise, sore throat, stiff neck, and a cough. The lymphadenopathy may be generalized, and the spleen is enlarged. (See Fig. 18-31.) The white cell count is elevated, and there are abnormal mononuclear cells in the blood and heterophil antibodies in the bloodstream. The pharynx is a brilliant red color, as is the soft palate (uvula), with a translucent edema in some instances. A morbilliform rash limited to the trunk may also be present. The eye signs are photophobia and conjunctivitis. There may also be jaundice. The disease may have widespread manifestations, with symptoms referable to the liver, heart, kidneys, and nervous system.

Influenza[20, 32]

Flu or influenza is an acute respiratory disease whose symptoms include fever, cough, sore throat, "runny" nose, and generalized muscular aches. Usually, the patients recover completely in a week or so, but have a lingering tiredness; however, in the aged or the chronically ill flu is a life-threatening disease.

Influenza is caused by a virus, which was identified by scientists in the 1930s. The three types of influenza virus are called types A, B, and C. The unpredictability of the flu has been known for centuries. In earlier times, when the disease reappeared in a ferocious manner after the absence of years, observers would assume that a new plague had struck. During the past century alone, there have been seven instances of pandemics (global spread) and numerous epidemics (confined more or less to one region). Flu outbreaks as a rule occur abruptly and spread rapidly through communities, peaking in about 3 weeks, and thereafter subsiding in 3 to 4 weeks.[32] The highest incidence is in children during these outbreaks, with 20% to 50% of the population likely to be affected. Every 10 years or so, new strains of influenza A virus cause pandemics.[32] In 1957 it was the Asian flu, and in 1968 the Hong Kong. Port Chalmers influenza, named for a town in New Zealand where it was isolated, was yet another variety of the pandemic strain that made its entrance in 1968. A new type called A-Scotland made its appearance in England in 1975. It is similar to the 1974 A–Port Chalmers flu strain. In January 1976 a new strain, the A-Victoria, named for Victoria, Australia, where it first appeared, arrived in the continental United States. All of these A types result from minor mutations in the makeup of the virus.

But as far as the body's immunological system is concerned, the new strain represents a new infection against which antibodies produced by previous strains of flu are comparatively ineffective. All the type A viruses differ from each other significantly in one surface antigen—the hemagglutinin—and, hence, in the protective antibodies which this chemical invokes in the body. At this writing, there is much concern over an appearance of swine influenza infection in humans. The swine influenza has been known to infect pigs and hogs since 1931, and the occurrence of influenza similar to the swine influenza in an outbreak in New Jersey is posing a major health problem.

Influenza caused by type B virus occurs in epidemic form, but the disease is generally much milder than influenza type A illness. Type C viruses are not connected with large epidemics.

The most frequent complication of influenza is a secondary bacterial infection in the lower respiratory tract. Pneumococci are the most commonly involved in these infections, but staphylococci, streptococci, and *Haemophilus influenzae* may also cause pneumonia, which may follow or accompany influenza.

Vaccines are the only preventive agents known at this time. They are not of value if the disease is in progress.[32] At the present writing, vaccines against the swine-type influenza are being prepared for mass vaccination of the population during 1976. This type of influenza is considered potentially dangerous to the health of the nation, similar to the great outbreak following World War I when thousands died.

Osteomyelitis[2]

Infectious diseases of the bone are called osteomyelitis. They may be localized or diffuse, and they may affect the periosteum, the cortex, or the marrow tissues in the cancellous portions of the bone. Any one of a number of pathogenic microorganisms may give rise to infection of the bone. Among the bacteria, *Staphylococcus aureus* and *S. albus* are more frequently causes of osteomyelitis than streptococci, pneumococci, and other forms of pyogenic bacteria. However, in infants under 2 years of age, streptococcic osteomyelitis occurs about twice as often as that caused by staphylococci.[2] The bacterium responsible for the infection may reach the localized site by way of the bloodstream or by direct extension from a neighboring focus of infection, such as a soft tissue abscess, sinus infection, periapical abscess of the tooth, or penetrating injury such as a fracture or laceration.

In acute hematogenous osteomyelitis (from bacterium) the bones affected in order of frequency are the femur, tibia, humerus, and radius. This type is most common in children. The metaphyseal ends of the diaphyses of long bones are affected first, as a rule. There is an initial exudative inflammation of the marrow tissue, leading to necrosis of the marrow and osseous parts. This soon spreads through the bone to reach the external surface of the cortex. The periosteum is dissected from the cortex by subperiosteal abscess, further impairing the blood supply. The infection tends to spread elsewhere in the medulla, and consequently a small or large portion of the bone is necrotic. In some instances the infection is localized in an abscess called Brodie's abscess, which is encased in a well-defined wall of fibrous or osseous tissue.

Pericarditis[24]

Pericarditis is a common condition that may be either acute or chronic (Fig. 14-5). It may result from rheumatic inflammation as part of pancarditis or from a variety of other infections, such as tuberculous, bacterial, viral, parasitic, or fungal, or it may be of uremic origin. It occurs with infectious diseases such as pneumonia, influenza, tonsillitis, and tuberculosis and with viruses of unknown origin. The infection may reach the pericardium by way of the lymphatics, blood, or direct extension from a neighboring focus of infection. The inflammatory process produces a serous exudate within the pericardial sac, which may at times be

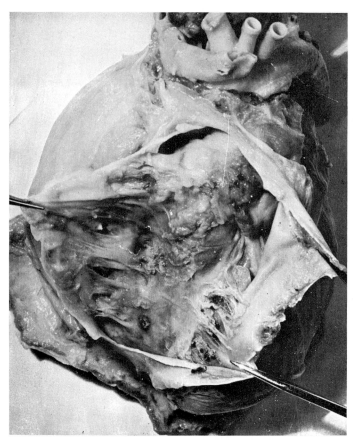

Fig. 14-5. Adhesive pericarditis. Pericardial sac has been opened, displaying fibrous bands joining visceral and parietal pericardium. (From Anderson, W. A. D., and Scotti, T. M.: Synopsis of pathology, ed. 9, St. Louis, 1976, The C. V. Mosby Co.)

sufficient to distend the pericardial cavity compressing the heart, great vessels, and lungs. Healing may result in the formation of a dense constricting scar around the heart. This scar prevents proper filling of the heart and causes the condition known as constrictive pericarditis or Pick's disease.

Reye's syndrome[8, 13]

Reye's syndrome is an encephalopathy associated with fatty degeneration of the viscera occurring in children as a rare sequel to influenza and other viral infections. Mortality ranges from 50% to 100%. Reye's syndrome following type B influenza may well be the most common potentially lethal virus-associated encephalopathy. It can occur, however, after other prodromal viral illnesses. The diagnostic criteria are prodromal viral illness, protracted vomiting within a week after onset of viral infection, with delirium and stupor beginning soon after onset of vomiting. There is an absence of focal neurologic signs. There are abnormalities of liver function, with elevated enzyme level, especially SGOT, and increased blood ammonia and prothrombin time. The patients may have hepatomegaly, widely dilated pupils that react to strong light, and hyperventilation. Hepatic coma develops in four stages—(1) stupor or delirium but response to strong stimuli; (2) coma but movements to avoid painful stimuli; (3) response to painful stimuli by extension of arms; spontaneous breathing, and pupils able react to light; (4) no response to stimuli and no reaction of pupils. Intracranial pressure develops rapidly in many cases. Cerebral edema is described as a prominent part of the syndrome. Electron microscopic studies demonstrate that the edema is within the oligodendrogliocytes, astrocytes, and myelin sheath.[13]

Rocky Mountain spotted fever[14, 20, 34]

Rocky Mountain spotted fever is caused by *Rickettsia rickettsii*, which is present in the salivary glands of the vector, the tick, and is injected into the skin at the time of the bite. Transmission of the rickettsiae from an attached tick to a human apparently takes 2 or more hours.[14] They enter the peripheral blood and are carried throughout the body. The reports of cases have been increasing since 1968, with a total of 668 recorded in 1973 in the United States, the highest on record for any year.[14] Originally the disease was believed to be confined to the western states, but in the 1930s it started to spread eastward, and into Canada, Mexico, Brazil, and Colombia. In most infested areas 1% to 5% of the tick population is infected by *Rickettsia rickettsii*. Ticks may be encountered at any time of the year, but the main season is generally between spring through early summer.

The first symptoms appear from 4 to 12 days after the tick bite or after it has been crushed on the skin.[34] The initial symptoms are fever, chills, severe headache, restlessness, and insomnia. Two to 5 days later, petechial hemorrhagic lesions appear, usually occurring first on the extremities around the wrists and ankles. Later the rash spreads over the entire body, including the face, palms of the hands, and soles of the feet. The rash results from the rickettsial invasion of the smooth muscle cells of the arteriolar walls as well as vascular endothelium. Headache is a prominent symptom, and neurologic manifestations are delirium, stupor, and coma in the more serious cases. Myocarditis and bronchopneumonia are complications. The spleen is usually enlarged and palpable.

One attack establishes a high degree of immunity. Vaccines are also available for prevention.

Smallpox[4, 20, 23]

Smallpox (variola) is an acute exanthematous fever of viral origin. It is characterized by an eruption of papules and vesicles or pustules on all parts of the skin and exposed mucous membranes. The period of incubation lasts about 12 to 15 days from exposure. It is mainly spread by direct personal contact. The skin lesions and secretions from the mouth and nose contain the virus. There are no smallpox carriers. Three types of smallpox are recognized—the discrete, confluent, and hemorrhagic. In the hemorrhagic form there is hemorrhage into and around the cutaneous lesions. Hemorrhages may also occur in the kidneys and lungs. This type has a poor prognosis. The term "alastrim" has been applied to the mild form. The term "verioloid" is used for infections modified by vaccination. In this form the cutaneous lesions are discrete, and the pustular stage is absent. Before vaccination provided protection, smallpox was as common as measles and much more fatal. Those who recovered from an attack were often disfigured for life, and some were blind. The disease is rare in the United States. In most countries of the world the disease is under control through vaccinations, but India, West Africa, and South America are exceptions. Travel abroad by United States citizens usually requires a smallpox vaccination of recent date. One attack confers immunity.

Syphilis[28, 29, 38]

Syphilis is an infection caused by the spirochete *Treponema pallidum*. This is the most serious venereal disease because of its devastating systemic effects. Syphilis is usually acquired through sexual intercourse, but the infection may be transmitted in blood transfusion and an infected mother can pass the infection to offspring in utero.

Anal and rectal syphilitic infections demonstrated by chancres occur in male homosexuals.[18] The increase of male homosexuality has contributed to the incidence of extragenital manifestations of venereal disease. Serologic examinations and rectal examination at regular intervals are important procedures in routine screening of homosexual patients.

In the first stage of acquired syphilis a chancre appears on the genital organs, usu-

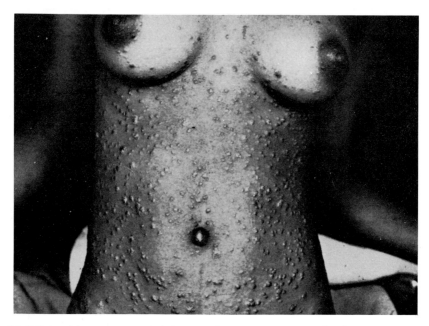

Fig. 14-6. Secondary cutaneous syphilis, papulosquamous. (From Olansky, S., and Rudolph, A. H.: In Top, F. H., editor: Communicable and infectious diseases, ed. 8, St. Louis, 1976, The C. V. Mosby Co.)

ally 10 to 30 days after contact with an infected person. The chancre is hard and varies from a small erosion to a deep ulcer. It is usually single, and in females it may be hidden in the vaginal vault. It is usually on the vulva in females and on the urethra in males. A regional lymphadenitis occurs during this stage. Chancres may also occur on the fingers, lips, and elsewhere on the body. The chancre heals within 4 to 6 weeks.

The secondary stage (Fig. 14-6) begins about 2 to 10 weeks after the appearance of the chancre. It is characterized by malaise, generalized lymphadenopathy, and a macular or papular eruption over the body. These eruptions also occur in the mouth, vulva, vagina, and rectum and are known as mucous patches. Gastrointestinal upset, iritis, and sore throat may also be symptoms of the secondary stage. The infections transmitted by blood transfusions are characterized by secondary stage symptoms. The lesions will subside spontaneously within a few weeks, but in untreated patients recurrent lesions may appear anytime from several months to 3 years later. This is the stage when the organisms enter the bloodstream.

The tertiary stage may not appear for 8 to 25 years after the initial infection. Nearly all tissues and anatomic sites may be involved in this stage, but the most seriously affected are the cardiovascular system, central nervous system, skeletal system, skin, and upper respiratory tract. Tissue destruction may be diffuse in this stage, and there may be gummas. (See Fig. 18-22, A.)

Syphilis is primarily a vascular disease, and the large arteries and the medium-sized and small muscular arteries may be involved, as well as the capillaries. Syphilitic aortitis is one of the most common and serious lesions of tertiary syphilis. (See Fig. 18-19, A.) Syphilis has also been responsible for more and different pathologic reactions in the central nervous system than any other single disease.[28] Regardless of

better control of neurosyphilis, it is responsible for about 33,000 patients in mental institutions in the United States.[28] Neurosyphilis occurs in about 20% to 25% of untreated cases and is more common in males than females.[28] In the central nervous system it occurs as meningovascular syphilis, paresis, and tabes dorsalis. (See Figs. 18-18, D, and 18-30, D.) Intracranial nerves may be damaged, causing deafness and visual disturbances. Paresis is the general paralysis of the insane and is a progressive type of cerebral degeneration. Tabes dorsalis is a late manifestation involving the spinal cord with severe neurologic symptoms.

Congenital syphilis (prenatal syphilis) is transmitted by the infected mother to the offspring in utero, usually during the first 2 years of the mother's infection. An overwhelming infection may result in death of the fetus and abortion, but if the fetus survives, the lesions are similar to those of tertiary syphilis in the acquired type.[38]

In infantile congenital syphilis, which lasts from birth to the second year, the lesions are mucocutaneous and osseous. The child has rhinitis with snuffles, and fissures may occur about the lips and anus. The long bones are usually involved and are deformed in some cases with the saber shin. There is an associated painful periostitis. Congenital neurosyphilis may result in mental retardation and internal hydrocephalus. Other manifestations are anemia, saddle nose, lymphadenopathy, and nephrosis. The late lesions of congenital syphilis develop after the second year but seldom after 30 years of age. These include Hutchinson's teeth, deafness, and interstitial keratitis in about 30% to 50% of the cases with vascularization of the cornea.[38]

Syphilis cannot be diagnosed solely on clinical manifestations, since it is a great mimic of many diseases. The diagnosis depends on demonstration of the organisms and specific antibodies. The tests most often employed are the VDRL (Veneral Disease Research Laboratory microflocculation slide test), the TPI (*Treponema pallidum* immobilization test), and TPCF (*Treponema pallidum* complement-fixation test).[38]

Tetanus[9, 29]

The etiologic agent of tetanus is *Clostridium tetani,* which is widely distributed in nature, particularly in cultivated and garden soil. It is commonly found in the feces of cattle and horses and, to a certain extent, in humans. Once an area is contaminated, the spores can exist indefinitely. This infection affects humans and many other mammals, particularly horses, mice, guinea pigs, and goats.[23] It is almost entirely a wound complication, particularly those that are punctured, lacerated, and contused. Necrotic tissue, foreign bodies, pus infections, and other irritants favor the development of tetanus. The infection is called lockjaw because of the painful spasms that occur in the muscles of the jaw and neck. The jaws may become immovable in severe and terminal cases. The spasms can spread to the voluntary muscles of the body, especially the back, producing opisthotonus. Tetanus is primarily an infection of the nervous tissue, with injury largely limited to the peripheral nerves and anterior horn cells. This incubation period varies from a few days to a month but is usually 4 to 14 days. Immunization against tetanus has contributed to a decreased incidence of the disease. Antitoxin, unlike that used in diphtheria, is limited in value, since tetanus toxin, once absorbed by the nervous tissue, is fixed to the tissue and no amount of antitoxin will neutralize or undo the damage that has already been done.

Tularemia[9, 36]

Tularemia (rabbit fever) is an infection caused by *Pasteurella tularensis,* a small gram-negative bacillus. It was first identified in the United States in 1911 in Tulare County, California, from which it derives its name. However, it is not confined to this area but occurs throughout the United States and in many foreign countries. Wild animals, particularly the jackrabbit, rabbit, and ground squirrel, are the organisms' chief natural reservoir. A variety of other animals, such as the muskrat, beaver, and even dogs and cats, may also be infected, and some insects and birds have also been known to contract the infection. A biting fly, called the deerfly, horseflies, and certain ticks are comon carriers. Humans become infected through the bite of an infected animal or carrier insect or from handling the carcass or eating undercooked meat of an infected animal. It is also possible to become infected by drinking water from streams inhabited by diseased animals, such as the beaver and muskrat.[36] Trappers, hunters, butchers, and laboratory workers are susceptible to infection from their direct contact with infected animals. About 180 cases are reported in the United States yearly; the mortality rate is about 4%.[9]

The organism needs no wound for entry into the body but is able to penetrate through apparently healthy skin. The infection may also be rubbed into the eyes with contaminated fingers. The incubation period is 3 to 5 days, and the onset is rather sudden with headache, chills, fever, and sometimes extreme exhaustion. The portal of entry can soon be identified by the development of an ulcer. Lymph nodes in the area of the ulcer are likely to become enlarged and are sometimes abscessed. Swollen lymph nodes may resemble the buboes of plague, a disease which has much in common with tularemia.

With ophthalmic lesions there is edema, marked hyperemia, itching, pain, and multiple small discrete yellowish nodules on the mucous membrane. Scarring of the cornea and blindness may result. Tularemia is a septicemic type of disease, and a variety of organs may be involved. The lungs may be involved with discrete nodules resembling those of tuberculosis, or there may be pneumonia. A granulomatous reaction simulating tuberculosis may also occur in the liver.

A number of tests are useful in establishing a diagnosis, such as cultures from local external lesions, blood, or in cases of pneumonia, from sputum. Material from lesions may also be inoculated into a guinea pig. Cultures are hazardous for laboratory workers from danger of contracting the infection. Skin tests are also useful as is the demonstration of specific agglutinins.[9]

Recovery is slow, but permanent immunity from further attacks results.

Typhoid[9, 23, 29, 37]

Typhoid fever is a communicable disease caused by the typhoid bacillus, *Salmonella typhosa*. The body discharges, urine and feces, of infected persons contain typhoid bacilli. If water, milk, or food becomes contaminated with these discharges, there is danger of spreading the disease. Some people who have recovered from typhoid fever and others who have again picked up typhoid bacilli after having had the disease are typhoid carriers. Flies may also carry the typhoid bacilli from infected material to food supplies.

The portal of entry is the gastrointestinal tract. The incubation period is usually 10 to 14 days, during which time the organisms have penetrated the intestinal mucosa and entered the lymphatic vessels and mesenteric nodes.[9] From here they are carried to the liver and then by way of the thoracic duct enter the bloodstream. The symptoms begin gradually, with a feeling of fatigue, some fever, cough, headache, and generalized aching. After the disease has become systemic, there is abdominal pain and tenderness, septicemia, splenic enlargement, and mental confusion. Rose colored spots may appear on the body in the second week of the illness, sometimes earlier, and sometimes later. The spots resemble petechial hemorrhages at first glance but will blanch on digital pressure, revealing them to be marked hyperemia. The rose spots disappear after a few days. The temperature is usually high for about 10 days. When the fever subsides, the symptoms slowly disappear.

The effects of bacterial injury are mainly in the intestinal tract, mesenteric lymph nodes, spleen, and liver. There is both splenomegaly and hepatomegaly. Lymph nodes in the region of the cecum are particularly swollen. Ulceration of the ileum may occur, with smaller ulcers in the colon. Leukopenia is characteristic of typhoid fever and is an important clinical sign. There are many complications such as septicemia, massive intestinal hemorrhage, peritonitis from perforation of the bowel, rupture of a mesenteric lymph node, with peritonitis, meningitis, endocarditis, or nephritis from focal metastatic infections. Infection of the gallbladder almost invariably occurs, and this organ is where typhoid carriers may be carrying the organisms.[9]

Confirmation of diagnosis may be made by laboratory tests that demonstrate typhoid bacilli in the blood, feces, and urine. A measure of immunity may be gained by a series of three injections; this immunity lasts for a year but can be renewed with booster shots. One attack of typhoid fever, as a rule, produces a lasting immunity.

Responses

Step 1: infection
Step 2: contagious
Step 3: 1. F; 2. T; 3. F; 4. T; 5. F
Step 4: 1. respiratory usual route (gastrointestinal in bovine tuberculosis; rarely placental, and cutaneous transmission in some types); 2. sexual contact (neonate's eyes rarely infected in birth process; rarely from handling infected material); 3. gastrointestinal; 4. skin; 5. gastrointestinal; 6. sexual contact; 7. respiratory tract; 8. respiratory tract; 9. gastrointestinal tract; 10. respiratory tract; 11. gastrointestinal tract; 12. respiratory tract; 13. skin; 14. skin; 15. respiratory tract; 16. respiratory tract
Step 5: 1. direct; 2. indirect; 3. intermediate host; 4. carrier (in any order)
Step 6: 1. direct; 2. indirect; 3. indirect; 4. direct; 5. carrier; 6. carrier; 7. direct (kissing has not been absolutely proved as a means of transference); 8. carrier;

9. carrier; 10. intermediate host; 11. direct; 12. intermediate host

Step 7: 1. meninges; 2. genital tract; 3. intestinal tract; 4. lungs; 5. respiratory tract; 6. stomach; intestines; 7. central nervous system; 8. lungs

Step 8: 1. X; 2. X; 4. X; 5. X; 8. X

Step 9: 1. T; 2. T; 3. F; 4. T; 5. T; 6. T

Step 10: 1. bacteria; 2. bacteria; 3. virus; 4. fungus; 5. protozoon; 6. virus; 7. bacteria; 8. bacteria; 9. bacteria; 10. bacteria; 11. bacteria; 12. virus; 13. rickettsia; 14. bacteria; 15. bacteria; 16. bacteria; 17. bacteria; 18. bacteria; 19. bacteria; 20. bacteria; 21. rickettsia; 22. virus; 23. virus; 24. fungus; 25. protozoon; 26. helminth; 27. helminth; 28. bacteria; 29. helminth; 30. virus; 31. helminth; 32. virus; 33. virus; 34. rickettsia; 35. virus; 36. fungus; 37. bacteria; 38. rickettsia; 39. helminth; 40. bacteria

REFERENCES

1. Baker, R. D.: In Anderson, W. A. D., editor: Pathology, ed. 6, St. Louis, 1971, The C. V. Mosby Co. (fungal infection).

2. Bennett, G. A.: In Anderson, W. A. D., editor: Pathology, ed. 6, St. Louis, 1971, The C. V. Mosby Co. (osteomyelitis).

3. Corman, L. C., and others: J.A.M.A. **230:** 568-570, 1974 (pharyngeal gonorrhea).

4. Downie, A. W.: In Rivers, T. M., and Horsfall, F. L., editors: Viral and rickettsial infections of man, ed. 3, Philadelphia, 1959, J. B. Lippincott Co. (smallpox).

5. Edmondson, H. A., and Peters, R. L.: In Anderson, W. A. D., editor: Pathology, ed. 6, St. Louis, 1971, The C. V. Mosby Co. (hepatitis).

6. Fekity, F. R.: In Beeson, P. R., and McDermott, W., editors: Cecil-Loeb textbook of medicine, ed. 13, Philadelphia, 1971, W. B. Saunders Co. (staphylococcus infection).

7. Hillman, M. R.: Am. Rev. Respir. Dis. **87:** 165, 1963 (vaccine protection).

8. Hochberg, F. H., Nelson, K., and Janzen, W.: J.A.M.A. **231:**817-821, 1975 (influenza type B–related encephalopathy).

9. Hopps, H. C.: In Anderson, W. A. D., editor: Pathology, ed. 6, St. Louis, 1971, The C. V. Mosby Co. (bacterial disease).

10. Howel, J. B. L.: In Beeson, P. R., and McDermott, W., editors: Cecil-Loeb textbook of medicine, ed. 13, Philadelphia, 1971, W. B. Saunders Co. (chronic bronchitis).

11. Klatskin, G.: In Harrison, T. R., and others, editors: Principles of internal medicine, ed. 4, New York, 1962, The Blakiston Division, McGraw-Hill, Inc. (carriers).

12. Marcial-Rojas, R. A.: In Anderson, W. A. D., editor: Pathology, ed. 6, St. Louis, 1971, The C. V. Mosby Co. (protozoal and helminthic diseases).

13. Medical News: J.A.M.A. **230:**1497-1498, 1974 (Reye syndrome)

14. Medical News: J.A.M.A. **230:**1504, 1974 (Rocky Mt. spotted fever).

15. Meyers, J. D., and others: Ann. Intern. Med. **81:**145-151, 1974 (parenterally transmitted hepatitis A associated with platelet transfusions).

16. Miale, J. B.: In Anderson, W. A. D., editor: Pathology, ed. 6, 1971, The C. V. Mosby Co. (infectious mononucleosis).

17. Millard, M.: In Anderson, W. A. D., editor: Pathology, ed. 6, 1971, The C. V. Mosby Co. (bronchitis).

18. Nazemi, M. C., and others: J.A.M.A. **231:** 389, 1975. (syphilitic proctitis in a homosexual).

19. Owen, R. L., and Hill, J. L.: J.A.M.A. **220:** 1305-1318, 1972 (rectal and pharyngeal gonorrhea in homosexual man).

20. Pinkerton, H.: In Anderson, W. A. D., editor: Pathology, ed. 6, St. Louis, 1971, The C. V. Mosby Co. (viral and rickettsial diseases).

21. Richter, M. N.: In Anderson, W. A. D., editor: Pathology, ed. 5, St. Louis, 1966, The C. V. Mosby Co. (leukemia in mice).

22. Robbins, S. L.: Pathology, ed. 3, Philadelphia, 1967, W. B. Saunders Co. (infectious diseases).

23. Rosenau, M. J.: Preventive medicine and hygiene, ed. 6, New York, 1940, Appleton-Century-Crofts (mode of entry and transference of infectious agents; immunity and infectious diseases).

24. Scotti, T. M.: In Anderson, W. A. D., editor: Pathology, ed. 6, St. Louis, 1971, The C. V. Mosby Co. (pericarditis).

25. Smadel, J. E.: Science **140:**153, 1963 (carriers).

26. Smith, J. W., and Mathewson, C., Jr.: West. J. Surg. **70:**225, 1962 (appendicitis).

27. Stollerman, G. H.: In Beeson, P. R., and McDermott, W., editors: Cecil-Loeb textbook of medicine, ed. 13, Philadelphia, 1971, W. B. Saunders Co. (streptococcus infection).

28. Thomas, E. W.: Med. Clin. North Am. **48:** 699, 1974 (neurosyphilis).

29. Top, F. A., Sr., and Wehrle, P. A.: Communicable and infectious diseases, ed. 8, St. Louis, 1976, The C. V. Mosby Co.

30. U.S. Department of Health, Education, and Welfare, Public Health Service Publication No. 157, Health Information Series 49, revised 1966 (amebiasis).

31. U.S. Department of Health, Education, and

Welfare, Public Health Service, DHEW Publication No. (CDC) 74-8271, 1974 (hepatitis).

32. U.S. Department of Health, Education, and Welfare, Public Health Service, DHEW Publication No. (NIH) 74-187, 1974 (influenza).

33. U.S. Department of Health, Education, and Welfare, Public Health Service Publication No. 211, Health Information Series 46, 1960 (meningococcal meningitis).

34. U.S. Department of Health, Education, and Welfare, Public Health Service Publication No. 319, Health Information Series 20, revised 1964 (Rocky Mountain spotted fever).

35. U.S. Department of Health, Education, and Welfare, Public Health Service, DHEW Publication No. (NIH) 72-307, Public Health Service Publication No. 1308, revised 1972 (shingles, herpes zoster).

36. U.S. Department of Health, Education, and Welfare, Public Health Service Publication No. 135, Health Information Series 44, revised 1962 (tularemia).

37. U.S. Department of Health, Education, and Welfare, Public Health Service Publication No. 282, Health Information Series 72, 1970 (typhoid fever).

38. von Haam, E.: In Anderson, W. A. D., editor: Pathology, ed. 6, St. Louis, 1971, The C. V. Mosby Co. (venereal diseases).

39. Wagner, R. R.: In Beeson, P. B., and McDermott, W., editors: Cecil-Loeb textbook of medicine, ed. 13, Philadelphia, 1971, W. B. Saunders Co. (herpes simplex).

40. Wiesner, P. J., and others: N. Engl. J. Med. **288**:181-185, 1973 (clinical spectrum of pharyngeal gonococcal infection).

CHAPTER 15

Congenital anomalies

Congenital anomalies or malformations exist at or before birth and are the result of a failure of a part or parts to unite or develop properly, usually during the embryologic existence. The most vulnerable period of embryonic life is considered to be the first 3 to 8 weeks, and most of the congenital disorders or defects representing an arrest in development of a part or parts or aberrations from normal pattern occur at this stage. Many of the defects, such as spina bifida, clubfoot, cleft lip or palate, amelia (absence of a limb or limbs), or other deformities in structure, are obvious at birth, but some such as Meckel's diverticulum, atresias of the esophagus and biliary system, and heart defects, are dis covered when the infant fails to thrive immediately after birth or later in childhood, or it may be a fortuitous finding.[5]

Nature as a rule faithfully follows an established blueprint for the construction of a human body, so that parents can be reasonably assured that their offspring will be born with all its necessary organs intact and functioning normally. However, confusion can creep in for a variety of reasons and disrupt the normal pattern. Even a slight interference with the morphogenetic process can cause imperfect development of a part or even absence of a part of the embryo. The absence of a limb or limbs (amelia) gained international recognition when a number of infants were born with knoblike or flipperlike appendages instead of normal legs and arms. The cause of this disorder was traced to the drug thalidomide, taken in pregnancy roughly between the twenty-eighth and the forty-second day of gestation when the arms and legs were being formed.

Eight weeks after conception the embryo (from a Greek word meaning to swell) becomes a fetus, which in Latin means the young one. All the major body systems are developed in the embryo in various stages. The normal fetus will further develop and synchronize all the systems until at the end of about 266 days or 9 months (from date of conception through embryonal and fetal stages) the infant is born free of malformations or deformities.

The embryonal and fetal parasitic existence in the womb has been made possible during this 9 months' stay by the remarkable organ, the placenta, which is a cakelike mass in the uterus that provides necessary nourishment and protection from harmful exogenous influences. Although the placenta normally safeguards the embryo or fetus from bacteria and other harmful agents, it cannot screen out all harmful organisms.

The German measles (rubella) virus can cross the placental barrier and cause damage to the developing fetus, when a woman contracts the disease early in her pregnancy.[13, 28] The first 3 months of pregnancy are the most dangerous period, but evidence exists that the fetus may also be affected when rubella occurs after this period. In the 1964 to 1965 epidemic some infants born to mothers who had rubella in the second trimester had hearing defects, were mentally retarded, or were of small stature.[28] The risk of serious malformation from maternal rubella in the first 8 weeks of pregnancy may exceed 50%, and the infants are more likely to have multiple anomalies. The affected babies may appear normal at birth and later develop a wide variety of defects. Until the 1964 to 1965 epidemic there were four categories generally included in the rubella syndrome[28]: (1) hearing loss; (2) eye defects, mostly cataracts, glaucoma, and unusually small size of the eyeball, lesions of the retina and clouding of the cornea unassociated with glaucoma; (3) cardiovascular defects, with patent ductus arteriosus, usually associated with pulmonary artery stenosis being the most common; and (4) abnormalities of the central nervous system —small head, mental retardation, delayed psychomotor development, cerebral palsy, and behavior disturbances, including infantile autism. In addition to these permanent defects a number of transient abnormalities were noted during this epidemic.[13] These included thrombocytopenic purpura, hepatomegaly and splenomegaly, hepatitis with jaundice, lymphadenopathy,[13] anemia with low white blood cell count, encephalitis, meningitis, injury of heart muscle evidenced by abnormal electrocardiographic tracings, and giant cell pneumonia of the newborn. Examination of aborted fetuses and infants born dead or dying soon after birth revealed the presence of the virus in almost all organs of the body.

The protozoon causing toxoplasmosis can also cross the placental barrier and cause destructive lesions of the central nervous system, eyes, and viscera. The lesions appear to result from maternal infection during the last trimester of pregnancy. Syphilis can also be transmitted to the developing offspring. (See the section on congenital syphilis in Chapter 14.) The effects of heroin on a fetus from an addicted mother are described in Chapter 12. In the early weeks of pregnancy, shingles may injure the developing fetus. The damage reported is similar to that often found in babies whose mothers had German measles (rubella) in early pregnancy. Ionizing radiation during pregnancy can also be harmful to a developing fetus, the type of defects depending on the stage of embryonic or fetal development at the time.

There is a tendency to confuse the inherited diseases with those that are true congenital disorders. For a disease to be inherited it must be transmitted by a gene or genes, whose characters are contained in the germ plasm of the parental sex cells. The distinction between congenital and inherited disorders will become clearer when you have studied the role of the gene in heredity, which is the subject of the next chapter.

A prerequisite for understanding congenital anomalies is a knowledge of normal anatomy and physiology; otherwise you cannot understand the extent and mechanism of the injury involved.

HEART[3, 4, 16, 23]

Congenital heart abnormalities are the result of inborn defects caused by failure of the heart or major blood vessels near the heart to develop normally during the period of growth before birth. About 30,000 to 40,000 infants are born yearly with this type of heart ailment, accounting for about 50% of all deaths caused by congenital defects in the first year of life. The etiology of most cases is unknown, but such maternal infections as German measles during the first trimester of pregnancy and nutritional disorders in early pregnancy may be contributing factors. The role of heredity as an etiologic factor in heart defects is not completely known, although there have been rare instances when similar defects were observed in siblings.

Some congenital heart defects are incompatible with life, so that the newborn lives only a few minutes or a few months. Some defects are so slight that they cause no trouble during the individual's lifetime;

some are only incidental findings at autopsy. The malformations of the heart are diverse, but surgery can now repair many of these crippled hearts, and the child can lead a normal or nearly normal existence, with the same life expectancy as those born with normal hearts.

To evaluate and understand the malfunctioning of a defective heart, you should have a clear understanding of the range of normal function of the heart in the newborn infant. Congenital heart defects occur in utero at some stage of development. To understand the normal heart of an infant, it is necessary to have a knowledge of fetal circulation, which differs materially from the infant's blood circulation after birth.

In the illustrations that accompany this chapter you will be able to compare a normal heart with a defective one in the major congenital disorders, and the mechanics of the damage in the latter should be readily apparent. By comparing the normal heart and circulation with that of the fetal circulation, again, you should be able to understand the difference in anatomic requirements for circulation of blood through the embryo and fetus and those for the normal heart after birth. The adjustments that must be made by the newborn infant in his circulatory system should also be apparent, for these directly affect the respiratory system and determine whether the systems will be adequate to sustain life.

Fetal heart development and circulation[2, 5]

The heart begins to form during the second week of embryonic life and by the eighteenth day it is beating, even if haltingly. In the earliest stages of development the circulatory system is a straight tube for the passage of blood in an undivided stream. This primitive organ is anchored in the body at the head (cephalid) by arterial trunks and at the tail (caudal) by the great veins. At this stage of development the embryo bears no resemblance to a human body, for there is mainly a bulbous end representing the head, with a tapering off to a tail or point. As the embryo develops, dilatations and sacculations occur in the walls of the tubes, and through convolutions or folds the partitions begin to form for the four chambers of the heart, complete with openings and valves for the direction of the blood flow through the heart. By the time the embryo is 8 weeks old, the heart will be developed. It is during these critical weeks for the embryo that deviations from the normal pattern may result in abnormal or arrested growth in the development of the heart as well as other organs.

One of the first requirements for life of the embryo is a system of circulation of blood so that oxygen and nutrients may be available. To understand the fetal circulation, you have to know something about the all-important role that the placenta plays as a go-between organ for the embryo or the fetus and the mother, exchanging oxygen, transmitting nutrients, and discarding wastes. The role of the circulatory system in the fetus in this respect is closely parallel to that of the neonate and adult, with notable exceptions, in anatomic variations for functioning. Contrary to popular belief the fetal circulation is not directly connected to the mother's bloodstream. It exists as a separate circulatory system, functioning through the umbilical vein and arteries in the cord—the lifeline from the fetus to the placenta. The mother also has a separate circulatory system in the placenta. The two systems, fetal and maternal, are walled off from each other. The walls of the blood vessels of the two systems are permeable, however, so that there can be an exchange of materials carried in the bloodstream of the mother and the fetus. The placenta acts as a barrier between the mother and the embryo or fetus for filtering out bacteria and damaging drugs, although selectively allowing transmission or exchange of materials. Actually the embryo or fetus is a parasite or a piece of foreign material as far as the mother is concerned, and would be rejected and cast off through her immunologic system if it were directly connected to her bloodstream. How the placenta can successfully subvert the mother's immunologic defenses is not known. The very secret of life and development of the fetus lies in the ability of the circulatory systems of the fetus and mother to act independently in separate chambers.

Pulmonary functions are absent in the fetus, so his source of oxygen is through diffusion in the placenta from maternal blood to fetal blood, and carbon dioxide is excreted by the reverse process. Some distinctive features of fetal circulation are obliterated after birth. The persistence of these after birth, with the exception of the umbilical cord (cut at birth), constitutes some of the serious congenital heart defects. These features are briefly as follows:

Ductus venosus is a fetal blood channel connecting the umbilical cord with the inferior vena cava, carrying oxygenated blood from the placenta. This becomes occluded at birth and is known as the ligamentum venosum.

Foramen ovale is an opening between the right atrium and the left atrium for shunting of blood. After birth, when the pulmonary circulation increases and more blood is returned from the lungs to the left atrium, the pressure rises in the left atrium, and the foramen ovale closes.

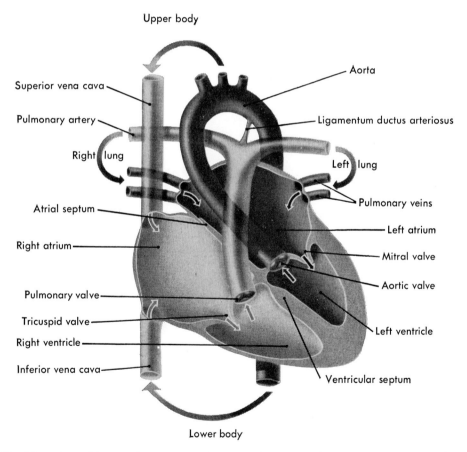

Fig. 15-1. Normal heart. The arrows indicate the direction of blood flow through the four chambers and great vessels. (From Nursing Education Service Bulletin No. 7, Ross Laboratories.)

Ductus arteriosus is a channel running from the pulmonary artery into the aorta for distribution of blood in part to the lower extremities and to the viscera of the abdomen and pelvis. The greater amount is sent to the hypogastric arteries and conveyed to the umbilical arteries for return to the placenta. When the umbilical cord is tied at birth, the placental circulation ceases, and the ends of the hypogastric arteries atrophy and are known as hypogastric ligaments.

Patent ductus arteriosus

At birth every infant has a patent ductus arteriosus, but when the lungs become inflated with air, this passageway is closed between the two major blood vessels, the pulmonary artery and the aorta (Fig. 15-1).

When this fails to occur, some oxygenated blood is passed back and forth needlessly to the lungs through this passageway, instead of going through the aorta and its tributaries to all parts of the body. Some oxygen will be lost to the tissues through this superfluous circulation to the lungs, and the aorta will not be carrying a full load of oxygen to body tissues. Growth will ultimately be retarded. The heart will be overworked in an attempt to balance the supply with the demand for oxygen, and compensatory cardiac enlargement will result. Since the heart depends upon the lungs for its supply of oxygen, the lungs become overworked in their effort to keep pace with oxygen demands and breathing becomes dyspneic on even slight exertion, with resultant fatigue. The extra workload

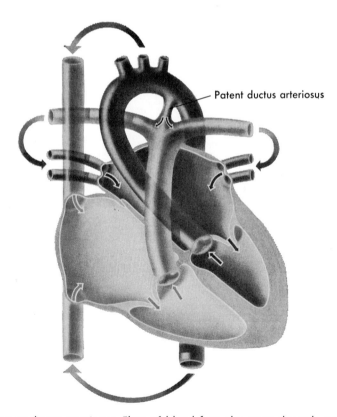

Fig. 15-2. Patent ductus arteriosus. Flow of blood from the aorta through a patent ductus to the pulmonary artery caused overloading of the pulmonary circulation. Left to right shunt—no cyanosis. (From Nursing Education Service Bulletin No. 7, Ross Laboratories.)

for supplying oxygen eventually weakens the lungs, and they become more susceptible to respiratory infections.

The damage in this defect is proportional to the extent and size of the persistent channel. The newborn infant may be asymptomatic, except for a systolic murmur. Later a typical machinery murmer may develop, usually with a thrill. Pulse pressures also vary, with Corrigan (jerky) or water-hammer radial pulsations. The diastolic pressure is lowered because of the flowoff of blood from the aorta into the pulmonary circuit. Pulmonary hypertension may also occur (Fig. 15-2).

Coarctation of the aorta

The aorta is normally a large vessel with a lumen adequate to carry sufficient oxy-

genated blood to the body tissues. In coarctation a marked thickening of the medial muscle layer pinches the lumen of the aorta, and the normal flow of blood is obstructed. The seriousness of the defect depends on the location of the constriction. In preductal coarctation the constriction of the aorta is terminal, before the entrance of the ductus arteriosus, which may remain patent during early life. In this type the unoxygenated blood from the right ventricle may pass through the patent ductus arteriosus into the aorta. Since normally all the blood passing into the aorta should be oxygenated, this adding of a portion of unoxygenated blood, which must be subtracted from total volume, represents some loss of needed oxygen for body tissues.

In postductal coarctation the stenosis of

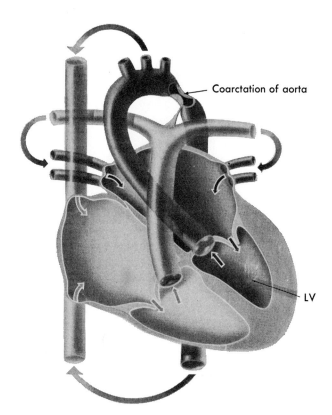

Fig. 15-3. Coarctation of the aorta with normally closed ductus. Narrowing of the inside of the aorta puts strain upon the pumping left ventricle *(LV)*. No shunt. (From Nursing Education Service Bulletin No. 7, Ross Laboratories.)

the aorta is directly beyond the ductus arteriosus, which generally closes normally. To supply the needed oxygenated blood to the lower body tissues, a collateral circulation bypasses the coarctation.

In both types of coarctation the left ventricular pressure and workload are increased to push blood through a narrow passageway. This results in hypertension in the upper extremities and hypotension in the lower extremities. Systolic murmurs are present in the majority of these patients.

Arterial pulsations in the lower extremities may be weak or absent as a result of reduction of the pulse wave by the constriction at the coarcted site. The child may be asymptomatic or may experience occasional fatigue, headache, leg cramps, and nosebleeds (Fig. 15-3).

Ventricular septal defects

Ventricular septal defects are abnormal openings between the right and left ventricles. They vary in size and may occur in either the muscular or membranous portion of the wall. The shunting of blood from the left to the right ventricle occurs during systole because of the higher pressure in the ventricle. The shunt may be reversed, that is, right to left, if pulmonary vascular resistance produces pulmonary hypertension. These patients experience cyanosis. If the ventricular septal defect is small and low, shunting of the blood is caused by normal pressure differential between the right and left chambers and the volume of blood flowing from the right ventricle is not markedly increased. Usually these patients are asymptomatic except for a heart

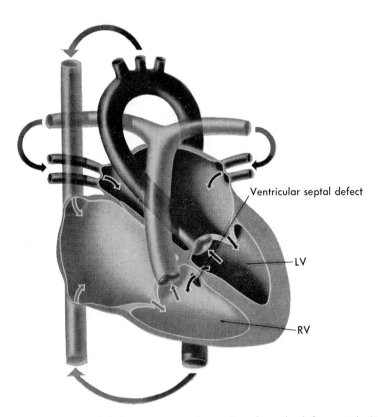

Ventricular septal defect

LV

RV

Fig. 15-4. Ventricular septal defect. Arrows indicate flow from the left ventricle (LV) to the right ventricle (RV), thus overloading the right ventricle, pulmonary circulation, and left heart. Left to right shunt—no cyanosis. (From Nursing Education Service Bulletin No. 7, Ross Laboratories.)

murmur in the first weeks of life. Small defects without symptoms appear to be compatible with a normal life expectancy.

With large membranous defects the oxygenated blood is shunted from the left to the right ventricle, and right ventricular hypertrophy may occur. The right ventricle is overworked because blood coming through the abnormal opening from the left ventricle, where pressure is higher, increases the volume of blood it must propel through the pulmonary circuit. The workload of the right ventricle is further increased by the resistance set up by vascular changes in the pulmonary arterial bed. In this type of membranous defect, if the septal opening is large, bidirectional shunting may occur. Symptoms of membranous interventricular septal defects are usually severe. Breathing is rapid; growth is retarded; and the infants have feeding difficulties. A blowing systolic murmur is heard over the third and fourth left intercostal space, frequently with a thrill. The sound of the closure of the pulmonary valve is intensified (Fig. 15-4).

Atrial septal defects

The atrial defects are abnormal openings between the atria. The shunt is usually from left to right, but occasionally this is reversed. There are three forms—patent foramen ovale, ostium secundum defect, and ostium primum defect.

Before birth the foramen ovale, a channel in the fetal heart between the right and left atria, shunts oxygenated blood from the right atrium directly into the left

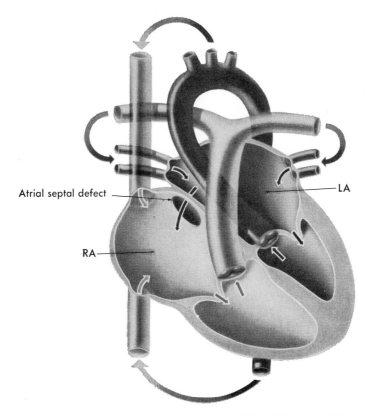

Fig. 15-5. Atrial septal defect. Arrow indicates flow of blood from the left atrium (LA) to the right atrium (RA), thus overloading the right heart, pulmonary circulation, and left heart. Left to right shunt—no cyanosis. (From Nursing Education Service Bulletin No. 7, Ross Laboratories.)

atrium, bypassing the right ventricle and thus the pulmonary circuit. At birth this channel should functionally close and during childhood slowly become obliterated. The malfunctioning of the foramen ovale (patent foramen ovale) is the result of a short valve, a perforated valve, or an enlarged opening at the valve site from incomplete closure. Usually there are no symptoms, but if the shunt is right to left, cyanosis is associated with increased right atrial pressure. In normal hearts the rise in pressure in the left atrium closes the foramen ovale at birth (Fig. 15-5).

The ostium secundum defect is located high in the atrial septum, consisting of one large or several small openings. The defect is the result of failure of the septum secundum to develop completely. There may be associated mitral valve stenosis. Symptoms consist of dyspnea and palpitation. The shunt may be right to left at birth, causing cyanosis. Later the shunt is left to right. Cardiac sounds may be irregular with a systolic murmur and thrill. The child fails to thrive, and exercise tolerance is poor. There may also be frequent episodes of pulmonary infections. The right atrium and right ventricle may become enlarged, as well as the pulmonary artery. This is the result of the increased workload of the heart.

The ostium primum defect is a large gap or opening at the base of the atrial septum. In embryonic life the septum primum divides the primitive atrium into the right and left chambers. If this septum fails to develop properly, a gap forms in the dividing wall of the atria. This type is frequently associated with mitral and tricuspid valve deformities, and there may also be a small, high ventricular septal defect. The shunt is left to right through the defect. Clinical symptoms are dyspnea and systolic murmur and thrill, with bilateral enlargement of the chambers of the heart.

The clinical manifestations of all the types of atrial defects are essentially the same, except for cyanosis, which is present only if the shunt is from right to left. All are dependent on the type and multiplicity of accompanying defects, such as valvular defects when the opening is in close proximity to the valves.

Subaortic stenosis

Subaortic narrowing or stenosis is caused by a fibrous ring below the aortic valve obstructing the blood flow from the left ventricle to the aortic outlet. The stenosis may also be valvular, involving the cusps of the valve with thickening and fusion. In some instances both the valvular cusps and subaortic stricture are involved. Any obstruction to the outflow of blood through the aortic valve increases the workload of the left ventricle and thus results in ventricular enlargement to accommodate the elevated pressure of blood. Depending on the size of the constriction, the infant or child may be asymptomatic. A systolic murmur with a palpable thrill, however, is usually heard at the second right interspace. The impaired cardiac output causes fatigue and syncope (fainting).

Atresia of the tricuspid valve

In atresia of the tricuspid valve there is no opening of the tricuspid valve through which the blood in the right atrium can enter the right ventricle. Blood from the right atrium passes directly through a septal defect into the left atrium and mixes with oxygenated blood from the lungs. This blood enters the left ventricle and is propelled into the systemic circulation. The lungs, however, may receive blood through a small ventricular septal defect, a patent ductus arteriosus, or the bronchial vessels. Other defects associated with tricuspid atresia include stenosis of the pulmonary valve, underdeveloped right ventricle, enlarged left ventricle, and patent ductus arteriosus. The infants are cyanotic from birth and have paroxysmal dyspneic attacks. The infant fails to grow properly and has clubbing of fingers and toes. Harsh systolic murmurs are heard along the left sternal border (Fig. 15-6).

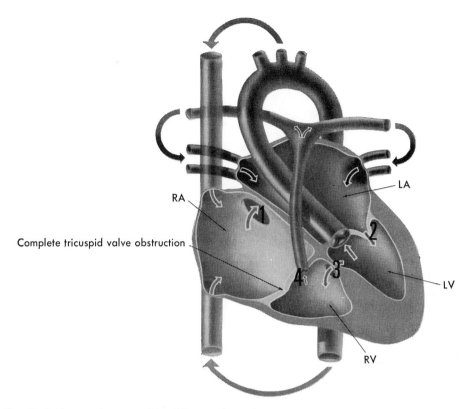

Fig. 15-6. Tricuspid atresia. Blood leaves the right atrium *(RA)* via an atrial septal defect (arrow 1), enters the left atrium *(LA)*, flows to the left ventricle *(LV)* through the mitral valve (arrow 2) and the ventricular septal defect (arrow 3) into the right ventricle *(RV)*, and into the small pulmonary artery (arrow 4). Atrial right to left shunt—cyanosis. (From Nursing Education Service Bulletin No. 7, Ross Laboratories.)

Tetralogy of Fallot

The word *tetra* comes from the Greek word meaning four. The tetralogy of Fallot is a combination of four heart defects— pulmonic stenosis, interventricular septal defects, dextroposition (displacement to the right) of the aorta or overriding aorta, and hypertrophy of the right ventricle. It is named after its discoverer, Louis Arthur Fallot, a French physician. A stenosis impedes the outflow of blood from the right ventricle into the pulmonary circuit, causing obstruction of the pulmonary valve. The right ventricle is overworked in pumping the blood through the narrow pulmonary valve and becomes enlarged. In the septum between the two ventricles is an abnormal opening, allowing unoxygenated blood in the right ventricle to mix with oxygenated blood in the left ventricle, thus decreasing the amount of oxygen the aorta carries to the body tissues for nourishment. The overriding aorta straddles the ventricles, arising at a point over the ventricular septal defect. It receives blood from both ventricles, which is a mixture of both oxygenated and unoxygenated blood.

With all these defects causing an oxygen supply incompatible with body demands for growth and nourishment and with the mixture of venous blood and arterial blood, there is cyanosis developing early in life and, later, retardation of growth. Other clinical manifestations include clubbing of

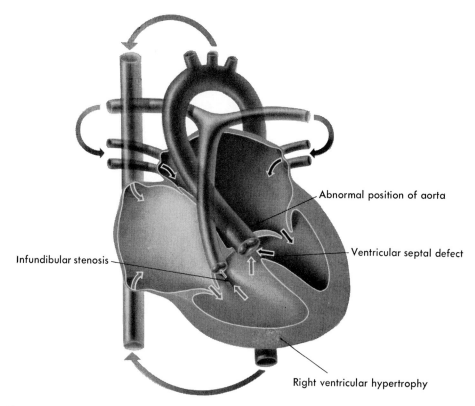

Infundibular stenosis

Abnormal position of aorta

Ventricular septal defect

Right ventricular hypertrophy

Fig. 15-7. Tetralogy of Fallot. Because of the obstructing infundibular pulmonary stenosis, blood flows through a ventricular septal defect into the abnormally placed aorta. Right to left shunt—cyanosis. (From Nursing Education Service Bulletin No. 7, Ross Laboratories.)

fingers and toes, systolic murmurs, and paroxysmal attack of dyspnea with loss of consciousness caused by cerebral anoxia. The aorta is prominent, the heart is small, and the right ventricle is hypertrophied (Fig. 15-7).

Transposition of the great vessels

In the normal heart the pulmonary artery is attached to the right ventricle, and the aorta arises from the left ventricle. Physiologically, their functions differ, with the pulmonary artery carrying unoxygenated blood to the lungs for reoxygenation, and the aorta carrying the freshly oxygenated blood to the body tissues. In transposition of the great vessels, as the name implies, the vessels are reversed, with the pulmonary artery being attached to the left ventricle and the aorta arising from the right

ventricle. This reversal allows oxygenated blood to be received from the lungs and carried back to them needlessly, thus depriving the body of oxygen. The aorta, with its attachment to the right ventricle, receives the blood returned from the body, which is low in oxygen content, and then sends it back through the aorta for redistribution to the body again. Thus oxygen deprivation for the body tissues is severe. Infants born with this defect can survive only if there are other heart defects, such as abnormal passageways (ventricular septal defects or atrial septal defects) or an abnormal vessel connecting the pulmonary artery with the aorta (patent ductus arteriosus). These defects counteract the effects of transposition by allowing oxygenated blood to reach the aorta. Transposition of the great vessels occurs in the

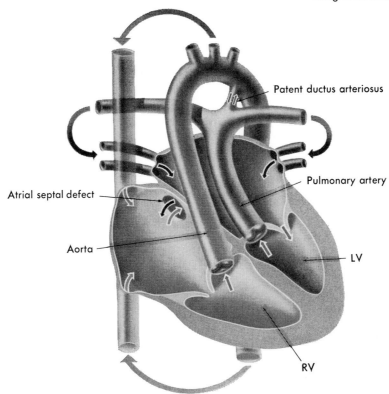

Patent ductus arteriosus

Atrial septal defect

Pulmonary artery

Aorta

LV

RV

Fig. 15-8. Transposition of the great vessels. Aorta arises from the right ventricle (RV), and the pulmonary artery from the left ventricle (LV). This example shows life supported by two bidirectional shunts—a patent ductus arteriosus and an atrial septal defect. Cyanosis. (From Nursing Education Service Bulletin No. 7, Ross Laboratories.)

embryo when there is a straight division of the bulbar trunk without normal spiraling.

These infants are deeply cyanotic at or shortly after birth. Breathing is rapid. If they survive, there is growth retardation and clubbing of fingers and toes. The majority of these patients die in infancy (Fig. 15-8).

Truncus arteriosus

Truncus arteriosus is caused by retention of the embryonic bulbar trunk, resulting from failure of the trunk to separate and to divide into an aorta and pulmonary artery. A single arterial trunk arises from both ventricles and overlies a septal defect. Both the pulmonary and systemic circulation are supplied from the same arterial trunk. This results in an admixture of oxygenated and unoxygenated blood from both

ventricles. Dyspnea and cyanosis occur with exertion. The first heart sound is accentuated, and there is a continuous murmur along the left sternal border, often accompanied by a thrill. A diastolic murmur may also be heard at the base of the heart. The child develops poorly and suffers from fatigue. Most patients die in infancy, but a few have survived to adulthood.

Anomalous venous return

In the normal circulation of blood through the heart and lungs the oxygenated blood is returned to the left atrium by the pulmonary veins. In anomalous venous return the oxygenated blood returns from the lungs by one or more pulmonary veins, emptying directly or indirectly through venous channels into the right atrium. If the anomalous venous return is complete, drainage of all the pulmonary and systemic veins empties into the right atrium. If the anomalous return of the pulmonary veins to the right atrium is only partial, the functions are the same as in septal defect of the atrium. If the defect is complete, an interatrial communication is necessary to allow blood to reach the left side of the heart for distribution to the systemic circulation. Patients with partial or complete anomalous venous return often have atrial septal defects, which shunt a mixture of unoxygenated and oxygenated blood to the left atrium and the systemic circulation.

Cyanosis is a common symptom with right-to-left shunting of blood in total anomalous pulmonary venous return. These patients also experience fatigue, dyspnea, tachycardia, and frequent upper respiratory infections. The left chest may protrude because of the marked right ventricular hypertrophy. The symptoms of partial anomalous pulmonary venous return are usually the same as those from atrial septal defects. Patients with complete anomalous return of pulmonary veins frequently die at an early age.

CENTRAL NERVOUS SYSTEM[8, 20, 25]

Among the many known or suspected causes of developmental disorders of the central nervous system are genetic disturbances (for example, trisomy 13-15, trisomy 18), maternal infections (for example, rubella), fetal infection (for example, syphilis), fetal hypoxia, irradiation, nutritional deficiencies and excesses, chemical agents, and mechanical trauma.

Gross developmental defects of the central nervous system include agenesis (absence of a part or parts), dysplasia (disarray from apparent abnormal growth), faulty closures, fusions, and other complex deformities. A malformation that primarily involves only the brain tissue is anencephaly, a condition where the forebrain and calvaria are absent because of defective organization of primordial tissue.

Another is porencephaly, which is abnormal cavitation within the brain substance and cavities that communicate with both the ventricles and the subarachnoid space. Both anencephaly and porencephaly are usually caused by maldevelopment of the brain in the embryo stage.

Closure and fusion errors for the most part are related to bony defects associated with various herniations, such as the myelocele, meningomyelocele, meningocele, encephalocele, spina bifida, and diastematomyelia.

Dysplasias are growth peculiarities affecting the size of the brain. The defects of macrogyria (unusually large gyri) and microgyria (very small gyri) would not be evident at birth as a gross developmental disorder. Microencephaly (a very small brain) and macroencephaly or megaloencephaly (a very large brain) might be evident at birth, especially if there is an associated hydrocephalus, as often occurs. Oxycephaly (tower-shaped skull) is associated with premature closure of the cranial sutures. Microencephaly and oxycephaly are associated with mental deficiency. Myelodysplasia may be caused by incomplete closure of the embryonic neural tube and is associated with spina bifida. Wasting of muscles below the knees and dissociated sensory loss over the legs occur. Micromyelia is an underdeveloped, small, or shortened spinal cord.

Hydrocephalus[20, 27]

The term hydrocephalus (Fig. 15-9) literally means water or fluid on the brain or in the head. It is an abnormal volume of cerebrospinal fluid in the intracranial cavity. Normally the fluid is formed and absorbed so that the volume remains constant while circulating freely in the skull and spinal cord. Obstructions to circulation and absorption result in hydrocephalus. Not all large heads are caused by hydrocephalus; they may be caused by a variety of conditions, some of a familial nature.[27]

The developmental defects that cause hydrocephalus include atresia, stenosis or absence of interventricular communication, failure of formation of the cisterna magna, and failure of cleavage of the pia-arachnoid. Associated malformations are spina bifida and the Arnold-Chiari malformation. Hydrocephalus may not always be caused by congenital anomalies.[20] It may be the result of hemorrhage before or at the time of birth, meningitis, or neoplasms, such as the medulloblastoma, that obstruct the cerebrospinal pathways. Toxoplasma has been incriminated as causing hydrocephalus.[20] It is transmitted in utero and in early pregnancy can interfere with the development of certain structures of the brain.

Hydrocephalus is divided into two types —internal and external. In internal hydrocephalus the cerebrospinal fluid accumulates under pressure, which is indicative of a disturbance in the absorption, formation, or circulation of the fluid. In the noncommunicating type of internal hydrocephalus there is obstruction within or at the outlets of the ventricles, preventing any or all of the cerebrospinal fluid from leaving the ventricles and entering the subarachnoid space. Obstructions may be caused by occlusion of the aqueduct of Sylvius or of Luschka's and Magendie's foramina, other developmental defects, inflammatory reactions, or neoplasms. About one third are caused by obstruction of Luschka's and Magendie's foramina. In the communicating type of internal hydrocephalus, abnormal accumulations of fluid are present even though the connections between the ventricular system and the subarachnoid space are patent. The obstruction is located in the subarachnoid cisternae at the base of the brain, within the subarachnoid space, or at both these sites. The obstruction may be caused by adhesions, failure of cleavage of the leptomeninges (cerebral), tumors, or abnormal absorption because of metabolic defects.[20, 27]

External hydrocephalus is relatively rare. In this condition most of the cerebrospinal fluid accumulates over the surface of the brain. It may be secondary to preexisting internal hydrocephalus. In this type the cerebrum and ventricles may be compressed by the excessive fluid.

The following symptoms and mechanisms of production refer only to internal hydrocephalus, since it is the prevalent type.

The ventricular system is greatly distended above the site of obstruction. This increased ventricular pressure causes thinning of the cerebral cortex and cranial bones. The cranial sutures are widely separated to accommodate the expanding pressure of the cerebrospinal fluid. The cerebral tissue may disappear, leaving only a thin membrane. Compression of the basal ganglia, brainstem, and cerebellum also occurs. The choroid plexuses usually become atrophied to some degree, and if the case is long standing, they are small, sclerotic, and degenerated. These latter findings represent those in cases that have come to autopsy.

At birth the head may be normal in size or only slightly enlarged, but within a

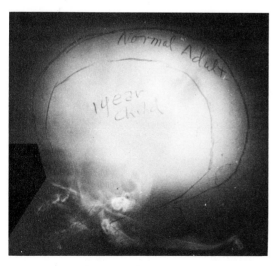

Fig. 15-9. Hydrocephalus in a 1-year-old infant. The superimposed lines show the normal size of a skull in a 1-year-old child and its expansion to that of a normal adult-size skull. (From Young, C. G., and Likos, J. J.: Medical specialty terminology, x-ray and nuclear medicine, St. Louis, 1972, The C. V. Mosby Co.)

period of 2 or 3 months it enlarges at a rapid rate because of tension from accumulation of cerebrospinal fluid (Fig. 15-9). Sutures gap widely, and the cortex of the brain is paper thin. The face shows marked alterations. The forehead is prominent, and the eyebrows and upper eyelids are drawn upward. The eyes are wide apart, and the bridge of the nose is depressed. In advanced cases the entire vault of the cranium is enlarged, with the scalp stretched almost to the bursting point, and the scalp veins stand out. The infant is unable to hold up his head because of its immense size and weight. In unarrested cases, as the head enlarges, the body fails to grow normally. There is gradual mental deterioration. Strabismus, nystagmus, and optic atrophy may also occur, with visual impairment. In the arrested or stationary cases, in which expansion has stopped, the sutures fill in, and the skull becomes rigid and thick. Mental retardation may or may not occur in these cases. A balance seems to be reached between the secretion of spinal fluid and its absorption.

Arnold-Chiari malformation[8, 20, 25, 26]

The Arnold-Chiari malformation is a defect of the hindbrain, which contains the cerebellum and medulla oblongata. These two structures are displaced downward in a tongue-like process and project through the foramen magnum. There may be caudal displacement of the fourth ventricle, with Luschka's and Magendie's foramina directing the flow of cerebrospinal fluid into the spinal subarachnoid space below the foramen magnum. At other times the fourth ventricle openings are obliterated. The cisterna magna may also be obliterated in part or totally by adhesion of the cerebellum to the medulla. Stenosis of the aqueduct of Sylvius may also be present. Various bony defects of the base of the skull and upper cervical vertebrae have been found in association with this malformation. It is a complex deformity in which nervous tissue defects are combined with bony and soft tissue defects. It is been attributed to traction resulting from fixation of the spinal cord at the site of a meningomyelocele, pressure from preexisting hydrocephalus, and malformation caused by dysplasia occurring at about the third month of fetal life.

Symptoms may include paralysis of the extremities, diplopia (double vision), and those symptoms that pertain to hydrocephalus or meningomyelocele, which usually accompany this defect.

Spina bifida[20, 25]

Spina bifida is a developmental anomaly characterized by incomplete fusion of one or more of the vertebral laminae. The anomaly is believed to develop about the fourth week of gestation, since closure of the neural tube is completed by the end of this time.

Spina bifida has occasionally been traced to heredity, but the majority of patients have no history of familial occurrence, maternal trauma, infection, or metabolic disturbance.

Spina bifida is classified into four types—spina bifida occulta, meningocele, meningomyelocele (myelomeningocele), and myelocele. The neural arch fails to fuse at the lumbar, lumbosacral, thoracolumbar, sacral, thoracic, or cervical regions, in this order of frequency.

Spina bifida occulta.[20, 25] In spina bifida occulta the dorsal arch may be a very thin slit separating one lamina from the spinous process, or the spines and laminae may be completely absent. Abnormalities of the spinal cord are involved in this defect. It may be attached to the lower end of the dural sac at the level of the second sacral vertebrae, or a fibrous stalk or band may be connecting the cord, its nerves, and its meninges to the overlying skin. The site in this instance may be indicated by a dimple of the overlying skin. A fistulous tract connecting the spinal cord and its meninges to the skin surface may exist. These are known as dermal sinuses.

Spina bifida may be asymptomatic. Neurologic disorders and other malformations or cutaneous or subcutaneous defects call attention to the defect. The progressive musculoskeletal manifestations are postural gait disturbances, and sensory impairment or paralysis of the lower extremities. There may be vesical and rectal sphincter disorders, with urinary dribbling and rectal incontinence. The malformations that often accompany spina bifida include hydrocephalus, cleft lip and cleft palate, congenital dislocated hip, clubfoot, strabismus, horseshoe kidney, hypospadias, and congenital scoliosis.

Meningocele and meningomyelocele.[8, 25] These defects are readily apparent at birth and are caused by defective closure of the neural tube and vertebral canal. The meningocele is a hernial sac or protrusion of the meninges or membranes covering the spinal cord. The sac contains only cerebrospinal fluid and the meninges. It may be present at any point along the spinal axis but is most often found at the neck or cervical region or the lumbar region.

The meningomyelocele is a visible sac along the spinal axis containing cerebrospinal fluid, meninges, and neural elements. The meningomyelocele usually communicates with the subarachnoid space, so there is a leaking sac. The spinal cord is frequently anchored to the dome of the sac, and the spinal nerves passing into the sac may be adherent to the walls or terminate in the sac. Since the spinal cord is the nerves' pathway from the brain, if the nerves are trapped in the sac and do not carry out their mission, denervation of certain areas of the body results. This may cause vesical and rectal sphincter loss of control and muscular imbalance of the lower extremities, including complete paralysis in some instances. Neurologic symptoms vary with the location of the meningomyelocele. If it is lumbosacral, the paralysis may be flaccid with loss of reflexes and absence of sensation of the lower extremities. If it is thoracic, spasticity with hyperreflexia may occur in one or both lower extremities. If it is cervical, the upper and lower extremities as well as the trunk are involved. If it is the lower cervical region, a peripheral type of motor weakness occurs in the arms with spasticity in the legs.

As a rule, the neurologic manifestations with meningocele are slight or even absent, since no nerve elements are involved in the sac. Meningomyelocele is a much more serious defect because nerve tissue is involved. The child may be retarded mentally and fail to develop physically because of interference with the nerves in the musculature.

Myelocele.[8, 20, 25] In myelocele, the extreme type of spina bifida, the neural tube has not closed. It consists of a disorganized mass of nervous tissue. At birth it is evident as a protuberant vascular tangle of nerve fibers and vascular tissue in the midline of the back, ranging from involvement of two or three vertebrae to involvement of the entire spine and cranium. It may be incompatible with life.

The term "rachischisis" is used to designate failure of the formation of the dorsal arch throughout the length of the vertebral column with exposure of the unclosed neural groove.

Cranium bifidum[20, 25]

Cranium bifidum includes cranial meningocele and meningoencephalocele, which are usually referred to as encephaloceles. The cranial meningocele is a protruding sac containing cerebrospinal fluid and meninges; when the brain tissue is present in the sac, the lesion is called meningoencephalocele. The sites where encephaloceles occur are the occipital, parietal, frontal, nasal, and orbital regions, in this order of frequency. They are various sizes and shapes, and varying amounts of cerebral tissue protrude through the defect. The entire ventricular system may be involved by communication with the cavity of the sac. The brain portions in the sac are usually hypoplastic or degenerated.

The patient's face characteristically has protruding eyes because of receding forehead and shallow orbits, prominent nose, and wide cheek bones. Infants with cranium bifidum present difficulties in feeding and handling and may have serious neurologic deficits.

Craniosynostosis[8, 20]

Premature union of cranial bones is known as craniosynostosis. It has been associated with heredity and may result from an abnormality of the mesenchymal tissues. In any case, there is deformity of the skull, which is called by a variety of names, according to the fusion of the sutures involved. In oxycephaly all the sutures fuse prematurely. The parietal and occipital bones ascend steeply, giving the head a dome or turret shape, caused by premature closure of the coronal sutures. When this occurs, the brain does not grow adequately, because expansion meets with firm resistance of solid bone. This results in mental and physical retardation.

The most frequent type of abnormal fusion of the sutures occurs when the sagittal suture joining the two parietal bones across the vertex of the head fuses prematurely. This suture is ordinarily unfused for a period of about 21 years to allow the brain to expand. If the sagittal suture is fused at birth, the head can only grow in an elongated or pointed fashion, with the forehead and back of the head expanding instead of broadening. This condition is called scaphocephaly or boathead.

In brachycephaly the coronal or crown suture fuses prematurely, giving the head a short and broad appearance. Both or only one coronal suture may be involved, but if only one side is involved, the forehead on the affected side will not grow. The forehead bone on the affected side is flat and small, and this results in elevation of the eyebrows and some recession of the eye on the affected side.

Craniosynostosis may result in significant cerebral or visual damage. The brain is compressed and cannot grow normally, and defects of vision occur. Without correction mental retardation results, although in isolated cases of sagittal synostosis the children have remained asymptomatic.

Diastematomyelia[18]

Diastematomyelia is a congenital abnormality of the spinal cord or cauda equina, in which the cord is divided longitudinally by a bony or cartilaginous septum attached to one or more vertebrae. It usually occurs in the lower thoracic or lumbar region. It is believed that during the development of the neural tube, the abnormal mesodermal cells protrude into neural tissue rather than become normally arranged around its periphery. Such migration of cells into the neural tube will eventually form a bony or cartilaginous spur. Since this spur or septum protrudes through the cord or cauda equina with resultant fixation, the cord is impaired in its normal ascent during longitudinal growth of the vertebral column. Spina bifida is quite commonly associated with this type of defect.

Clinically, cutaneous lesions, such as nevi, abnormal tufts of hair, dimpling of skin, lipomas, telangiectases, and dermal sinus tracts, may be found in the midline of the back, usually overlying the bony defect. In most cases innervation to the lower extremities is impaired, resulting in abnormal gait when the child is learning to walk. Sphincter control, both vesical and rectal may be disturbed. There may also be atrophy of the lower extremities and various types of foot deformities. The deep tendon reflexes may be hyperactive, diminished, or absent. These are caused by interruption of nerve supply to muscles in the lower extremities.

Congenital dermal sinus tracts[25]

Congenital dermal sinus tracts are anomalies in which epithelial-lined tracts extend inward from the skin surface to connect with the central nervous system and its meninges at any point along the cerebrospinal axis. This anomaly develops during the third to the fifth week of intrauterine life when the neuroectoderm normally separates from the epithelial ectoderm along the dorsum of the embryo. When complete separation of the nervous and epithelial tissue occurs, persistent epithelial defects in the form of small tracts or tubes are formed. These tracts are most frequently in the lumbosacral and occipital areas. They are often referred to as pilonidal sinuses when in the coccygeal area and are a constant threat to episodes of infection as long as they exist. The tracts may extend from the skin surface to the skull, vertebrae, meninges, brain, or spinal cord, depending on location. If accompanying cysts form within the cranium or spinal cord, compression of the brain or spinal cord results, blocking the flow of cerebrospinal fluid. If the cystic expansion is intracranial, the symptoms are those of tumor or obstructive hydrocephalus. If the cystic expansion is intraspinal, weakness of the lower extremities, sphincter disturbances, and tendon reflex abnormalities occur.

GENITOURINARY TRACT[1, 21]

Significant anomalies of renal structures are usually characterized by pain in the flank, accompanied by fever and a rise in the white blood cell count caused by superimposed infection. Many of them are asymptomatic and are an incidental finding at surgery, physical examinations, or at autopsy.

Complete renal agenesis is incompatible with life. Unilateral renal agenesis is the absence of one kidney, or one kidney may be present but only in nonfunctioning, rudimentary form. Arrested development of the mesonephros in the embryo is the underlying factor. In unilateral hypoplasia or dwarfed kidney there is usually complete absence of a normal parenchyma. In this case, part of the metanephric blastema fails to make contact with the ureteral bud in the embryo. In renal ectopia (Fig. 15-10)

usually only one kidney is misplaced. In crossed ectopia the kidneys may be abnormally fused, the small one to the larger one. The most common ectopic kidney lies in the bony pelvis on the sacral prominence. The ectopic kidney is subject to hydronephrosis and pyelonephritis.

In duplication of the pelvis and ureter, splitting or reduplication of the ureteral bud occurs in the embryo. There may be complete bilateral splitting on one or both sides. Incomplete splitting results in branched ureters with double pelves. When bilateral duplication is complete, there are four ureteral openings in the bladder. Ectopic ureteral openings may be present in these cases, occurring near the urinary meatus in the female and resulting in con-

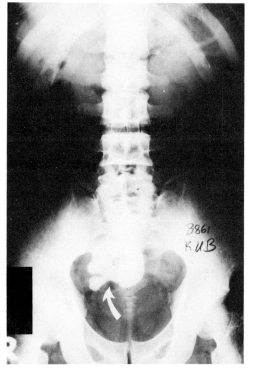

Fig. 15-10. Ectopic kidney with staghorn calculus. The kidney (arrow) is misplaced in the pelvis. (From Young, C. G., and Likos, J. J.: Medical specialty terminology, x-ray and nuclear medicine, St. Louis, 1972, The C. V. Mosby Co.)

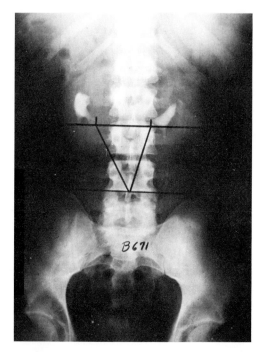

Fig. 15-11. Horseshoe kidney. The lower poles are fused. This gives the configuration of a horseshoe. (From Young, C. G., and Likos, J. J.: Medical specialty terminology, x-ray and nuclear medicine, St. Louis, 1972, The C. V. Mosby Co.)

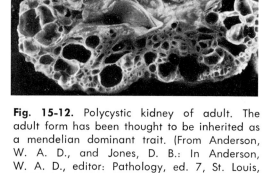

Fig. 15-12. Polycystic kidney of adult. The adult form has been thought to be inherited as a mendelian dominant trait. (From Anderson, W. A. D., and Jones, D. B.: In Anderson, W. A. D., editor: Pathology, ed. 7, St. Louis, 1977, The C. V. Mosby Co.)

tinuous dribbling of urine. In the male the opening may be in the prostatic utricle or in the seminal vesicles. With ectopic openings the complications are hydronephrosis, pyelonephritis and urinary calculi.

Horseshoe kidney[1]

Horseshoe kidney (Fig. 15-11) occurs when a fusion of the adjacent lower poles of the kidneys forms a shape like a horseshoe facing upward. The fushion may be only a fibrous band, or actual renal tissue may be involved. The pelves of the two kidneys are entirely separate. In the embryo the fusion is that of the renal blastema. Often this anomaly is associated with other congenital anomalies, such as spina bifida. Unilaterally fused kidneys (crossed renal ectopia) are rare. The kidneys in this instance lie on the same side of the vertebral column, with one ureter crossing the midline. These kidneys are subject to infections, such as pyelonephritis, and to hydronephrosis.

Polycystic kidney[1]

Polycystic kidney (Fig. 15-12) is usually a bilateral deformity, with multiple cysts representing dilated renal tubules or capsular spaces that have failed to communicate with the renal pelvis. The cysts progressively enlarge and compress the normally functioning renal parenchyma. The cysts vary in size from small ones to those that coalesce to form large cavities. The defect may be discovered in children, or it may escape notice until adulthood when it becomes symptomatic. Renal impairment is the result of this anomaly, with gradual compression and obliteration of nephrogenic tissue. Symptoms include nephritis, renal insufficiency, and finally uremia. Occasionally the cysts may become secondarily infected.

Hypospadias[1]

Hypospadias in the male or female represents an abnormal urethral opening. It can occur in a variety of sites, such as urovaginal in women and walls of the penile channel in men. Such deformities are complicated by urinary leakage or difficulty in urination.

True hermaphroditism and pseudohermaphroditism[9]

Intersexual anomalies of the gonads of an individual may be of one or both sexes. The two main types of ambisexual development are *true hermaphroditism* and *pseudohermaphroditism*. The cause has been attributed to sex chromosomal imbalance. The laboratory examination of chromosomes may show male or female chromosomes, depending upon the dominance of one sex type of chromosome over the other. Some cases of pseudohermaphroditism are caused by adrenal hyperplasia.

In true hermaphroditism an individual may have an ovotestis (both gonadal elements in a single organ) but without other gonadal elements in some cases; bilateral ovotestes; an ovotestis in combination with either an ovary or a testis; or an ovary and a testis. Although both types of gonads are represented to some degree in all these cases, usually neither is completely functional. However, exceptions have been reported. External genitalia may occasionally be male or female but are usually of an indifferent type. There may be an enlarged clitoris, a small penis showing some degree of hypospadias, a bifid or cleft scrotum, or an enlarged labia simulating the bifid scrotum. It is not possible to predict on an anatomic basis whether the individual will be male or female at puberty.

In pseudohermaphroditism an individual has the gonad of one sex and, to a variable extent, internal and external genitalia of the opposite sex. Congenital adrenal hyperplasia is the most common cause of female pseudohermaphroditism. These individuals show precocious male secondary sexual development at an early age, 1 to 4 years. Male pseudohermaphodites possess testes, variously located, but they do not form spermatozoa. External genitalia commonly simulate the male but may simulate females. The secondary sexual characteristics are predominantly male in most of these cases.

Hydrocele[1]

Hydrocele is the abnormal accumulation of serous fluid in the sac of the tunica vaginalis. In the congenital type, direct communication with the abdominal cavity is the result of failure of the funicular process to close.

Cryptorchidism[21]

In cryptorchidism the testicle is retained anywhere along the route of descent. Incomplete descent is found quite frequently in infants. The cryptorchid testicle is always smaller than normal after puberty. The undescended testicle may be atrophied.

ALIMENTARY TRACT[11, 22]

Many congenital anomalies develop in the alimentary tract because of its extensive length and diverse functions. The most common type of defect is one that creates an obstruction. They are usually compatible with life after corrective surgery. Some anomalies, such as imperforate anus, may be apparent at birth, but most are not diagnosed until after specific signs and symptoms occur. A knowledge of normal anatomy and physiology of the gastrointestinal tract is essential before you can correlate abnormal development with functional disturbances.

Congenital biliary atresia[10, 17, 19]

Congenital biliary atresia is one of the most serious malformations encountered in infants and young children, and death usually occurs within the first 2 years of life. Jaundice is a prominent symptom. The majority of neonates who are jaundiced beyond the second week of life have been shown to have congenital biliary atresia. Infants are not jaundiced at birth, since bilirubin is cleared through the placenta by the mother.

In congenital biliary atresia the intrahepatic and extrahepatic biliary ducts are involved. There may be atresia or hypoplasia of the biliary duct system. The severity of this anomaly or anomalies (if more than one duct is involved) and the unfavorable prognosis of patients can be appreciated when you consider the importance of the bile secreted by the liver for use in the intestinal tract for emulsification and absorption of fats.

When drainage from the biliary ductal system into the duodenum is not possible, the infant or child develops jaundice. In this connection it should be stated that jaundice develops from other causes, both obstructive and nonobstructive of the biliary system in the neonate. In congenital biliary atresia the child develops a progressive biliary cirrhosis, associated with enlargement of the liver and spleen, ascites, and portal hypertension. Esophageal varices also develop with recurrent episodes of bleeding, which may terminate in death. The respiratory distress is caused by the elevation of the diaphragm by the abdominal distention. Although the death rate is high, new techniques in surgery are now responsible for correction of the defect in some patients, depending on the extent of damage.

Congenital hypertrophic pyloric stenosis[22]

Congenital hypertrophic pyloric stenosis is hypertrophy of the circular muscle about the pylorus, the gateway from the stomach to the duodenum. This napkin ring narrowing or constriction of the pylorus produces obstruction to the flow of gastric contents into the intestines. It has been known to occur in more than one member of a family, but it is most often classified as a congenital developmental defect.

Symptoms do not usually occur in the first 2 weeks of life, but about 1 or 2 months after birth. The symptoms are projectile vomiting, marked dehydration, excessive hunger because of food loss, loss of weight or failure to gain, progressive constipation caused by obstruction, scanty urination, left to right passage of gastric peristaltic waves during or after feeding. The hypertrophied pylorus may be palpated.

Annular pancreas[6, 15]

The pancreas lies in the bend of the duodenum, with two portions extending around the second part of the duodenum, one anteriorly and one posteriorly. Because of a developmental defect, these sometimes fuse and form an encircling ring of pancreatic tissue that produces compression and stenosis of the duodenum. This results in an intestinal obstruction. Since the second part of the duodenum is stenosed, the first part will dilate and thicken. The common bile duct that connects the biliary system with the duodenum for passage of bile may become partially blocked. A number of coexisting congenital anomalies have been reported, such as monogolism, congenital heart disease, Meckel's diverticulum, malrotation of the cecum, and esophageal atresia.

Symptoms are usually noted within the first 2 weeks of life, but if the duodenal obstruction is slight, they may not arise until adulthood. The prominent symptoms are recurrent vomiting, which may contain bile if the biliary system is involved; malnutrition from vomiting; and jaundice.

New evidence shows that congenital constricting bands or congenital annular bands can be traced to a tear in the amnion occurring at a strategic time in embryonic development.[6] Strands from the amnion and chorion wrap themselves around fetal parts when this occurs.[6]

Esophageal atresia[22]

Esophageal atresia is caused by failure of the esophagus to develop as a continuous passage to the stomach in the embryo. If this defect exists, passage of food to the stomach is obstructed. The different types are classified according to anatomical location. Both upper and lower segments of the esophagus may be closed or blind; the upper segment may open into the trachea, introducing ingested food into the air passages, and the lower portion may end in a blind pouch. The most common type, occurring in about 90% of cases, is the ending of the upper segment of the esophagus in a blind pouch near the level of the bifurcation of the trachea, with a lower segment from the stomach connected to the trachea by a short fistulous tract. In another less common type both upper and lower segments of the esophagus are connected by a common fistulous tract to the trachea. This type also allows ingested food to enter the air passages instead of the stomach.

In all cases when ingested food gains entrance to the air passageway, excess mucus is aspirated, and if the defect is complete so that no food can reach the stomach, the fluid returns through the nose and mouth when the infant is fed. When there is a fistulous tract from the stomach to the trachea, air is forced through the fistula into the stomach and alimentary tract, causing acute gaseous abdominal distention. An obstruction to the esophagus in some cases may be incompatible with life.

Malrotation with periduodenal bands and volvulus[22]

Malrotation is a congenital anomaly in which the cecum is incompletely rotated. Usually the mesentery or peritoneal fold is not attached to the posterior abdominal wall. This developmental defect occurs in the embryonic stage. Periduodenal bands may be fixing the cecum to various structures in the right upper quadrant, or there may be volvulus of the midgut associated with abnormal positions of the cecum. The cecum may be abnormally lying on the duodenum, in which case pressure will cause obstruction. In cases of abnormal positions of the cecum a normal posterior fixation of the intestines is lacking, and there is only a rudimentary attachment near the origin of the mesenteric artery. The intestinal mass from the duodeno-jejunal junction to the midtransverse colon is thus supported by an incompletely anchored mesentery. This mass can twist around the rudimentary attachment of the mesentery, angulating and obstructing the alimentary tube at the duodeno-jejunal junction and the transverse colon. The mass by partially or completely occluding the superior mesenteric artery may cause an infarction of the entire midgut.

Symptoms are usually present in neonates but may not occur until childhood or even adulthood. In infants there is vomiting after feedings, which often contains bile. Abdominal distention occurs first in the epigastrium but later extends to include the mid and lower intestinal areas. Dehydration results from loss of fluids through vomiting as well as through loss of pancreatic juice, bile, and gastric secretions. With volvulus and infarction of the midgut, there may be scanty stools, possibly containing blood, or diarrhea. Older children complain of abdominal pain, nausea following meals, and vomiting.

Congenital megacolon (Hirschsprung's disease)[11]

Congenital megacolon is a neuromuscular defect in the rectum, rectosigmoid, or lower part of the sigmoid, but it may also occur at higher levels. It is caused by a defect in the innervation of the intrinsic musculature of the bowel wall. Normally, nerves in the intrinsic musculature produce coordinated peristaltic movements that propel waste products toward the anus. The defect in innervation can be caused by an absence or a reduction of ganglion cells supplying the muscles of the intestinal wall or by a disorder of the sympathetic and parasympathic nerve fibers in this area. When the waste material reaches the defective area, it is not passed along normally because of loss of peristaltic waves, and the bowel above the defect becomes hypertrophied and dilated. This produces abdominal pain, distention, and constipation.

The symptoms may be present at birth, or they may appear during the first week of life. At birth there is failure to pass meconium, a dark green mucilaginous mixture of amnion and intestinal gland secretions present in the intestines of a full-term fetus. Acute intestinal obstruction can occur from the accumulation of fecal masses palpable through the thin abdominal wall. There is weight loss, failure to grow, and malnutrition.

Intestinal atresia[11]

In intestinal atresia the intestinal tract is completely obstructed, usually in the ileum, because of improper development during the second or third month of fetal life. The lumen of the intestine may be blocked completely, or the intestine may end in a blind sac. There may also be multiple blind sacs with segments of the intestine joined to each other by threads, giving the appearance of a string of link sausage.

Symptoms occur in the first few days of life, consisting of vomiting, scanty stools, and abdominal distention. Later there is dehydration and fever. Surgery is the only definitive treatment.

Inguinal hernia[11]

Inguinal hernia is more prevalent in premature infants than in full-term infants. The defect results from imperfect closure of the processus vaginalis peritonei at the internal inguinal ring. Loops of intestine descend through this opening into the inguinal canal and scrotum and become tightly caught. Blood supply is cut off or diminished. The hernia may be unilateral or bilateral. It is much more prevalent in males than females. Symptoms include colicky pain, vomiting, constipation, abdominal distention, and a mass in the inguinal or scrotal region in the male.

Imperforate anus[11,12]

Imperforate anus is a congenital absence of the normal anal opening. Arrest or abnormality of development of the anal canal occurs in about the seventh to eighth week of fetal life. The external anal sphincter develops in a normal position, but the rectum may stop developing at any point along its course. The rectum may end blindly or it may communicate with the perineum anterior to this muscle. It may also communicate with the urethra or bladder in the male or with the vagina in the female. The common types include a persistent anal membrane with no anal opening; a rectal pouch ending blindly at some distance above the anus in which fistulous tracts between the rectum and perineum or genitourinary system may be found; a normal anus and anal pouch ending blindly in the hollow of the sacrum; or stenosis or stricture of the anus.

The symptoms are rarely observed shortly after birth but develop as general symptoms of bowel obstruction, characterized by absence of a stool and abdominal distention. If there is only stenosis of the anus, the symptoms may not develop for a year or more and are characterized by abdominal distention and obstipation.

Meckel's diverticulum[11]

Meckel's diverticulum is a rather common anomaly, occurring in 2% of the population.[21] It is particularly likely to lead to complications in children. The anomaly is caused by incomplete obliteration of the omphalomesenteric duct, which is a narrow tube in the embryo uniting the umbilical yolk sac with the midgut of the embryo. It develops between the fifth and sixth weeks of fetal life. When the duct persists, it is usually connected with the ileum near the ileocecal valve and produces obstruction by the twisting of a loop of the bowel at this site. A fibrous band may attach the end of the diverticulum to the umbilicus, mesentery, abdominal wall, or abdominal viscera. The mucosal lining may resemble that of the ileum, jejunum, duodenum, or stomach. There may also be aberrant islands of pancreatic tissue. If gastric mucosa is present, ulceration with hemorrhage may occur, secondary to secretion of hydrochloric acid and pepsin from the ectopic mucosa. Intussusception may also be a presenting symptom. Other symptoms are periumbilical pain with mild tenderness of the abdomen and hemorrhage from the bowel if the obstruction is severe. Symptoms, however, often do not occur until adult life. The blind pouch created by the persistence of the omphalomesenteric duct, representing Meckel's diverticulum, is prone to form a reservoir for the collection of undigested foods, leading to infection or diverticulitis.

ORAL CAVITY AND FACE[7, 24]

The two most common congenital anomalies of the oral cavity and face are the cleft palate and cleft lip. Cleft lip (cheiloschisis), a fissure or fissures in the upper lip, and cleft palate (palatoschisis), a congenital fissure or fissures in the hard and soft palate or in the soft palate alone, may exist as single deformities or both may be present in the same infant at birth. Cleft lip or cleft palate, or both, may be associated with chromosomal aberrations. Cleft palate with cleft lip is seen in trisomy 13-15 (chromosomal triplication). In this syndrome, severe central nervous system defects, eye defects, congenital heart disease, polydactyly, clubbed feet, and microcephaly are present in addition to harelip and cleft palate. The patients usually die before the age of 6 months unless they are chromosomal mosaics (for example, an individual with an altered genetic constitution from abnormal segregation of chromosomes, such as 45, 46, or 47 chromosomes). In mosaicism the clinical manifestations of a disease caused by chromosomal aberration appear relatively mild. Cleft lip and

cleft palate also occur in cases of trisomy 18. Symptoms of this syndrome are severe mental retardation, congenital heart disease, deformed feet and hands, and low-set malformed ears. The patients die before 1 year of age. Another sex chromosome variation in which cleft palate occurs is the XXXXY syndrome (49 chromosomes in males).

The prolabium (exposed part of the upper lip), premaxilla, and nasal septum develop between the fifth and eighth weeks of embryonic life. It is assumed that the facial structures fail to fuse during this period. The hard and soft palates develop from the seventh to the twelfth weeks of embryonic life. During this period the lateral palatal processes of the maxilla grow upward obliquely, arching over the tongue and fusing in the midline. This growth takes place in stages, anterior and posterior, until it is complete at the uvula by the twelfth week. If these processes fail to fuse completely, a cleft of the palate occurs, involving both soft and hard palate or the soft palate alone.

Cleft lip and cleft palate

Cleft lip may be unilateral, bilateral, complete, incomplete, or mixed. Incomplete closure may represent only a notch in the red border of the lip, which may or may not extend beyond the border. The nostril is often wider than normal on the affected side. The wings or alae of the nose are flattened. Complete cleft lip may be unilateral (to one side of the center) or bilateral (involving the lip on both sides of the middle portion). If it is unilateral, the alveolar process may be notched but more commonly is completely separated. The maxilla on the defective side is underdeveloped, and the nasal septum is attached and deviated to the palatal process on the opposite side. The nostril is broadened on the affected side with flattened ala. If it is bilateral complete, the middle portion of the lip or prolabium is isolated in the midline between the nose and what would normally be the upper lip. It is attached to the basal structures of the nose. The nose is usually broadened, with wide nostrils and alae widely separated.

Cleft lips often involve the palate and may be unilateral complete or bilateral complete. The cleft in unilateral complete cleft lip and palate extends through both soft and hard palates, involving the alveolus between maxilla and premaxilla on one side. There is a direct communication between the oral and nasal cavity on the affected side. The cleft in bilateral complete cleft lip and palate extends through both palates and also through the alveolus on each side of the premaxilla. The communication between the nose and oral cavity involves both nasal chambers.

The isolated cleft palate may be an incomplete submucous cleft in the soft palate, or it may be one extending through the entire soft and hard palate to the incisive foramen. The soft palate alone may be involved, but a cleft cannot occur in the hard palate alone. The soft palate clefts are widest in the middle and are narrow at the uvula.

The obvious difficulty presented by these defects is inability of the infant to take nourishment properly. Fluids regurgitate through the nose in cleft palate defects, and the infant has difficulty in swallowing and breathing. The defects are corrected by cheiloplasty or palatoplasty (plastic surgery of lip and palate, respectively).

STEP-BY-STEP EXERCISES

Step 1. Indicate those statements that best describe congenital anomalies or malformations.

1. They exist before birth. ___
2. They occur as a consequence of infection or injury during the first few months after birth. ___
3. Congenital heart anomalies result from failure of the heart or major blood vessels to develop normally before birth. ___
4. The rubella virus can cross the placental barrier and injure the embryo during the first trimester of pregnancy if there is maternal infection. ___
5. Toxoplasmosis, a protozoon infection, can do no harm to the developing offspring if the mother has the infection. ___
6. The placental barrier shields the unborn from all maternal infection. ___
7. Some congenital anomalies are compatible with life. ___

Step 2. Congenital anomalies may occur in the central nervous system, genitourinary system, gastrointestinal system, and the heart and major blood vessels. Complete the blanks with the name of the organ or system in which the following anomalies occur.

1. Patent ductus arteriosus _____
2. Polycystic kidney _____
3. Congenital biliary atresia _____
4. Horseshoe kidney _____
5. Tetralogy of Fallot _____
6. Ventricular or atrial septal defects

   _____
7. Imperforate anus _____
8. Coarctation of the aorta _____
9. Hirschsprung's disease _____
10. Arnold-Chiari malformation _____
11. Esophageal atresia _____
12. Spina bifida _____
13. Meningocele _____
14. Cryptorchidism _____
15. Congenital hypertrophic pyloric stenosis _____
16. Truncus arteriosus _____

Step 3. Complete the blanks in the following statements.

1. Absence or closure of a normal body orifice, such as may occur in the

gastrointestinal anomalies, is called

_____ .

2. An abnormally closed anus is called

an_____ _____ .

3. Failure of the heart channel, ductus arteriosus, to close normally is

called _____ _____ _____ .

4. When the lumen of the aorta is pinched or constricted, this is called

_____ .

5. Abnormal openings between the atria

are called _____ _____ _____ .

6. A very small brain is called

_____ .

7. An abnormal increase in volume of cerebrospinal fluid in the intracranial

cavity is called _____ .

8. A hernial sac or protrusion of the

meninges is called _____ .

9. Premature union of the bones of the

cranium is called _____ .

10. Fusion of the lower poles of the kidneys creating a certain shape is

called_____ _____ .

11. A testis retained anywhere along the

line of descent is called _____ .

12. Cheiloschisis is a term for _____

_____ .

13. Palatoschisis is a term for _____

_____ .

Responses

Step 1: 1. X; 3. X; 4. X; 7. X
Step 2: 1. heart; 2. genitourinary system; 3. gastrointestinal system; 4. genitourinary system; 5. heart; 6. heart; 7. gastrointestinal system; 8. heart; 9. gastrointestinal system; 10. central nervous system; 11. gastrointestinal system; 12. central nervous system; 13. central nervous system; 14. genitourinary system; 15. gastrointestinal system; 16. heart
Step 3: 1. atresia; 2. imperforate anus; 3. patent ductus arteriosus; 4. coarctation of the

aorta; 5. atrial septal defects; 6. microcephaly; 7. hydrocephalus; 8. meningocele; 9. craniosynostosis; 10. horseshoe kidney; 11. cryptorchidism; 12. cleft lip; 13. cleft palate

REFERENCES

1. Anderson, W. A. D., and Jones, D. B.: In Anderson, W. A. D., editor: Pathology, ed. 6, St. Louis, 1971, The C. V. Mosby Co. (congenital anomalies of the genitourinary tract).
2. Anthony, C. P., and Kolthoff, N. J.: Textbook of anatomy and physiology, ed. 9, St. Louis, 1975, The C. V. Mosby Co.
3. American Heart Association: If your child has a congenital heart defect, New York, 1963, The Association.
4. American Heart Association: Evaluation and management of congenital cardiac defects, New York, 1960, The Association.
5. Arey, L. B.: Developmental anatomy, Philadelphia, 1954, W. B. Saunders Co.
6. Field, J. H., and Krag, D. O.: J. Bone Joint Surg. **55A:**1035, 1973 (congenital annular bands).
7. Gorlin, R. J., and Vickers, R. A.: In Anderson, W. A. D., editor: Pathology, ed. 6, St. Louis, 1971, The C. V. Mosby Co. (cleft lip and cleft palate).
8. Greenfield, J. G., and others: Neuropathology, London, 1958, Edward Arnold (Publishers) Ltd. (malformations of the central nervous system).
9. Hertig, A. T., and Gore, H.: In Anderson, W. A. D., editor: Pathology, ed. 6, St. Louis, 1971, The C. V. Mosby Co. (hermaphroditism).
10. Holder, T. M.: Am. J. Surg. **107:**458, 1964 (atresia of extrahepatic bile duct).
11. Horn, R. C., Jr.: In Anderson, W. A. D., editor: Pathology, ed. 6, St. Louis, 1971, The C. V. Mosby Co. (alimentary anomalies).
12. Kiesewetter, W. B., Turner, C. R., and Sieber, W. K.: Am. J. Surg. **107:**412, 1964 (imperforate anus).
13. Kilbourne, E. D.: In Beeson, P. B., and McDermott, W., editors: Cecil-Loeb textbook of medicine, ed. 13, Philadelphia, 1971, W. B. Saunders Co. (congenital rubella).
14. Knight, V.: In Beeson, P. B., and McDermott, W., editors: Cecil-Loeb textbook of medicine, ed. 13, Philadelphia, 1971, W. B. Saunders Co. (congenital toxoplasmosis).
15. Lacy, P. E.: In Anderson, W. A. D., editor: Pathology, ed. 6, St. Louis, 1971, The C. V. Mosby Co. (annular pancreas).
16. Lev, M.: In Anderson, W. A. D., editor: Pathology, ed. 6, St. Louis, 1971, The C. V. Mosby Co. (congenital heart disease).

17. Longmire, W. P., Jr.: Ann. Surg. **159**:335, 1964 (congenital biliary hypoplasia).
18. Matson, D. D., and others: Pediatrics **6**:98, 1950 (congenital clefts of spinal cord).
19. Miller, S., Fonkalsrud, E. W., and Longmire, W. P., Jr.: Arch. Surg. **92**:813, 1966 (congenital biliary atresia).
20. Minckler, J.: In Anderson, W. A. D., editor: Pathology, ed. 5, St. Louis, 1966, The C. V. Mosby Co. (nervous system anomalies).
21. Mostofi, F. K., and Leestma, J. E.: In Anderson, W. A. D., editor: Pathology, ed. 6, St. Louis, 1971, The C. V. Mosby Co. (cryptorchidism).
22. Nursing Education Series No. 4, Columbus, Ohio, 1959, Ross Laboratories (alimentary tract obstructions of infancy).
23. Nursing Education Series No. 7, Columbus, Ohio, 1961, Ross Laboratories (congenital heart abnormalities).
24. Nursing Education Series No. 11, Columbus, Ohio, 1962, Ross Laboratories (cleft lip and cleft palate).
25. Nursing Education Series No. 14, Columbus, Ohio, 1964, Ross Laboratories (abnormalities of the central nervous system).
26. Peach, B.: Arch. Neurol. **12**:613, 1965 (Arnold-Chiari malformations).
27. Ransohoff, J., Shulman, K., and Fishman, R. A.: J. Pediatr. **56**:399, 1960 (hydrocephalus).
28. U.S. Department of Health, Education, and Welfare, Public Health Service, DHEW Publication No. (HSA) 75-5107, reprinted 1975 (rubella).

CHAPTER 16

Heredofamilial diseases

In the classification of diseases and in understanding their etiology a distinction must be made between those that are strictly inheritable according to genetics; those that are familial, representing predilection or predisposition for certain disorders; and those that are congenital or prenatal disorders, resulting from malformations or other abnormalities that have occurred in utero and are not explainable on a genetic basis. In the previous chapter the diseases existing at or before birth have been discussed. A large number of inherited metabolic disturbances were discussed in Chapter 7. In addition, in Chapter 13 on hypersensitivity and immunity, a number of diseases of a familial nature were discussed.

MECHANISM OF HEREDITY IN TRAITS AND DISEASES

The term hereditary is derived from the Latin word *hereditas,* meaning heirship. Heredity is the genetic relationship between succesive generations. Genetics is the science that deals with the origin and transmission of physical and mental qualities from parent to offspring.

In a study of this type with limited scope, it is not possible to detail all the intricate factors involved in the physical and genetic bases of heredity. For a better understanding of these principles and their evolvement the student is referred to textbooks on biology and genetics. Briefly, however, the general principles can be explained to elucidate the mechanisms involved in the inheritnce of diseases and of abnormalities.

The modern scientific study of heredity began with Gregor Johann Mendel (1822 to 1884), a teacher of natural science and an abbot of a monastery in Austria. In 1865 he outlined the principles of heredity from his study on the hybridization of peas.[10] These studies were based on his findings in the cross matching of peas and the records he kept of successive generations concerning changes in structure on a predictable basis. The essential factors of Mendel's discovery are the segregation and independent assortment of unit characters. He showed that inheritance is subject to certain laws (now known as Mendel's laws) and that if the pedigrees of the progenitors are known, the type of offspring produced by such mating can be predicted with a high degree of accuracy. Mendel's law that unit characters are capable of being inherited independently of one another is one of the most important concepts of heredity.

It has been a little over a century since Mendel gave us the laws of heredity, and the theoretic basis of genetics has undergone revision and expansion since that time. The progress in the past 10 to 15 years has been not only in the area of ordinary mendelian transmission of heredity, but also in discovering the molecular or chemical basis of heredity and uncovering the chromosomal basis of many congenital disorders. These discoveries have resulted in important advances in the clinical knowledge of the cause of many inherited diseases and in the methods of treatment for many of them. The remarkable advances that have been made in the unravelling of the genetic code of transmission of disease started with the discovery of the molecular structure of DNA (deoxyribonucleic acid), which is the basic hereditary material found in every living cell.[1] James Watson and Francis Crick, in 1953, worked out the theory of how DNA transmits information and produces copies of itself for each succeeding generation.[1] One of the greatest mysteries of nature has always been how a tiny fertilized human egg starting as a single cell can grow into a human being, with its billions of highly differentiated cells in a multitude of organs with diverse functions and the ability to reproduce itself. All these complexities of structure and function started to work the instant life began with the fertilized egg, and it all began with DNA.

Every individual is the result of a union of two germ cells, the ovum from the female and the sperm from the male. Within the single cell formed from this union is a nucleus containing 46 pairs of chromosomes (each parent contributed 23 pairs), 44 autosomes and 2 sex chromosomes, the XX in the female and the XY in the male. Each chromosome contains about 25,000 genes, which in turn are made of DNA segments. Each cell has the exact amount and kind of DNA as the original cell, but each cell has a different job to do in the production of a person. Only a specified part of the cell's DNA is used. It is DNA that transmits instructions from one cell to another and from one generation to the next. One half of it in a fertilized egg was contributed by the male sperm and the other half by the female ovum. DNA has the unique ability to split in two and make exact copies of itself. This chromosome or DNA duplication occurs during a phase of mitosis (division of cells) of the original single egg cell and the continuous subdivision of daughter cells. It is thus that a human being winds up at birth with about

10 trillion cells with the hereditary traits or characteristics laid down by DNA, derived from one parent or the other. You are, therefore, a blueprint of your ancestry. The diseases you inherit will be on the basis of dominant, recessive, or sex-linked inheritance,[19] as explained in Fig. 16-1.

In genetics, only when an individual has two identical recessive genes can they produce their effects.[6] The individual with two genes exactly alike is said to be homozygous for a trait or character. In dominant inheritance of a trait or disease the capability of expression is carried by only one of a pair of homologous chromosomes; in other words, only one of the genes has to be present in an individual to produce given effects. An individual with one dominant and one recessive gene is heterozygous for an abnormality or trait. In dominant inheritance the abnormality or the trait may be carried through each successive generation. In sex-linked inheritance the genes are transported on the X chromosomes (female sex chromosomes). The defect appears in the male sex only but is transmitted by the female. The males in the family will not transmit the defect to their sons but will transmit it through normal females of the family. The mechanisms for transmitting sex-linked disease are explained in Fig. 16-1.[6, 20]

Many hereditary diseases have a definite racial distribution. Sickle cell anemia affects Negroes primarily, although it is also found in people of the Mediterranean and Middle and Near Eastern areas. Hemolytic disease of the fetus and newborn caused by Rh blood factor occurs primarily in whites and is uncommon among blacks and very rare in some Asian populations. Cystic fibrosis and phenylketonuria (PKU) are found mainly in the white race and occur only rarely among blacks. PKU is also rare among Jews of Eastern and Central European ancestry, whereas Tay-Sachs disease is found mainly in these groups. Thalessemia, a hereditary blood disease, is most prevalent among peoples of the Mediter-

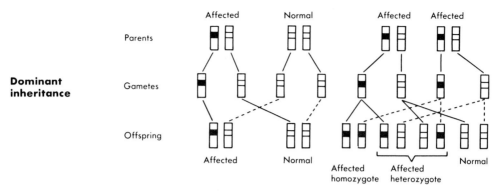

Dominant inheritance

In dominant inheritance, most of the affected individuals are heterozygous for the abnormality; that is, the chromosomes contain one normal gene and one abnormal gene, and the trait is carried through each successive generation. Diseases transmitted by dominant inheritance include hereditary spherocytosis, achondroplasia, Huntington's chorea, and renal glycosuria.

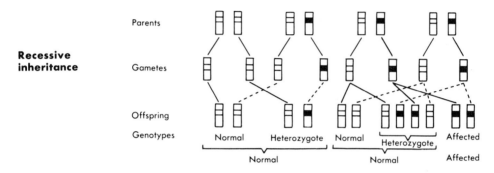

Recessive inheritance

For a recessive trait to become manifest, the individual must be homozygous for the abnormal gene. Among the numerous conditions transmitted by simple recessive inheritance are sickle cell anemia, phenylketonuria, fructosuria, galactosemia, glycogen storage disease, familial cretinism with goiter, erythropoietic porphyria, and ceruloplasmin deficiency, or Wilson's disease.

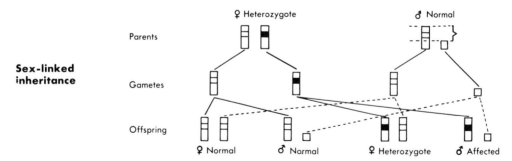

Sex-linked inheritance

Sex-linked genes are transported on the X chromosome. When a female heterozygous for a recessive sex-linked disease marries a normal male, four types of offspring may be produced: a normal female having two normal X chromosomes, a normal-appearing female carrier having one normal X chromosome and one X chromosome with the abnormal gene, a normal male having the mother's normal X chromosome, and an affected male having the mother's abnormal X chromosome. Examples of recessive sex-linked disorders are color blindness and hemophilia.

Fig. 16-1. Inheritance of disease in man. (After Hsia; from Therap. Notes **69**:237, Sept., 1962, Parke, Davis & Co.)

ranean region and Southeast Asia or persons of such ancestry.

Consanguineous marriage or marriage between relatives may be particularly hazardous for the offspring from the hereditary standpoint of diseases or abnormalities. Closely related persons are likely to carry the same alleles, and their offspring are thus much more apt to be homozygous for any abnormal genes the parents possess. Inbreeding tends to secure the homozygous combinations and brings to the surface latent or hidden recessive characters. The hazards of consanguineous marriage are also particularly evident if the objectionable hereditary characters or traits are dominant.[20]

Medical research of recent years has made much progress in the study of chromosomal aberrations, which are almost invariably associated with congenital abnormalities. Three striking examples of chromosomal aberrations are mongolism, gonadal dysgenesis (Turner's syndrome), and seminiferous tubule dysgenesis (Klinefelter's syndrome).[9] Mongolism is discussed later. Persons with Klinefelter's syndrome have 47 chromosomes, or the XXY karyotype.[2] The XXY individual tends to be excessively passive, and a few have an IQ below 100.[9] XXY male karyotypes occur in a ratio of 1 in 1000 live births.[9] Testicular tubular dysgenesis and azoospermia are present. Gynecomastia, mental deficiency in some, and a eunuchoid appearance may also be part of the syndrome. Persons with Turner's syndrome have a total of 45 chromosomes with only one X chromosome, resulting in an XO karyotype instead of XX.[2] The XO female karyotype occurs in 1 per 10,000 female births.[9] Manifestations of Turner's syndrome[2] are short stature, varying features of hypogonadism after puberty, with amenorrhea, lack of breast development, and delayed closure of epiphyses.[19] Red-green color blindness, mental deficiency, cardiovascular anomalies, hypertension, deafness, and a variety of other abnormalities may also be present.[2] The hall-

mark of diagnostic findings is the short fourth metacarpal or metatarsal, or both, occurring in about two thirds of the patients.

In the combined studies of 46,150 live births in Canada, Scotland, Denmark, and New England, the incidence of chromosomal abnormalities was 1 in 400 for newborn boys and 1 in 680 for girls.[9] The theory that men with the XYY chromosome abnormality have a special proclivity to crime has been debated since 1960, but in recent studies it was not established that the extra Y chromosome is a cause of violence in a personality. Mosaics are persons who for some reason have two different populations of cells with different karyotypes in their bodies.[9]

A widespread technique to determine the female or male chromosomal makeup is the examination of cytologic smears of buccal mucosa for sex chromatin (Barr bodies).[2] The normal female has a pair of X chromosomes (XX) and 44 autosomes, and one sex chromatin body is present in the interphase nucleus (resting or metabolic). These individuals are called chromatin-positive. The normal male has an X and Y sex chromosome present in each diploid cell and is designated XY. Of his 46 chromosomes, 44 are autosomes and one is an X sex chromosome and one is a Y sex chromosome. No sex chromatin or Barr body is present in the interphase nucleus, and he is called a chromatin-negative individual.

Mutations are inheritable abnormalities of quality, form, and function caused by the alteration of the basic hereditary material in one gene. Genetic abnormalities usually originate as mutations. Genes are remarkably stable and are transmitted to successive generations with great regularity. An individual is the sum result of the combined effect of all his genes, and he will therefore vary when one of these genes is altered. A mutant gene must reside in a germ cell before it can be inherited. Mutants, however, may arise at any time in the development of the individual, since genes may also be altered in any somatic cell, but such body changes are not transmitted. This type of alteration must not be confused with the abnormal distribution of chromosomes in pathologic embryonic development. Induced genetic mutations, called mutagens, are the result of chemical or physical agents. The best known mutagens are produced by penetrating ionizing radiation, such as x rays, gamma rays from radium or other radioactive material, and the neutrons from nuclear reactors. The chemical mutagens are the result of compounds such as nitrogen mustard, mustard gas, and formaldehyde, among others.

How much of our physical and mental makeup is influenced by heredity and how much by environment is the subject of much controversy. There can be no doubt that both play important roles in the final molding of the individual's body and mind. In connection with this question, it is well to remember that we do not inherit traits of character themselves, but the power to react in a certain manner under certain conditions. Many inherited characters will or will not be realized, depending upon whether the environment is properly constituted.

FAMILIAL PREDISPOSITION TO DISEASES

Many extremely common diseases are not considered to be hereditary as explained strictly on a genetic basis (inheritance of dominant or recessive genes), but experimental evidence and family pedigree studies do indicate that a susceptibility to many diseases is inherited. Among the diseases in which there is evidence of susceptibility are carcinoma of the stomach, coronary atherosclerosis, diabetes mellitus, epilepsy, gout, varicosities, hypertension, and rheumatoid arthritis. It is difficult to diagnose diseases as having a familial basis unless the evidence is clear cut; even the reappearance of a disease in successive generations does not prove that it has been transmitted or is even transmissible. Many environmental factors enter into the occurrence of disease, such as faulty diet, bad hygienic habits, and even cultural traits. These conditions may exist in several generations and would seem to run in families, but if environmental factors were equal in all the generations under study, diseased conditions might be the product of continued faulty diet or hygienic factors. The interrelationships between genetic and environmental factors are therefore often difficult to assess.

The study of twins, identical and fraternal, has shed some light on the inheritance of disorders or the familial tendency toward certain diseases. In studies of mental illness and feeblemindedness, identical twins are very likely to show the same defect. In family histories of dementia praecox (schizophrenia), evidence indicates a constitutional predisposition toward the disease, possibly on a hereditary basis of recessive genes. Manic depressive illness is also prone to occur in families, and again a predilection to development of the disease on a familial basis has been implicated.[16]

Experimental evidence plus family histories clearly indicate that hypersusceptibility and other anaphylactic conditions usually show a familial history of these conditions transmitted through several generations. These diseases are asthma, hay fever, urticaria, migraine, angioneurotic edema, and other allergic manifestations. The inherited susceptibility to allergic sensitization is probably the most important factor in development of allergic disorders. The individual does not inherit sensitivity to a specific substance but a predisposition to become sensitive to various substances such as foods and inhalants.[13, 16]

REPRESENTATIVE HEREDOFAMILIAL DISEASES
Familial polyposis of the colon[5, 15]

Familial polyposis (Fig. 16-2) is rather uncommon, but since it is often silent until malignancy occurs, it is discussed here. The incidence of carcinoma occurring in these polyps is almost 100% in untreated

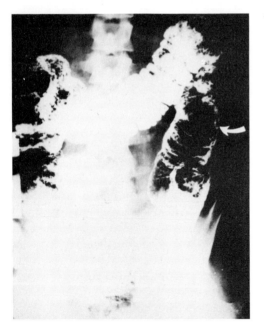

Fig. 16-2. Familial polyposis. Arrow points to the multiple polyps of the colon. (From Young, C. G., and Likos, J. J.: Medical specialty terminology, x-ray and nuclear medicine, St. Louis, 1972, The C. V. Mosby Co.)

cases.[15] In this disease the bowel mucosa, especially of the large intestine, is totally covered by numerous small polyps, which are usually pedunculated or sessile. These polyps begin to develop immediately after birth.[15] They may extend through the entire intestinal tract and involve the mucosa of the stomach. It is a heredofamilial disease, transmitted as an autosomal dominant, making its existence known in the second and third decades of life. Discovery is often by chance, when bleeding and, rarely disturbances in bowel function develop. Most cases are not discovered until malignancy of the intestine has occurred or there is metatasis to other visceral organs, such as the liver. This is one type of cancer that develops in young adults and even adolescents. Familial polyposis is diagnosed by sigmoidoscopic examination and barium enema studies, plus a history of familial incidence (Fig. 16-2).

The Peutz-Jeghers syndrome, another type of polyposis or multiple polyps, is not prone to malignancy. These polyps are almost always pedunculated and occur throughout the stomach and intestines. The disorder is transmitted as a simple mendelian dominant and occurs in childhood. Roughly one half of the children of an affected parent will be afflicted.[5] A characteristic symptom of this type of multiple polyps is a peculiar brownish pigmentation of the skin and mucosa of the mouth. Other symptoms include hemorrhage and intussusception.

Sickle cell anemia[16, 24]

Sickle cell anemia is an inherited disease transmitted by a recessive trait affecting Negroes primarily but it is found also in people of the Mediterranean and Middle and Near Eastern areas. It is one of several hereditary blood diseases caused by abnormal hemoglobin. The change in the molecular structure of the hemoglobin causes the red blood cells to twist into the shape of a sickle, giving the disorder its name. The hemoglobin is known as sickle hemoglobin or hemoglogin S. The sickle shape of the blood cells prevents them from passing freely through many of the small blood vessels. This accounts for their frequently piling up and forming blood clots that block the flow of blood to local tissues with consequent tissue damage. Almost any organ may be involved, but the liver, spleen, bones, kidneys, and brain are frequent sites of the damage. The abnormal red blood cells of sickle cell anemia are considerably shorter-lived than normal red blood cells. The chronic anemia present in sickle cell patients is partly caused by the higher rate of destruction of the red blood cells. Bone marrow may also fail to produce red blood cells normally for brief periods of time, resulting in an acute severe anemia superimposed on a chronic one. Since the discovery of the sickle hemoglobin by Dr. Linus Pauling in 1949, more than 100 abnormal hemoglobins have been described.

Persons who are carriers of sickle cells but do not have the disease are said to have sicklemia or the sickle cell trait. A person with a sickle cell variant has both the sickle hemoglobin and another abnormal hemoglobin in his red blood cells. Sickle cell anemia, sickle cell trait, and sickle cell variants are sometimes collectively termed sickle cell disease. Sickle cell variants are named after the abnormal hemoglobin or the blood disease present, for example, sickle cell–hemoglobin C disease, sickle cell–hemoglobin D disease, and sickle cell–thalassemia disease. The course of the disease is usually milder than that of sickle cell anemia. Sickle cell–hemoglobin C disease is associated with increased risk of complications in pregnant women and maternal mortality. Diagnosis of the different variants is dependent upon demonstration of the types of hemoglobin present in the blood by hemoglobin electrophoresis.

The carrier state, sometimes termed sicklemia, is generally a benign condition with no clinical manifestations. Under special circumstances a crisis can occur, such as during anesthesia; flying at high altitudes in unpressurized aircraft; strenuous physical exercise, particularly at high altitudes; infections; anemia; and alcoholic intoxication. There may be spontaneous bleeding into the urinary tract as evidenced by bloody urine. Unless a complication occurs, persons with a sickle cell trait are usually not aware of their carrier state, and they require no treatment. The silent carrier state is detected by blood tests used in screening for sickle cell anemia.

Typically the patient with sickle cell anemia will be the offspring of parents who have the sickle cell trait. Each child born to parents with the sickle cell trait has one chance in four of having sickle cell anemia, one chance in two of being a carrier of the trait, and one chance in four of having neither the trait nor sickle cell anemia. If only one parent has the trait, none of the children will have sickle cell anemia, but each of the children has one chance in two of being a carrier. If one parent has sickle cell anemia and the other one has neither the disease nor the trait, their offspring will carry the trait but will not have the disease.

Sickle cell anemia is not apparent at birth, but the infants destined to be later diagnosed as having sickle cell anemia (between second and fourth year in the majority of cases) will have bizarre symptoms, including irritability, colic, distended abdomen, bouts of fever, poor appetite, vomiting, slow growth, pale complexion, and jaundice. Some infants may have symmetrical swelling of both hands and feet. In older children and adults the crises are more readily recognized. An infection such as a sore throat or cold may precede or accompany a crisis. Intervals between crises vary, but there may be periods of relative freedom from symptoms, despite a moderate degree of anemia. The signs and symptoms of a crisis are fever, weakness, jaundice, increase in pallor, loss of appetite, pain in the chest, arms, legs, back, and abdomen. Joints may be swollen and painful. In a crisis there may also be headache, drowsiness, convulsions, stiff neck, nosebleed, bloody or dark urine, inability to speak, or a state of shock. There may also be lymphadenopathy, splenomegaly, hepatomegaly, heart murmurs, and an enlarged heart. If the spleen is enlarged, at high altitude infarction may occur. People with sickle cell anemia are often poorly developed with short trunk and long arms and legs. The disease is not associated with mental retardation. Infections, particularly of the respiratory tract, are common and often are the cause of death. Other leading causes of death are heart failure, kidney failure, and shock. Many children with sickle cell anemia die in early life, and most patients until recently did not live beyond 40 years of age. Pregnant women with sickle cell anemia may have serious complications.

Since sickle cell anemia is hereditary and

there is no cure, the only means of primary prevention is the screening of the population at risk for carriers and providing genetic counseling. Several simple and inexpensive tests now available for screening purposes identify not only those with sickle cell anemia but also those with the trait or variants.

Hemophilia[4, 14, 26]

Hemophilia is inherited through a sex-linked recessive trait. The female is the carrier, and the male is symptomatic. A defect in the blood-clotting mechanism causes spontaneous bleeding in the joints, muscles, mucous membranes, and kidneys. In moderately severe cases, mild trauma will cause superificial bleeding, and in mild cases a slight trauma will produce bruising. Factor VIII (AHG–antihemophilic globulin) is deficient, and the severity of the disease depends on the AHG level. If the AHG level is below 5%, severe bleeding may occur spontaneously; if it is between 20% to 50%, excessive bleeding occurs only with trauma or surgery. The AHG level is similar in affected members of the same family.[4, 14]

Not all the male members of a family will have hemophilia, even though the mother is carrying the defective gene. This defective gene can skip generations, and for this reason from 30% to 50% of hemophilic patients are unable to give a familial history of a bleeding tendency. Hemophilia affected the royal families of Europe. Queen Victoria was a carrier, and her son Leopold died of hemophilia; two of her daughters who where carriers took the disease either directly or through their children into the royal houses of Germany, Russia, and Spain.

Cystic fibrosis of the pancreas[7, 8]

Cystic fibrosis of the pancreas is a generalized inherited disease, transmitted as a mendelian recessive trait with clinical consequences only in homozygotes. It is characterized by increased viscosity of mucous secretions of the pancreas, tracheal and bronchial glands, intestinal glands, and mucous salivary glands. (See Fig. 18-1, A.) Electrolyte concentrations, particularly of sodium and chloride, are also increased, especially in the secretions of the exocrine and parotid glands, and in secretions of other glands. The nature of the biologic defect is unknown. It is a disease of early childhood, but recently it has been found in adolescents and adults.

The clinical manifestations are a chronic cough, wheezing, a thick tenacious sputum, and frequent respiratory tract infections. These symptoms are considered to be the hallmark of the disease. The damage to the bronchi is irreversible. Progressive pulmonary involvement leading to pulmonary insufficiency and eventual death occurs as a consequence of complications such as atelectasis, lung abscesses, cor pulmonale, pulmonary hypertension, emphysema, pneumothorax, hemoptysis, and asphyxia. Pancreatic insufficiency is characterized by abdominal distention, large, bulky, foul-smelling stools, diarrhea, and abdominal cramps. Pancreatic insufficiency can occur without the pulmonary manifestations. Children may also exhibit meconium ileus, cirrhosis of the liver, and collapse from heat exhaustion. The paranasal sinuses may be chronically involved as evidenced by postnasal drip, polyp formation, and a nasal voice. Approximately one half of the children die before the age of 10 years and the majority before the age of 30 years. The pulmonary involvement determines the fate of the patient.

Muscular dystrophy[12, 15, 25]

A group of diseases fall under the heading of muscular dystrophies. (See Figs. 18-27, 18-30, and 18-32.) All are characterized by degeneration and injury to individual muscle cells. One type is called progressive muscular dystrophy because of the progressive character of the wasting of the muscle. In muscular dystrophy the voluntary skeletal muscles are weakened, usually equally on both sides of the body. The internal muscles, such as the diaphragm, are not affected. Muscular dystrophy has long been recognized as a disorder that affects several in one family. In most forms an inherited characteristic transmitted from either parent is responsible. Muscular dystrophy is found throughout the world. In the United States, 200,000 persons are estimated to be more or less disabled with the disease.[25] The affected children rarely live to adulthood. The disease attacks all ages, and many patients will eventually spend time in a wheel chair. In adults the ailment may continue for 20 to 30 years or more, but some become helpless in a few months.

The dystrophies are divided into a number of clinical forms, depending upon the genetic pattern of inheritance and the extent of muscular damage. No classification is universally accepted today. The most prominent type is called severe generalized familial muscular dystrophy, but it is also known as Duchenne's muscular dystrophy and pseudohypertrophic muscular dystrophy. This type begins in infancy, with the toddler becoming at first clumsy, still later weak, and eventually helpless. In the slightly older age group the walk becomes a waddle, and the child has difficulty in getting to his feet when sitting. The calf muscles are hypertrophied, with fat replacing muscle fibers, but these muscles are abnormally weak despite the appearance of huskiness. The arms hang limply because shoulder girdle muscles are weakened. In the last stages the affected muscles are completely wasted, and the child is very thin. This type runs a rapidly fatal course, terminating in death usually before adult life. Males are affected more often than females. It is inherited as a sex-linked mendelian recessive.[12, 15, 25]

In the mild restricted muscular dystrophy, males and females are affected equally. It is inherited as a mendelian dominant. It is slowly progressive in the wasting of muscles. Both infants and adults are affected. The juvenile type has the names of limb-girdle, Erb, or Leyden-Moebius muscular dystrophy.[12, 15]

In the facio-scapulo-humeral muscular dystrophy, also known as Landouzy-Dejerine, the weakness starts in childhood or early adult life, with both sexes equally affected. The muscles of the face, shoulder girdle, and upper arm are affected, with gradual weakening.

Dystrophia myotonica is a progressive muscular involvement of distal muscles. It usually begins in the third decade and runs a prolonged course. It is familial in occurrence. The muscles most prominently affected are those of the hand, lower arm, and legs.[12]

The etiology has been variously attributed to an embryonic defect, faulty potassium metabolism, metabolic protein deficiency, and inability to utilize creatine. One view accepted by several is that the condition is an inborn metabolic defect in metabolism of creatine and creatinine. This is based on the biochemical changes of an increased excretion of creatine and a decreased excretion of creatinine in the urine, accompanied by increased levels of creatine in the plasma. The creatinine levels in the plasma are usually normal.[12]

Friedreich's ataxia[3]

Friedreich's ataxia is one of the most common hereditary diseases of the nervous system. It is characterized clinically by progressive disturbance of equilibrium and motion. Myelin degeneration occurs in the spinocerebellar tracts and posterior columns. The spinal cord is reduced in size. The trait may be either dominant or recessive. The onset is in childhood or before the age of 20 years.

The chief early symptoms are ataxia of gait and pes cavus. Later, clumsiness of the hands, dysarthria, and nystagmus appear. The knee and ankle jerks are lost early. Kyphosis, often with chest deformity, develops as the disease progresses. The course is relentless, and most patients are unable to walk within 5 years after onset. Blindness sometimes occurs, usually from optic nerve atrophy but less often from cataract. The intelligence becomes impaired. In a few families the disease has been associated with deaf mutism or progressive deafness. Death may result from pneumonia or cardiac failure. Death usually occurs during the third decade.[3]

Down's syndrome or mongolism[12, 17, 18, 23]

Down's syndrome or mongolism is a genetic disease characterized by physical defects or deformities and mental deficiency. Down's syndrome (trisomy 21) is evidenced by extra chromosomal material in pair 21. It is most often caused by nondisjunction in the male or female gamete during meiosis, which is a special type of cell division occurring during the maturation of sex cells by which the normal diploid set of chromosomes is reduced to a single set through two rapid successive stages in which the nucleus divides twice but the chromosomes only once.

The afflicted child has mongoloid facies and senile features. There is moderate to severe mental retardation. The skull may be flattened anteroposteriorly. Gaze may be upward and outward, with epicanthal folds. The nose is short and flat bridged, and the tongue protrudes. The neck is broad and short, and the abdomen is prominent. The genitalia are underdeveloped. Phalanges are short. Mongolism may be associated with a variety of other defects of the eyes, ears, heart, and extremities. A valuable radiographic diagnostic sign is the widening and flaring of the ilia, called the "elephant ear" appearance. This sign is particularly pathognomonic of mongolism.

Several factors involve high risk for women giving birth to a child with Down's syndrome.[23] Advanced maternal age comprises the largest group of high risk factors. The risk for a woman between the ages of 40 and 45 is about 1:100 and 1:40 for the age group of 45 and over. The recurrence risk for Down's syndrome (trisomy 21) is about 1% up to the age 35 if a previous

child has been afflicted with the disease. The risk of producing a child with Down's syndrome is about 20% if the mother carries a translocation that involves the D/21 chromosomes (D chromosomes include 13, 14, and 15).[23] A translocation occurs when a piece of one chromosome breaks off and attaches to a different chromosome, for example, either 13, 14, or 15, might break off and rejoin with 21 (with loss of little pieces).[23] If the father carries a similar translocation, the risk for some unknown reason is only about 2%. Rarely, if either parent carries a balanced 21/21 translocation, the risk increases to 100%. Fathers as well as mothers who possess chromosomal mosiacism with a 21 trisomic cell population are risks for having more than one child with mongolism. If a pregnant woman is afflicted with Down's syndrome, her risk of giving birth to a mongoloid infant is 50%.[23]

Antenatal diagnosis of Down's syndrome is now possible through the technique of amniocentesis. This test consists of obtaining amniotic fluid through the insertion of a needle into the amniotic cavity. The fetal cells withdrawn from this fluid represent the fetal chromosome and genetic complement. This technique has also been used in the past for study of the biochemistry of amniotic fluid and for antenatal diagnosis of sex.

At the present time other antenatal diagnostic techniques are being developed and perfected, although now in the experimental stage.[11] They may become extremely useful in diagnosis of anencephaly and other congenital abnormalities that cannot be detected with amniocentesis. Amniography is an x-ray technique. A contrast material is injected into the amniotic fluid, and the dye material mixes with the amniotic fluid and provides a contrast to the fetus, with the resulting x ray depicting the outline of the fetus. Ultrasonography is a procedure employing the techniques of ultrasound.[11] It is often used to locate the placenta prior to amniocentesis. Fetoscopy involves visualization of the fetus utilizing a fiberoptic endoscope.[11]

Huntington's disease (Huntington's chorea)[12, 21, 27]

Huntington's chorea is now more often known by the name of Huntington's disease (HD), as recommended by neurologists, since this name embraces other forms of the disease than chorea. It was named after an American doctor, George Huntington, who made extensive studies of its occurrence in families. It is a progressive degenerative disease of the basal ganglia and cerebral cortex and is dominantly inherited.

Men and women are both affected, and either can have a defective gene for HD. Those with a defective HD gene will develop Huntington's disease symptoms if they live long enough, but the tragedy of the disease is that they can pass on the defect to any of their offspring even before they have symptoms. The HD gene is an autosomal dominant, which means that the gene is located on a chromosome other than the sex chromosomes. If either parent has the defective gene, all offspring have a 50:50 chance of inheriting the disease. The symptoms of the disease usually do not become obvious until the patient is nearly 40 years old, but if milder symptoms of the disease have not appeared by the age of 35, the chance that the person will develop HD grows less with each year of later life. The typical picture of Huntington's disease is a combination of mental and physical symptoms, any of which may appear before the other. Early symptoms may be confused with nervousness, but as the disease progresses, the uncontrollable chorea may be obvious from the abnormal involuntary movements, such as jerking, twisting, and muscle spasms of the limbs, trunk, and face. The word *chorea* is a Greek word for dance. These excessive, jerking, chorea-type movements may not be the first symptoms of the disease, because HD may begin with distressing personality changes, such as irritability; carelessness in appearance, habits, promises, and responsibilities; poor judgment; loss of memory; and indifference. As the physical or mental symptoms become more severe with progression of the disease, the physical jerking may lead to speech loss or difficulty and trouble with swallowing. Mental symptoms may progress to severe mental illness. The length of life after symptoms appear varies from a few years to 15 years. The patients usually succumb to progressive weakness and complications such as pneumonia or heart failure. The exact number of people with HD is unknown, but it is estimated that about 10,000 to 14,000 Americans have HD symptoms. However, this figure may be misleading since there are missed diagnoses and deliberately concealed cases to avoid discrimination of family members in many ways, such as childbearing, insurance, and employment.

The diagnosis is made from a family history and signs and symptoms. Loss of nerve cells in various areas of the brain account for symptoms, and at present there is no biochemical or microscopic test for Huntington's disease that would make a diagnosis possible. Nor is there a cure. The best way to combat the disease is by dissemination of information about it. Individuals of HD families should be informed of their risk before the age of reproduction and again during marriage counseling. Tragedies have resulted because children were not informed of the risks when a parent had HD, or they were misinformed about the true diagnosis.

Retinitis pigmentosa[22]

Retinitis pigmentosa is an inherited disease that usually manifests its first symptoms in adolescents or children as night blindness. Over a lifetime it is progressive and gradually decreases the person's ability to see at night and also hampers side vision, resulting in "tunnel vision." The changes are in the retina, the innermost layer of the eye, and they consist of decreasing activity of the rods and cones, which are the specialized light-receiving cells of the retina. The rods are particularly affected and since they are used for peripheral vision, this causes the tunnel vision. The night vision is damaged as a result of the inability to detect shades of black and white in dim light, which is also a property of the rods in normal vision. Blood supply to the retina is diminished because the deteriorated light-receptor cells no longer respond to stimuli. The loss of blood supply further lessens the retina's ability to function. It is believed that an abnormality in the biochemistry of the eye or the body's metabolism is the cause. Some scientists believe that retinitis pigmentosa is primarily caused by a change in the pigment-producing tissue of the retina or by changes in the small blood vessels that supply nourishment to the outer layers of the retina. The exact cause, however, is not known.

At the present time there is no treatment that can halt the progress of the disease in a person who has a defective gene. In some cases the disease does not progress to complete blindness, and many patients retain a reading vision throughout their lives, but it may be restricted to a small central part of the visual field.

The disease is usually diagnosed by an ophthalmologist by the use of an ophthalmoscope, through which he can see the many black pigment deposits scattered throughout the retina and along the edges. Rarely, however, the pigment may be absent. By the use of an electroretinograph (ERG), retinitis pigmentosa may be distinguished from other diseases of the retina. This instrument records electrical impulses that the retina gives off when light strikes it, and in the case of retinitis pigmentosa, these impulses are extremely weak.

STEP-BY-STEP EXERCISES

Step 1. Complete the blanks in the following statements.

1. The genetic relationship between suc-

cessive generations is called _____.
2. The science that deals with the origin and transmission of physical and mental qualities from parent to offspring

is called _____.
3. The basic hereditary material found

in every living cell is _____.
4. There are 44 autosomes and 2 sex chromosomes in a cell formed from the union of an ovum and a sperm. The sex chromosomes in a female are

_____; in a male _____.
5. Recessive genes produced their effects only when an individual has two of them that are identical. This indi-

vidual is said to be _____ for a trait.
6. In dominant inheritance of a trait or disease only one of a pair of homologous chromosomes has to be present in an individual to produce given effects. This individual with one dominant and one recessive gene is

said to be _____ for an abnormality or trait.
7. When a disease is transported on the X chromosome of the female and the defect appears in the male sex only,

it is said to be _____ inheritance.

Step 2. Many common diseases, while not hereditary, develop in families on the basis of familial predisposition or susceptibility.

Indicate which of the following diseases might have a familial predisposition or susceptibility.

1. Asthma __
2. Gout __
3. Hayfever __
4. Pneumonia __
5. Diabetes mellitus __
6. Epilepsy __
7. Carcinoma of the kidney __
8. Rheumatoid arthritis __

Step 3. Mark the following statements *T* for true or *F* for false.

1. Malignancy is likely to occur in untreated familial polyposis. ___
2. Sickle cell anemia is a common type of anemia occurring equally in all races. ___
3. A common view of the etiology of muscular dystrophy is that it is an inborn metabolic defect. ___
4. Mongolism can occur as a result of chromosomal aberration. ___
5. Huntington's chorea, a progressive degenerative disease of the basal ganglia and cerebral cortex, has an onset early in the life of a child. ___

Responses

Step 1: 1. heredity; 2. genetics; 3. DNA (deoxyribonucleic acid); 4. XX; XY; 5. homozygous; 6. heterozygous; 7. sexlinked

Step 2: 1. X; 2. X; 3. X; 5. X; 6. X; 8. X

Step 3: 1. T; 2. F; 3. T; 4. T; 5. F

REFERENCES

1. Crick, F. G. C.: Sci. Am. **207:**66, 1962 (genetic code).
2. Gorlin, R. J., and Vickers, R. A.: In Anderson, W. A. D., editor: Pathology, ed. 6, St. Louis, 1971, The C. V. Mosby Co. (Klinefelter's syndrome; Turner's syndrome).
3. Greenfield, J. G., and others: Neuropathology, London, 1958, Edward Arnold (Publishers) Ltd. (Friedreich's ataxia).
4. Hoak, J. C., Connor, W. E., and Warner, E. D.: J. Iowa Med. Soc. **54:**331, 1964 (hemophilia).
5. Horn, R. C., Jr.: In Anderson, W. A. D., editor: Pathology, ed. 6, St. Louis, 1971, The C. V. Mosby Co. (familial polyposis).
6. Hsia, D. Y.: Inborn errors of metabolism, Chicago, 1959, Year Book Medical Publishers, Inc.
7. Kowlessar, O. D.: In Beeson, P. B., and McDermott, W., editors: Cecil-Loeb textbook of medicine, ed. 13, Philadelphia, 1971, W. B. Saunders Co. (cystic fibrosis of the pancreas).
8. Lacy, P. E., and Kissane, J. M.: In Anderson, W. A. D., editor: Pathology, ed. 6, St. Louis, 1971, The C. V. Mosby Co. (cystic fibrosis of the pancreas).
9. Medical News: J.A.M.A. **230:**655-659, 1974 (karyotyping).
10. Mendel, G. J. (translation by W. Bateson): J. R. Hort. Soc. **26:**1, 1901 (Mendel's study of hereditary transmission).
11. Milunsky, A.: The prenatal diagnosis of hereditary disorders, Springfield, Ill., 1973, Charles C Thomas, Publisher.
12. Minckler, J.: In Anderson, W. A. D., editor: Pathology, ed. 5, St. Louis, 1966, The C. V. Mosby Co. (progressive muscular dystrophy; mongolism).
13. Peacock, L. B.: J. Med. Assoc. State Georgia **50:**479, 1961 (familial susceptibility to diseases).
14. Ratoff, O. D.: Arch. Intern. Med. (Chicago) **112:**92, 1963 (hemophilia).
15. Robbins, S. L.: Pathology, ed. 3, Philadelphia, 1967, W. B. Saunders Co. (familial polyposis; muscular dystrophy).
16. Rubin, M. I.: In Nelson, W. E., editor: Textbook of pediatrics, ed. 7, Philadelphia, 1959, W. B. Saunders Co. (inherited susceptibility to diseases).
17. Shaw, M. W.: In Beeson, P. B., and McDermott, W., editors: Cecil-Loeb textbook of medicine, ed. 13, Philadelphia, 1971, W. B. Saunders Co. (mongolism).
18. Smith, D., and Wilson, A.: The child with Down's syndrome (mongolism), Philadelphia, 1973, W. B. Saunders Co.
19. Sorsby, A.: Practitioner **183:**133, 1959 (chromosomal inheritance).
20. Stern, C.: Principles of human genetics, ed. 2, San Francisco, 1960, W. H. Freeman and Co., Publishers.
21. U.S. Department of Health, Education, and Welfare, Public Health Service, DHEW Publication No. (NIH) 57-49, revised 1974 (Huntington's disease).
22. U.S. Department of Health, Education, and Welfare, Public Health Service, DHEW Publication No. (NIH) 73-408, 1974 (retinitis pigmentosa).
23. U.S. Department of Health, Education, and Welfare, Public Health Service, DHEW Publication No. (NIH) 74-538, 1975 (antenatal diagnosis and Down's syndrome).
24. U.S. Department of Health, Education, and Welfare, Public Health Service, DHEW Publication No. (HSM) 73-5108, 1974 (sickle cell anemia).
25. U.S. Department of Health, Education, and Welfare, Public Health Service Publication No. 996, Health Information Series 106, 1963 (muscular dystrophy).
26. Wintrobe, M. M.: Clinical hematology, ed. 5, Philadelphia, 1961, Lea & Febiger (blood factors, hemophilia, etc.).
27. Yahr, M. D.: In Beeson, P. B., and McDermott, W., editors: Cecil-Loeb textbook of medicine, ed. 13, Philadelphia, 1971, W. B. Saunders Co. (Huntington's chorea).

CHAPTER 17

Role of endocrine glands in disease

The endocrine system is composed of ductless glands that release their secretions into the blood. The secretions are known as hormones. The disorders or dysfunctions of the endocrine glands represent excessive, deficient, or untimely secretions of a hormone. These disorders may be caused by a primary disease of a gland, or they may be secondary to a disease state in another organ, such as secondary hyperparathyroidism of renal failure. All the hormones circulate in the blood, and thus their effects are felt throughout the body because of their impingement on most of the organs and systems. The hormones are necessary for growth, development, and normal metabolism, and in the case of the gonads they are necessary for reproduction. The role of the hormones in the maintenance of a stable internal environment necessary for life and their failure in this capacity establishes for them a rightful place in discussion of disease mechanisms.

The functions and disorders of the following endocrine glands are discussed in this chapter: pituitary, thyroid, parathyroids, adrenals, and gonads (ovaries and testes). The thymus and pineal body are not discussed, since their functions are not clearly delineated or understood. Diabetes mellitus, in which there is a faulty production of insulin secreted by the islands of Langerhans in the pancreas, has been discussed elsewhere.

PITUITARY BODY (HYPOPHYSIS CEREBRI)[2, 3, 5]

The pituitary body or gland actually consists of two glands—the adenohypophysis or anterior pituitary gland and the neurohypophysis or posterior pituitary gland. The major functions of the anterior lobe are to control the functions of other endocrine glands and to regulate body growth (Fig. 17-1). The major hormones secreted are adrenocorticotropic hormone (ACTH), regulation of adrenocortical hormones except aldosterone; thyrotropic or thyroid-stimulating hormone (TSH), regulation of thyroid activity; gonadotropins (FSH, follicle-stimulating hormone; LH, luteinizing hormones; and ICHS, male analogue of LH); somatotropic or growth hormone (STH or GH); and melanocyte-stimulating hormone (MSH), stimulation of pigmentation of the skin (Fig. 17-1). The posterior lobe of the pituitary gland secretes two hormones—antidiuretic hormone (ADH) and oxytocin. The antidiuretic hormone stimulates water reabsorption by the distal and collecting tubules of the kidneys and also stimulates smooth muscle of blood vessels and intestine. If the ADH secretion is inadequate, diabetes insipidus occurs. This disease has been discussed in Chapter 9. Oxytocin stimulates powerful contractions of the uterus during delivery and causes milk ejection from the lactating breast.

PITUITARY

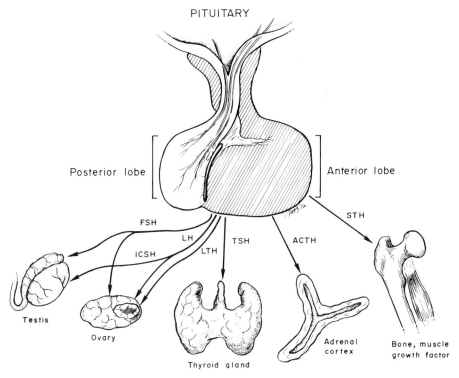

Fig. 17-1. The pituitary gland, showing target organs of anterior pituitary hormones.

Hyperpituitarism[2, 3, 5]

Hyperpituitarism causes excessive secretions of growth hormone, as manifested in the diseases of gigantism and acromegaly.

Gigantism.[2, 3, 5] Gigantism is caused by excessive secretion of growth hormone, beginning before ossification is completed; possibly caused by an acidophil adenoma of the pituitary gland. Pituitary giants may reach a height of 7 or 8 feet. It has been speculated that Goliath, the Biblical giant slain by David with a slingshot, was a pituitary giant.

The abnormal growth often begins in infancy or at puberty. The patients may have normal or retarded mental development. Sexual development and muscular strength, which may be excessive for a time, eventually are decreased, even below normal. The diameter of the skull is increased and the tables are thickened. Cranial sutures may remain open. The epiphyseal union of the long bones is retarded by several years, with the length of the long bones being increased. The tuberosities of long bones are exaggerated, and the vertebral bodies may show wedging, osteoporosis, or eburnation on radiographic examination. There is splanchnomegaly. The increased size of the hypophysis is accompanied by the symptoms of headache and visual disturbances. Acromegalic characteristics may develop in these patients. Gigantism is a rare disorder that has been considered to be a childhood counterpart of acromegaly.

Acromegaly.[2, 3, 5] Once the epiphyseal lines are closed at puberty, no further longitudinal growth can take place. Thus, if excessive amounts of growth hormone are secreted, appositional enlargement occurs in the bones, but all the tissues share in the overgrowth. The facial features are coarsened, and the lips and nose are particularly large. The mandible is also particularly large, and the hands and feet are

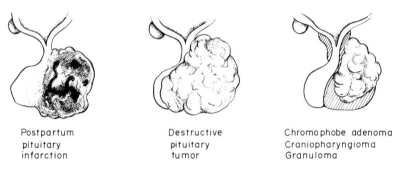

Postpartum
pituitary
infarction

Destructive
pituitary
tumor

Chromophobe adenoma
Craniopharyngioma
Granuloma

Fig. 17-2. Lesions responsible for anterior lobe insufficiency.

enlarged and spadelike. Hypertrophy of the larynx and vocal cords causes a deepened voice. Overgrowth of bones causes spinal deformity, with the joints being more susceptible to degenerative lesions. Early in the disease the gonads may be large, but they later tend to shrink because of loss of gonadotropic hormones. Sexual functions tend to fail or diminish with progression of the syndrome. Women cease to menstruate, and men lose libido and potency. Milk secretion or galactorrhea has been observed in some acromegalic women.

In most cases acromegaly is caused by an acidophil adenoma of the pituitary gland. Patients are usually over 30 years at the time of diagnosis.

Hypopituitarism[2, 3, 5]

Hypopituitarism is caused by destruction of the anterior pituitary or a deficiency of hormones of the anterior lobe of the pituitary (Fig. 17-2). When the entire anterior pituitary is destroyed, it is called panhypopituitarism. In hypopituitarism, however, the deficiency can be mild to severe. The destruction of the anterior pituitary is accompanied by secondary atrophy of the gonads, thyroid, and adrenal cortex. The most common cause of pituitary insufficiency in adults is pituitary tumor, such as the chromophobe adenoma. The most common cause of severe hypopituitarism in adults is probably postpartum necrosis of the gland, often referred to as Sheehan's disease. The pathogenesis of this condition

is in dispute, but the common denominator recognized is obstetric accident, with severe and prolonged puerperal circulatory collapse.

Other lesions responsible for pituitary insufficiency are fibrosis, granulomas (syphilitic or tuberculous), ischemic necrosis following acute infection, fracture of the base of the skull, and septic cavernous sinus thrombosis. (The cavernous sinus is located at the side of the body of the sphenoid bone.)

Simmond's disease and pituitary dwarfism, forms of hypopituitarism, are discussed below.

Simmond's disease.[2, 3, 5] Simmond's disease is a result of chronic pituitary insufficiency. Necrosis of the anterior lobe of the pituitary gland occurs in this condition. It may be a postpartum condition, or it may be caused by head injuries or granulomas.

The most noteworthy clinical manifestation is loss of axillary and pubic hair. Complaints are weakness, loss of energy, loss of libido in men, and decreased libido and amenorrhea in women. There is anhidrosis (lack of sweating), and the skin is smooth and dry. The facies have a myxedematous appearance. Hypochromic or normochromic anemia may be a feature. When it occurs in children, puberty is delayed.

The basal metabolic rate (BMR) and blood pressure tend to be lowered. Urinary gonadotropins and corticosteroids are decreased. The earliest and most frequent manifestation is the result of failure of growth hormone and gonadotropin secretion. The secondary gonadal failure is followed by thyroid deficiency and later adrenocortical deficiency.

Pituitary dwarfism.[2, 3, 5] Lesions involving the pituitary in childhood cause dwarfism, but stunted growth may be found in various chronic diseases, such as primary gonadal dysgenesis. Dwarfism caused by pituitary insufficiency is rare and may result from tumors of the anterior lobe. Failure of children to grow in dwarfism associated with tumors of the anterior lobe or intracellar cysts may be accompanied by thyroid, adrenocortical, and gonadal insufficiency. In true pituitary dwarfism the children fail to develop sexually and in stature. The skeleton is small and delicately formed, retaining childhood proportions. The chest is flat and narrow, and the hair is soft and silken. In the very young, dentition and ossification may be delayed for years. The pituitary dwarf retains his intelligence.

Adenomas[2, 3, 5]

Adenomas of the pituitary gland (Fig. 17-2) are classified into three types according to the nature of the predominant cells. These are chromophobe adenoma, acidophil adenoma, and basophil adenoma, but there may also be a mixture of cells. Adenomas may arise in any part of the anterior pituitary. They grow slowly but may extend into the cranial cavity to involve the optic chiasm and tracts, the hypothalamus or midbrain, and even the frontal and temporal lobes. The mechanical effects are those of pressure on adjacent structures. The endocrine effects are hyposecretion or hypofunction of the gland, with a remote endocrine effect being hypogonadism. Chromophobe adenomas are the most common and attain the largest size. They are usually found in adults between the ages of 30 and 50 years. Acidophil adenomas are the next largest group of pituitary adenomas, and they are usually smaller than the chromophobe adenomas. As a rule they are confined to the sella turcica. Acidophil

adenomas may be associated with acromegaly or gigantism. Basophil adenomas are rare, and they are the smallest of all the pituitary adenomas.

The craniopharyngioma has been discussed in Chapter 6.

THYROID GLAND[4, 20, 24]

Thyroid activity is controlled primarily by thyrotropic hormone or thyroid-stimulating hormone (TSH) (Fig. 17-1). The thyroid gland through its hormones, thyroxine (T_4) and triiodothyronine (T_3), influences or controls the rate of basal and general metabolism; that is, it controls the rate at which chemical changes in the living cells build or destroy protoplasm. It creates the energy by which we live and move and assimilate new material. Adequate amounts of thyroid hormone are essential for normal growth and development. Since thyroid hormone accelerates oxidative processes in body cells, the level of the oxidative processes can be measured by determining the level of basal or resting metabolism as evidenced by respiratory exchange of oxygen. This test is called the *basal metabolic rate* or the *BMR*.

The important constituent of the thyroid hormone is iodine. The iodine is bound to protein in the blood and is called *protein-bound iodine* or *PBI*. The amount of PBI in the blood can be measured by laboratory procedures and is widely used as a test of thyroid functioning.

After oral or intravenous administration of radioactive iodine (iodine 131) in diagnostic studies, the amount of iodine taken up by the thyroid gland is called *radioactive uptake (RAU)* or *radioactive iodine uptake (RAIU)*. The amount excreted in the urine and the amount present in blood samples can also be measured. Radioactive studies of the thyroid can determine whether the thyroid gland is functioning normally by using scintillation counters to determine the percentage of uptake by the thyroid. An overactive thyroid gland clears the iodine or iodide from the bloodstream

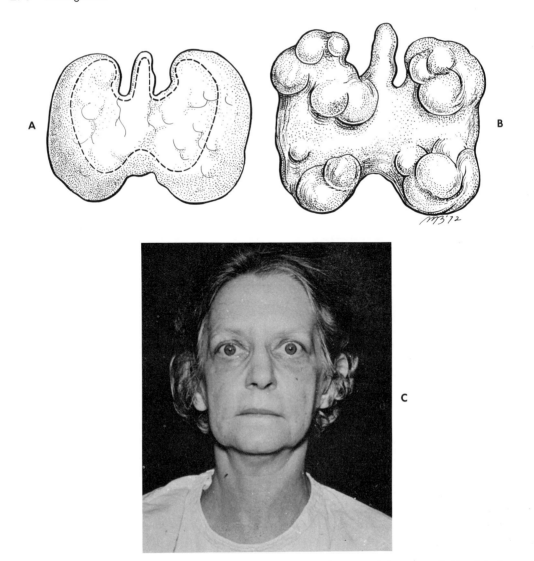

Fig. 17-3. Thyroid lesions in hyperthyroidism. **A,** Hyperplasia. **B,** Adenomas. **C,** Exophthalmos (clinical sign) and goiter. (**C** from Anthony, C. P., and Kolthoff, N. J.: Textbook of anatomy and physiology, ed. 9, St. Louis, 1975, The C. V. Mosby Co.)

at a much faster rate and in larger quantities than the normal thyroid. An underactive thyroid just reverses this clearance of iodide from the bloodstream.

Hypersecretion of thyroid hormone is referred to as *hyperthyroidism.* Hyposecretion of thyroid hormone is called *hypothyroidism.*

Some diseases representing dysfunctioning of the thyroid gland are described as follows.

Goiter[1, 4, 11, 20, 24, 29]

Thyroid hyperplasia or goiter (Fig. 17-3, *A* and *C*) results from failure of the normal rate of manufacture of thyroid hormone. Among the causes of this failure are iodine deficiency, enzymatic defects, goitrogens, and antithyroid compounds. By far the most common type of goiter is caused by iodine deficiency. Goiter occurs in endemic form in inland geographic areas such as the Great Lakes region and in mountainous regions where the iodine content of the soil and water, and therefore the diet, is extremely low. Seafood and leafy vegetables grown along the seacoast are important sources of iodine. Iodized table salt used in unrestricted diets supplies an ample amount of iodine.

In some patients, goiters develop that are not caused by iodine deficiency. Goiters may occur in persons who have received prolonged iodine therapy. They also occur in newborn infants of mothers who have received prolonged iodine therapy during pregnancy. The mechanism of thyroid enlargement in patients with iodine therapy is not well understood. However, it is believed to be related to interference with the conversion of iodide to the necessary organic combining form by large amounts of iodide. It has been reported in people who have been treated for long periods with medications containing many times the normal iodine requirements. These persons were suffering from chronic respiratory disease. Reversion to normal after discontinuance of the iodine medication occurs in most of such patients.

Genetic enzymatic defects in thyroid synthesis have also resulted in goiters. In this type of goiter the iodine may be adequate in supply, but it cannot be trapped or sufficiently concentrated in the gland. The iodide trap block may also cause goiters produced by certain pharmacologic agents, such as potassium thiocyanate or potassium perchlorate.

A number of chemicals, so-called goitrogens, impede thyroid hormone synthesis. Some of the naturally occurring goitrogens are cabbage, rutabaga, kale, turnips, and possibly peanuts, carrots, and strawberries. Infants fed on soybean milk formulas without iodine supplementation have been found to have goiters. Antithyroxinogenic compounds include sulfonamides, phenylbutazone, chlopromazine, cobalt, antimony, colchicine, nitrogen mustard, and aminothiazole. The clinically tried antithyroid compounds such as propythiouracil and other thiocarbamides, appear to inhibit thyroid hormone synthesis at several stages.

Goiters that develop because of iodine deficiency are thought to occur most often during periods of unusual demand for thyroid hormones. They are more common among girls at puberty and may also develop in boys during that same period.

Symptoms of iodine-deficiency goiter are usually minimal if there is no hypothyroidism. However, if the thyroid is markedly enlarged, pressure symptoms such as dysphagia, cough, and a choking sensation may occur. Cosmetic considerations have motivated surgery, but thyroidectomy is also desirable because of the higher incidence of neoplasm in longstanding goiter, particularly the nodular type. Thyroid enlargement is so common in endemic areas that it is almost considered normal.

If patients with nontoxic goiters caused by iodine deficiency or block at the iodide trap are given thyroid medications, involution of the goiter may occur. In the absence of treatment, however, where secretion of the thyroid-stimulating hormone continues for months or years, there will be a marked variation in the cellular response of the acinar cells. Some tissues may form nodules, which may become encapsulated and form adenomas, classified histologically according to their appearance as embryonal, trabecular or solid, tubular, microfollicular, macrofollicular, colloid, and hyperplastic.

The toxic adenoma (Fig. 17-3, B) is uniformly hyperplastic. It has an iodine-concentrating capacity far beyond that of adjacent normal thyroid tissue. Because of hyperfunction, this adenoma can produce symptoms of hyperthyroidism. Patients with this hyperplastic adenoma are usually over 40 years of age and have various cardiac symptoms or complaints. These include palpitation, dyspnea, fibrillation, and perhaps frank heart failure.

Hyperthyroidism (Graves' disease)[4, 16, 20, 24]

In hyperthyroidism (Fig. 17-3) secretion of thyroid hormone or activity of the thyroid gland is increased. It is usually characterized by a goiter and exophthalmos (Fig. 17-3, C), and there may be thyrotoxicosis.

Thyroid storm or crisis is an overwhelming or uncompensated form of thyrotoxicosis.[16] It appears commonly after surgery when the thyrotoxic patient has been prepared inadequately or the diagnosis of hyperthyroidism was not made preoperatively. It appears most commonly, however, during an intercurrent and stressful medical illness, such as uncontrolled diabetes or ketoacidosis, infection, or trauma. The clinical manifestations are those of severe hypermetabolism with fever ranging from 100° F to 106° F, and warm, flushed skin.[16] Sweating may be profuse and the pulse rate is rapid. Atrial fibrillation may be present. Shock may ultimately occur. If there is underlying cardiac disease, pulmonary edema may be present. There may also be profuse diarrhea with nausea and vomiting. Liver abnormalities are common, with frank jaundice. Involvement of the central nervous system is manifested by psychoses, convulsions, agitation, or coma.[16]

In Graves' disease the thyroid is vascular, and an audible bruit may be heard, usually over the superior pole of the right or left lobe.

Patients with hyperthyroidism or Graves' disease have a variety of cardiac symptoms and signs. Females are more likely to show an increased heart rate than males. Cardiac output is increased, with a decrease in circulation time. Exertional dyspnea and palpitation are common. Auricular fibrillation and occasionally auricular flutter are found in a few of the cases. Enlargement of the heart, however, is unusual unless there has been previous heart disease. Symptoms of nervousness, excitability, restlessness, and emotional instability are almost always a part of the picture. Tremors of the hands and the extended foot are also common. (See Fig. 18-32, F.) Muscular wasting and weakness are present, particularly of the muscles of the extremities and back. Muscular wasting is most apparent in the temporal muscles and shoulder girdle. The skin is velvety, warm, and moist. The patient perspires easily. Although there are no morphologic changes in the gonads, some females in the childbearing age complain of irregularity of menses with a decreasing amount of menstrual flow. Amenorrhea may also occur. In some males there may be a varying degree of gynecomastia, which is more likely to occur if there is concomitant exophthalmos. This may range from subareolar thickening to a swelling comparable to that of the adolescent female breast.

Exophthalmos may vary in degree from minimal to very severe. In most patients it is mild. Retraction of lids and a stare of widening of the palpebral fissures are common. Other signs include infrequent blinking, tremor of closed lids, absence of wrinkling on upward gaze, weakness of convergence, and palsy of extraocular muscles. A lid or a globe lag may also be present. Severe symptoms include proptosis with protrusion of the eyeball, edema of the upper and lower lids, and frequently a chemosis or conjunctival edema. Exophthalmos may be progressive and be so rapid and extensive that the patient cannot close his eyes. This leads to ulceration of the cornea, infection, and even loss of an eye.

Cretinism[4, 20, 24]

Cretinism is a congenital deficiency of thyroid function. In rare instances it may be caused by failure of development, but it usually occurs in areas of iodine-deficiency goiter. Cretinism is characterized by retarded mental, physical, and sexual development. Sporadic cases of cretinism occur in children born of healthy mothers, but these are believed to be caused by genetic metabolic errors.

The cretin has a dwarfed stocky build, with short legs and muscular incoordination. Development of the head is faulty, with a short forehead, broad nose, wideset eyes, and a short, thick neck. The eyelids are puffy and wrinkled. The mouth is open, with thick lips and often a protruding tongue. The abdomen and umbilicus are also protuberant. Eruption of decidous teeth is delayed and irregular. The skin is dry, thick, and coarse. Deafness or deaf-mutism is a common occurrence with cretinism in endemic areas. The outstanding feature of cretinism is, however, mental retardation.

Myxedema[4, 20, 24]

Childhood or juvenile myxedema occurs because of thyroid dysfunction after birth. These children are usually spared the serious mental retardation of the cretin. Most have a history of normal growth and development with normal dentition up to the time of the development of myxedema. The juvenile myxedematous patients' bodies are disproportionately longer compared with the lower extremities, and they tend to become dwarfs. Sexual development does not occur.

Adult myxedema is a form of hypothyroidism that occurs most frequently in adults between the ages of 30 and 60. It is four times as common in females as in males. (See Figs. 18-4, *C*, and 18-15, *C*.) The condition may be a primary thyroid disorder or secondary to deficiency of the pituitary hormone (pituitary myxedema).

The typical facies and voice alone are often sufficient to make a preliminary diagnosis. The face and eyelids are edematous, the tongue is thick, the speech is slow or slurred, and the voice is deep and coarse in the female. Both mental and physical activities are slow. The hair is dry and brittle. The skin is coarse, dry, scaling, and cold. Although the cheeks and nose may be flushed or erythematous, elsewhere the skin is often slightly yellowish, apparently caused by carotinemia resulting from retarded conversion of carotene to vitamin A. Perspiration is diminished. There may also be muscular weakness, ascites, and prolonged recovery of reflexes. The heart is enlarged, with poor heart sounds and oc-

casional precordial pain. The pulse is slow. Frequently there is hypertension. Urea clearance tests indicate some depression of renal function. Anemias, such as aplastic anemia, may accompany the disease, but true pernicious anemia may be a coincidental complication.

In pituitary myxedema the hair is finer and softer than in primary myxedema. Pubic and axillary hair are lost. The heart is small, and there is hypotension. Amenorrhea is present in females. The skin is not so dry as with primary myxedema.

Thyroiditis[4, 20, 24]

In acute thyroiditis the thyroid gland may become temporarily enlarged and tender as a complication of bacterial or viral infection. This inflammation of the thyroid is characterized by fever, which may be quite high and spiking. Malaise is extreme, and a firm, very tender, enlarged thyroid gland may be palpated.

Noninfectious chronic thyroiditis includes Hashimoto's struma, lymphocytic thyroiditis, granulomatous thyroiditis, Riedel's struma, and nonspecific chronic thyroiditis.

Hashimoto's disease is believed by some to be an autoimmune disease, since antibodies to thyroid antigens have been discovered in patients with this disease. The clinical manifestation is that of an enlarged thyroid, and the symptoms of hypothyroidism may be the first indications. It is much more frequent in women than men, but does occur occasionally in young children. It is most common in those between the ages of 30 and 50 years. In children the destruction of the thyroid can lead to thyroid failure and growth retardation. The thyroid may be enlarged up to five times its normal size, with a weight of 30 to 50 grams. In adults the enlarged thyroid gland may be asymptomatic, but some patients complain of dysphagia or pressure symptoms.

In *Riedel's struma* or *thyroiditis*[19] a mass of dense, infiltrative fibrotic tissue replaces the thyroid gland. The mass extends into the trachea and surrounding strap muscles. The presenting symptoms are choking or difficult swallowing. This disease is much more frequent in women than in men, and the usual age of onset is 40 years. The thyroid may be moderately enlarged and firm and densely adherent to the trachea.

Lymphocytic thyroiditis is also called juvenile or adolescent thyroiditis. It is characterized by enlargement of the thyroid gland. It has been suggested that this type of thyroiditis is a variant of Hashimoto's thyroiditis, which affects younger people.

Nonspecific chronic thyroiditis is the most common type of thyroiditis, and it is often confused with Hashimoto's struma. The thyroid gland is smaller than in Hashimoto's struma, weighing considerably less. There is a chronic inflammatory reaction, believed to be the result of infectious, chemical, immunologic or vascular injury.

Granulomatous thyroiditis is also called *de Quervain's thyroiditis* or *subacute thyroiditis*. The gland is moderately enlarged and hard.

PARATHYROIDS[18]

The parathyroid glands produce a hormone concerned with the metabolism of calcium and phosphorus and the maintenance of normal levels of these elements in the blood.

Hypoparathyroidism[18]

In hypoparathyroidism, functioning of the parathyroid glands is decreased. It is usually caused by accidental removal of some or all of the parathyroid tissue during a thyroidectomy. In rare instances it occurs idiopathically, with replacement of the parathyroids by fat, or the parathyroids have been unidentifiable in those cases that have come to autopsy. A few cases have been reported with widespread moniliasis. In hypoparathyroidism the serum phosphorus is high and the serum calcium is low. Little or no calcium is excreted by the kidneys in the urine.

Symptoms are a marked increase in neuromuscular excitability with tetany. Tetany, however, can occur from hypocalcemia caused by rickets, osteomalacia, steatorrhea, and alkalosis that may result from hyperventilation. Cataracts frequently occur, as well as loss of hair and skin lesions. Bones are more dense than normal. Brain tissue may also be calcified.

Hyperparathyroidism[18, 26]

In hyperparathyroidism, functioning of the parathyroid glands is increased. It may be caused by a benign or malignant neoplasm of the parathyroid tissue, rarely by hyperplasia of the parathyroid glands, or by diffuse hyperplasia of parathyroid tissue secondary to disturbance of calcium and phosphorus metabolism elsewhere in the body; it may be found in cases of renal rickets, renal failure, or osteomalacia. Almost all the cases of primary hyperparathyroidism are caused by neoplasms of the functioning parathyroid tissue. Usually the neoplasm is a benign adenoma limited to one parathyroid gland or a part of it, but occasionally there may be multiple adenomas and more than one gland involved. The adenomas secrete increased amounts of parathyroid hormone. As a result of hyperfunction, the serum calcium is elevated at the expense of the bones and the serum phosphorus is depressed by the increased urinary excretion. When the condition is well established, it is called generalized osteitis fibrosa cystica or von Recklinghausen's disease. As a result of decalcification of the bones, there are multiple bending deformities of the long bones as well as of the spine and thorax. The bones fracture easily. Muscular weakness develops. Giant cell tumors and cysts of bone occur. The renal changes are the result of metastatic calcification. Calcium deposition in the kidneys results in tubular obstruction and necrosis. Renal calculi are present in a majority of the patients and may be the basis for the presenting symptoms. Calcium deposition also occurs in the blood vessels, mainly the media. Metastatic calcification has also been found in the lungs and stomach. Calcium deposition is particularly abundant in those cases in which renal function fails and phosphate retention results in a high concentration of both calcium and phosphorus in the blood.[6]

Hyperparathyroidism is the most common and generally accepted cause of hypercalcemia.[6, 22] Symptoms of hypercalcemia in hyperparathyroidism are malaise, muscular weakness, bradycardia, depression, anorexia, polyuria, polydipsia, nausea and vomiting, abdominal pain, and constipation. There may also be bone tenderness, hyperextensible joints, depressed reflexes, and reduced muscle tone. The eye signs are deposits in the conjunctiva of small glasslike, clear particles at the edges of the eyelids. These cause irritation, burning, and increased lacrimation, all of which in turn cause inflammation of the conjunctiva. The calcium deposits in the cornea may be slender, elongated, heavy, gray opacities on the nasal or temporal edge.[22]

Hyperparathyroidism is characterized by a variety of symptoms and by involvement of many bodily systems. Skeletal abnormalities with pain, are the second most frequently occurring symptom, the first being renal calculi. The bone pain is sometimes confused with arthritis, because many of these patients are believed to have arthritis as well as hyperparathyroidism. Involvement of joints in hyperparathyroidism has been reported, with the lesions being periosteal resorption of bone near the articular surfaces, calcification of periarticular and synovial membranes, and calcification of articular cartilages. Patients with hyperparathyroidism are also prone to repeat bouts of acute pancreatitis.

A secondary hyperparathyroidism known as renal rickets is more common in children than in adults. The children have growth disturbances that may result in dwarfism. Skeletal deformities are present with changes in the shafts of bones and particularly in the epiphyseal cartilages. These cartilages may be entirely pushed away from the normal position at the end of a bone shaft, or they may be twisted or bent. The skull is greatly thickened. Renal rickets appear to be in response to low serum calcium.[6]

ADRENALS[7, 8, 15, 23]

The adrenal glands, situated over the superior pole of each of the kidneys, are composed of an inner core, the medulla, and an outer shell, the cortex. The cortex is essential to life and makes up about 80% of the entire weight of the gland. The major functions of the adrenal cortex are regulation of the carbohydrate, electrolyte, protein, and water metabolism, and regulation of body defense mechanisms. "The steroid hormones produced by the adrenal cortex may be grouped broadly into corticoids, adrenal androgens (17-ketosteroids), aldosterone, estrogens, and progesteroids."[8] With the exception of aldosterone the growth, structure, and secretory activities of adrenal cortical hormones are entirely regulated by the hormone corticotropin (Fig. 17-1), produced by the anterior pituitary gland. The major hormones secreted by the adrenal medulla are epinephrine (adrenaline) and norepinephrine (noradrenaline). The major function of the adrenal medulla is the stimulation of organs under the control of the sympathetic nervous system for reaction of the body to acute or transient stress.

A generalized abnormality of the adrenal cortex is present in a number of disorders. An excess, imbalance, or deficiency of adrenal corticoids will cause disease (Fig. 17-4). The abnormalities may be inherent in the adrenal cortex itself, or they may be secondary to a disorder of the anterior pituitary. The major disorder of the adrenal medulla is a pheochromocytoma.

Chronic primary adrenocortical insufficiency (Addison's disease)[7, 23]

Chronic primary adrenocortical insufficiency is caused by adrenocortical defi-

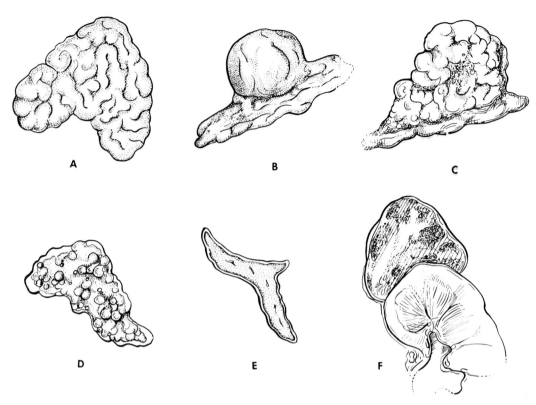

Fig. 17-4. Adrenal lesions in adrenocortical insufficiency. **A,** Hyperplasia of adrenal cortex. **B,** Adenoma of adrenal cortex. **C,** Carcinoma of adrenal cortex. **D,** Tuberculosis of adrenal glands (Addison's disease). **E,** Atrophy of adrenal cortex. **F,** Hemorrhage destruction of adrenal gland, as occurs in Waterhouse-Friderichsen syndrome, classically associated with meningococcemia. (See also Fig. 14-1.)

ciency or hypocorticalism. It is better known as Addison's disease (Fig. 17-4, *D*), after its discoverer, Thomas Addison. The disorder is relatively rare in the United States. It is a slowly progressive disease; destructive atrophy of the adrenal cortex occurs in about 55% of the cases in the United States.[7] About 40% are caused by tuberculosis, but this correlates with the incidence of this disease in the population.[7] When tuberculosis of the adrenal glands is bilateral, both the adrenal cortex and medulla are progressively destroyed. The remaining cases, with the exception of those caused by surgery, are attributed to a variety of diseases, such as metastatic carcinoma, histoplasmosis, torulosis, amyloidosis, venous thrombosis, and hemo-chromatosis.[7] Recently an autoimmune destructive process has been implicated. Autoimmune lesions are alterations in antigen-containing tissues caused by the interaction of autoantibodies and antigens. Circulating adrenal complement-fixing antibodies have been demonstrated in some patients with Addison's disease. Regardless of etiology, complete destruction of the adrenal cortex is incompatible with life unless appropriate hormonal therapy is instituted. All the hormones secreted by the adrenal cortex become deficient in Addison's disease.

The first symptoms experienced by the patient are usually those of weakness and easy fatigability. The facial expression is one of weariness; talking may be an effort.

The symptoms are not as noticeable after a night's rest, but as the day progresses, mental lethargy and physical weakness increase. Muscular weakness is greater in those who have poor muscular development. There is increased irritability, nervousness, and emotional instability, and periods of depression with a clinical picture of neurasthenia or psychoneurosis. The first abnormality noted may be acute prostration caused by a relatively minor infection. The acute adrenal insufficiency (Fig. 17-4, *F*) is characterized by profound weakness and stupor. There is vasomotor collapse, usually preceded by a period of increasing anorexia, nausea and vomiting, and increasing hypotension. Chemical derangements in acute adrenal insufficiency are azotemia, hyponatremia, and hypochloremia. Serum concentrations of potassium, magnesium, and phosphorus are elevated.

Marked pigmentation of the skin and mucous membranes is present in well over 90% of the patients with adrenal deficiency of spontaneous origin but is strikingly less in those patients who have had subtotal or total adrenalectomy. Usually these patients have been on cortisone therapy from the onset of their illness. Some pigmentation is nearly always present in primary adrenal insufficiency. The pigmentation is usually diffuse, with deposition of melanin pigment accentuated on exposed areas of the skin, and more marked at nipples, friction areas, and in skin creases and scars; the mucous membranes of the gums also show pigmentation. There is darkening of the hair, vitiligo, and freckling. Emaciation and dehydration may occur, but all patients will have a history of recent weight loss.

Hypotension is a symptom in all cases. However, those with previous hypertension may have a drop in pressure to near normal limits. The heart is small.

Hypoglycemic manifestations are hunger, headache, weakness, sweating, trembling, blurring of vision, diplopia, and disorientation, or the patient may become unconscious. These attacks are more likely to occur in the early morning or several hours after a meal rich in carbohydrates, which represents a reactive hypoglycemia. These symptoms may occur with relatively small reductions in blood sugar.

The growth of body hair is decreased in both sexes, but more so in females, who may show complete absence of axillary hair.

Addison's disease must be differentiated from panhypopituitarism, which is characterized by some of the symptoms of Addison's disease. In panhypopituitarism, hypotension is usually mild. Skin pigmentation is nearly always absent. The corticotropin deficiency in panhypopituitarism is reflected in other target glands, the thyroid and gonads. When the condition dates from childhood, dwarfism occurs. There is no dehydration as occurs in primary adrenal deficiency. Hypothyroidism results from a deficiency of thyrotropic hormone. The skin has a fawn color and a tendency to be dry and wrinkled. The deficiency of gonadotropins causes amenorrhea or azoospermia. Acute adrenal insufficiency may occur in both Addison's disease and in secondary adrenal insufficiency caused by panhypopituitarism.[7]

Cushing's syndrome (hypercortisolism)[7, 15, 21, 23]

In hypercortisolism, secretory activity of the adrenal cortex is excessive. The condition is named after the famous neurosurgeon, Harvey Cushing, who found basophil tumors of the hypophysis in his patients. These tumors, however, are often absent. An overactive pituitary and a chromophobe adenoma may secrete ACTH in abnormally large amounts. These pituitary abnormalities produce bilateral hyperplasia of the adrenal cortex (Fig. 17-4 *A*), with the increase in production of cortisol responsible for the signs and symptoms of Cushing's syndrome. Adrenal tumors that produce Cushing's syndrome are adrenocortical adenomas and carcinoma of the adrenal cortex (Figs. 17-4, *B* and *C*).

In Cushing's syndrome, abnormal fat

distribution is caused by the effect of cortisol on fat metabolism. The rounded or moon face is characteristic. There is a buffalo hump behind the shoulders, with enlarged supraclavicular fat pads. The abdomen is pendulous. The arms and legs by contrast to the rest of the body appear almost thin. The skin is thin and almost paperlike, and because of stretching and the disappearance of elastic fibers, purple striae appear over the abdomen, buttocks, upper thighs, and breasts and may even appear on the upper arms. The skin bruises easily, with ecchymoses occurring from minor or trivial trauma. Wound healing is poor. There is muscular wasting and weakness and early development of osteoporosis. These symptoms are caused by the catabolic effect of excess cortisol with protein loss. The bone symptoms, however, are caused by loss of protein matrix of bone and calcium through increased urinary excretions. This results in compression fractures of the vertebrae, rib fractures, and the dorsal kyphosis encountered in these patients. The patient may even become bedridden because of muscular weakness and vertebral fractures. Other symptoms include hypertension and diabetes, latent or overt. Arteriosclerosis may develop rapidly. There may be impotence in the male and amenorrhea in the female. Some patients may have only a pronounced lability of mood, but others may have a definite psychosis, which can range from depression to mania. It is of interest here to note that one of Harvey Cushing's first patients was an inmate of an institution for the insane.[7]

Adrenogenital syndrome[7, 23]

The adrenal cortex normally secretes a number of androgenic or masculizing compounds, and when these are secreted in excess, there will be changes in sex characteristics. Puberty praecox occurs with hyperplasia of the adrenal cortex, and with benign or malignant adenoma in children. In boys there is increased strength and rapid growth of sex organs. In girls, the clitoris becomes enlarged, and there is a male distribution of hair, and the voice deepens.

An adult female with this disturbance becomes masculinized. The musculature of the arms and legs becomes heavy. There is generalized hirsutism and a receding hair line or baldness. The breasts are small, and the clitoris is enlarged. The uterus atrophies. There may be a loss of heterosexual sex drive. Menstruation and ovulation cease. The skin is thick and resilient.

In males adrenal cortical tumors usually develop after the age of puberty, and gynecomastia and loss of sexual potency occur. The external genitalia are small. There may be weight gain and loss of the normal masculine facies and psyche. Pubic hair is decreased.

Primary hyperaldosteronism (Conn's syndrome)[8]

Primary hyperaldosteronism is caused by excessive aldosterone secretion by the adrenal. Primary aldosteronism is associated with adrenocortical adenoma in the majority of the cases, and with carcinoma, multiple adenomas, and cortical hyperplasia of one adrenal in the remainder. In those under 20 years of age, most cases of hypersecretion of aldosterone are associated with either nodular cortical hyperplasia or bilateral diffuse hyperplasia of the adrenal cortex. In Conn's syndrome of hyperaldosteronism, there is hypokalemic alkalosis, renal potassium loss, and hypertension. This combination of symptoms may be cured by removal of aldosteronomas (aldosterone-secreting adenoma of the adrenal). A secondary type of aldosteronism occurs as a result of renal artery narrowing or malignant nephrosclerosis. Primary hyperaldosteronism or Conn's syndrome is characterized by weakness, tetany, paresthesia, polydipsia, polyuria, and transient paralysis.

GONADS[10, 12, 14]

The gonads are the ovaries in women and the testes in men.

Ovary[12, 14]

The ovary has a twofold physiologic function: (1) the development and release of ova and (2) the elaboration of estrogen and progesterone. These activities are carried on from the menarche to menopause. In the sexually mature woman the cyclic production of steroid ovarian hormones is regulated by the secretion of gonadotropins (FSH—follicle stimulating hormone; LH—lutenizing hormone) (Fig. 17-1) from the anterior lobe of the pituitary gland under the neuroendocrine control of the hypothalamus. A number of conditions may result from pathologic aberrations of the normal ovarian cycle. Failure of ovulation (amenorrhea) causes sterility. Amenorrhea is discussed below.

Amenorrhea.[12-14, 25, 28] Amenorrhea is the absence of menstruation. It can be either primary or secondary. In primary amenorrhea there is absence of menarche. The menarche usually occurs between the ages of 12 and 15 years and if it is delayed beyond this time, it can be the sign of endocrinologic disorders. Certain aberrations of sex chromosomes in women are associated with primary amenorrhea. These may be either abnormalities of the number of sex chromosomes or morphologic abnormalities of one X chromosome. The abnormalities of sex chromosomes are demonstrated in a tumor called gonadoblastoma.[12, 27] There is a lack of sexual development and eunuchoidal features with masculinization. The patients have a male sex chromatin pattern, 46/XY or sex chromosome mosaicism, XO/XY. The tumor contains germ cells–Sertoli-granulosa cells and Leydig-theca cells or a mixture of both male and female germ cells.

The most common type of secondary amenorrhea is, of course, pregnancy. It is usually the first diagnosis considered. Patients with secondary amenorrhea have at some time menstruated. It may be caused by endocrine disorders. Gonadotropins, follicle-stimulating hormones (FSH) and luteinizing hormones (LH) of the adeno-hypophysis, are responsible for the growth and development of the gonads and the maintenance of their normal functions. These hormones are secreted cyclically, starting at puberty. FSH stimulates the development of the estrogen-producing graafian follicle, bringing it to maturation. Luteinizing hormones then cause ovulation and the beginning of the corpus luteum formation. The luteotropic hormone (LTH) is responsible for the maintenance of the corpus luteum and probably for its production of estrogen and progesterone. The estrogen and progesterone produced in response to these pituitary hormones are responsible for the endometrial changes leading to menstruation. Disturbances of the functions of the adenohypophysis in regard to those hormonal secretions can have profound effects. A deficiency of gonadotropic hormones leads to amenorrhea in such conditions as pituitary hypogonadism, in which there is failure of development of secondary sex organs and characteristics. The breast, uterus, and normal pubic hair are affected, and the menses fail to appear. An excess of the growth hormone in active acromegaly is also associated with amenorrhea. Amenorrhea also occurs with chromophobic, acidophilic, or basophilic tumors of the pituitary as well as with craniopharyngioma. Other endocrine disorders in which amenorrhea may occur are Cushing's syndrome (p. 277) and the adrenogenital syndrome (p. 278).

Some local gynecologic diseases that may cause amenorrhea are tuberculosis that has spread from the fallopian tubes to involve the uterus and ovaries, gonorrheal salpingitis, and polycystic ovaries or the Stein-Leventhal syndrome. In the Stein-Leventhal syndrome[17] the follicle cysts are lined by theca cells, and the thickening of the ovarian capsule may prevent rupture of the cysts and formation of corpora lutea. Arrhenoblastoma, a tumor of the ovary that produces male hormones, also causes amenorrhea. It has a marked effect on the patient's sex characteristics. An imperforate hymen may cause false amenorrhea or cryptomenorrhea resulting from obstruction of the lower genital tract.

Testes[10]

The primary role of testicular hormones is to develop and maintain the male accessory sex organs and to develop the masculine secondary sexual characteristics. The substances with these properties secreted by the testes are androgens, the most potent and important of which is testosterone. The testes are under the direct control of the secretions of the anterior pituitary gland—the follicle-stimulating hormone (FSH), interstitial cell–stimulating hormone (ICSH), or luteinizing hormone (LH). The FSH stimulates growth of seminiferous tubules and is necessary for maturation of spermatozoa. Luteinizing hormones induce the Leydig cells to secrete testosterone and androsterone and also aid in promoting the final stages of spermatogenesis.

Diseases affecting the gonads that are discussed elsewhere are Klinefelter's syndrome (p. 256), Turner's syndrome (p. 256), and true hermaphroditism and pseudohermaphroditism (p. 245).

Hypogonadism[9]

Hypogonadism is abnormally decreased functional activity of the gonads. Ovarian hypogonadism may result from hypofunction of the pituitary; it may be caused by postnatal castration; or it may be congenital. It is characterized by anorexia and amenorrhea, poor development of the genitalia and sex characteristics, and scanty axillary and pubic hair. Testicular hypogonadism may be caused by anterior pituitary insufficiency; it may be caused by the absence of testicular tissue; or it may result from disturbed formation of the tubules or Leydig's cells. It is characterized by sexual immaturity, a hypoplastic penis, absent or small testes, and lack of axillary, pubic, and facial hair. There may be gynecomastia (abnormal development of

breasts in a male). In hypogonadism the bones in the hands and feet may be abnormally long and slender because of delayed epiphyseal closure and prolonged growth. This is sometimes seen in eunuchoid males. Hypogonadism secondary to hypopituitarism may be caused by a pituitary or suprasellar tumor.

STEP-BY-STEP EXERCISES

Step 1. The ductless glands comprise the endocrine system. The secretions they release into the blood are known as hormones. The effects of the hormones are felt throughout the body. Diseases or dysfunctions of the endocrine glands result when the secretions of the hormones are excessive, deficient, or untimely. These diseases or dysfunctions may be caused by primary disease of a gland, or they may be secondary to a disease process in some other organ.

On the basis of the above comments, indicate those statements that best apply to secretions of the endocrine glands.

1. Hormones are released into the bloodstream by endocrine glands. __
2. The effects of hormones are confined entirely to the endocrine glands secreting a specific hormone. __
3. Diseases or dysfunctions of endocrine glands are caused by excessive, deficient, or untimely secretions of hormones. __
4. An endocrine disorder is always caused by a primary disease of a gland. __

Step 2. Hormones are necessary for growth, development, and normal metabolism. Their role in maintaining a stable internal environment is necessary for life.

On the basis of this statement would you say that hormones contribute to the vital physiologic values that must be maintained for good health?

Yes __ No __

Step 3. Complete the blanks in the following statements relating to the pituitary gland.

1. The pituitary gland actually consists

of two parts, referred to as _____

_____ and _____ _____ .

2. The major hormones secreted by the pituitary gland for control of other endocrine glands or for growth of the body and pigmentation of skin are:

a. Adrenals _____

b. Thyroid _____

c. Gonads _____ (_____ ;

_____)

d. Body growth _____

e. Pigmentation of skin _____

Step 4. Complete the blanks in the following statements relating to the thyroid gland.

1. The two hormones of the thyroid gland are _____ and

_____ .

2. The important constituent of thyroid hormone is _____ . It is bound to protein in the blood and is referred to as _____

_____ or _____ (initials).

3. A test using radioactive material to determine function of the thyroid gland is called _____ _____ .

Step 5. Complete the blanks in the following statements relating to the adrenals.

1. The inner core of the adrenal gland is called the _____ .

2. The outer shell is called the _____ .

3. The major hormones secreted by the inner core are _____ and

_____ .

4. The hormones secreted by the outer shell are called _____ _____ .

Step 6. A hormone concerned with the metabolism of calcium and phosphates and the maintenance of normal levels of these elements in the blood is produced by the _____ glands.

Step 7. The gonads of the male are the _____ ; the gonads of the female are the _____ .

Step 8. The following are diseases of endocrine glands. Complete the first blank with the name of the involved gland; in the second blank indicate whether the disease is caused by excessive or deficient secretion of a hormone, or its content as in goiter.

1. Hyperpituitarism _____ ;

_____

2. Gigantism _____ ; _____

3. Cretinism _____ , _____

4. Acromegaly _____ ; _____

5. Hypoparathyroidism _____ ;

_____

6. Simmond's disease _____ ;

_____

7. Addison's disease _____ ;

_____

8. Hyperparathyroidism _____ ;

_____

9. Adrenogenital syndrome _____ ;

_____

10. Primary myxedema _____ ;

_____

11. Cushing's syndrome _____ ;

_____

12. Goiter (common form) _____ ;

_____ _____

Step 9. Complete the blanks in the following statements.

1. Absence of menstruation is referred to as _____ .

2. The disorder caused by extensive secretion of androgenic or masculiniz-

ing compounds by the adrenal cortex is referred to as the _____

_____.

3. The disease caused by excessive aldosterone secretion is called _____ _____ or _____ syndrome.

4. Increased secretion of thyroid hormone is called _____. This occurs in _____ disease.

5. A _____ is a medullary adrenal tumor.

Responses

Step 1: 1. X; 3. X
Step 2: Yes
Step 3: 1. adenohypophysis or anterior lobe; neurohypophysis or posterior lobe; 2. a. adrenocorticotropic or ACTH; b. thyrotropic or thyroid-stimulating hormone (TSH); c. gonadotropins (follicle-stimulating hormone [FSH]; luteinizing hormone [LH]); d. somatotropic or growth hormone (STH or GH); e. melanocyte-stimulating hormone (MSH)
Step 4: 1. thyroxine; triiodothyronine; 2. iodine; protein-bound iodine or PBI; 3. radioactive uptake (RAU) or radioactive iodine uptake (RAIU)
Step 5: 1. medulla; 2. cortex; 3. epinephrine or adrenaline and noradrenaline or norepinephrine; 4. steroid hormones
Step 6: parathyroid
Step 7: testes; ovaries
Step 8: 1. pituitary; excessive; 2. pituitary; excessive; 3. thyroid; deficiency; 4. pituitary; excessive; 5. parathyroids; deficiency; 6. pituitary; deficiency; 7. adrenals; deficiency; 8. parathyroids; excessive; 9. adrenals; excessive; 10. thyroid; deficiency; 11. adrenals; excessive; 12. thyroid; iodine deficiency
Step 9: 1. amenorrhea; 2. adrenogenital syndrome; 3. primary hyperaldosteronism or Conn's; 4. hyperthyroidism; Graves'; 5. pheochromocytoma

REFERENCES

1. Atwood, E. B., Cassidy, C. E., and Aurbach, G. D.: J.A.M.A. **174:**459, 1960 (goiter).
2. Christy, N. P.: In Beeson, P. B., and McDermott, W., editors: Cecil-Loeb textbook of medicine, ed. 13, Philadelphia, 1971, W. B. Saunders Co. (diseases of the pituitary).
3. Currie, A. R.: In Anderson, W. A. D., editor: Pathology, ed. 6, St. Louis, 1971, The C. V. Mosby Co. (diseases of the pituitary).
4. De Groot, L. J.: In Beeson, P. B., and McDermott, W., editors: Cecil-Loeb textbook of medicine, ed. 13, Philadelphia, 1971, W. B. Saunders Co. (diseases of the thyroid).
5. Erzin, C.: Clinical symposia, July-Sept., Summit, N. J., 1963, Ciba Pharmaceutical Co. (the pituitary gland).
6. Foertsch, J. H.: J. Okla. State Med. Assoc. **56:**322, 1963 (hyperparathyroidism and hypercalcemia).
7. Forsham, P. H.: Clinical symposia, Summit, N. J., April-June, 1963, Ciba Pharmaceutical Co. (abnormalities of the adrenal cortex).
8. Forsham, P. H.: Clinical symposia, Summit, N. J., April-June, 1963, Ciba Pharmaceutical Co. (the adrenal gland; aldosterone).
9. Gordon, B. L., editor: Current medical terminology, Chicago, 1963, American Medical Association (hypogonadism).
10. Grumbach, M. M.: In Beeson, P. B., and McDermott, W., editors: Cecil-Loeb textbook of medicine, ed. 13, Philadelphia, 1971, W. B. Saunders Co. (testes).
11. Harrison, M. T., Alexander, W. D., and Harden, B. M.: Lancet **1:**1238, 1963 (goiter).
12. Hertig, A. J., and Gore, H.: In Anderson, W. A. D., editor: Pathology, ed. 6, St. Louis, 1971, The C. V. Mosby Co. (female genitalia; ovarian lesions).
13. Jacobs, P. A., and others: Lancet **1:**1183, 1961 (amenorrhea).
14. Kase, N.: In Beeson, P. B., and McDermott, W., editors: Cecil-Loeb textbook of medicine, ed. 13, Philadelphia, 1971, W. B. Saunders Co. (ovaries; ovarian lesions).
15. Liddle, G. W.: In Beeson, P. B., and McDermott, W., editors: Cecil-Loeb textbook of medicine, ed. 13, Philadelphia, 1971, W. B. Saunders Co. (adrenals).
16. Newmark, S. R., Himathengkam, T., and Shane, J. M.: J.A.M.A. **230:**592-593, 1974 (hyperthyroid crisis).
17. Nesbitt, R. E. L., Jr., and Shelley, T. F.: Nebr. State Med. J. **48:**113, 1963 (Stein-Leventhal syndrome).
18. Oertel, J. E., and Anderson, W. A. D.: In Anderson, W. A. D., editor: Pathology, ed. 6, St. Louis, 1971, The C. V. Mosby Co. (parathyroids).
19. Raphael, H. A., and others: Mayo Clin. Proc. **41:**375, 1966 (Riedel's struma).
20. Rawson, R. W.: The thyroid gland, Clinical symposia, Summit, N. J., April-June, 1965, Ciba Pharmaceutical Co. (thyroid diseases).
21. Ross, E. J., Marshall-Jones, P., and Friedman, M.: Q. J. Med. **35:**149, 1966 (Cushing's syndrome).

22. Schneider, S. H.: Ariz. Med. **30**:183, 1963 (hyperparathyroidism; hypercalcemia).

23. Sommers, S. C.: In Anderson, W. A. D., editor: Pathology, ed. 6, St. Louis, 1971, The C. V. Mosby Co. (adrenals).

24. Sommers, S. C.: In Anderson, W. A. D., editor: Pathology, ed. 6, St. Louis, 1971, The C. V. Mosby Co. (thyroid).

25. Stander, R. W.: J. Indiana State Med. Assoc. **53**:1873, 1960 (amenorrhea).

26. Steinbach, H. L., and others: Am. J. Roentgenol. Radium Ther. Nucl. Med. **86**:329, 1961 (primary hyperparathyroidism: correlation of roentgen, clinical, and pathologic features).

27. Teter, J.: Am. J. Obstet. Gynecol. **84**:722, 1962 (gonadoblastoma).

28. Therapeutic Notes, March, 1962, Parke-Davis Co. (amenorrhea).

29. Weaver, D. K., and others: Arch. Surg. **92**: 796, 1966 (nodular goiter).

SYMPTOMATOLOGY

abdominal distention
abdominal rigidity
abnormal uterine bleeding
anhidrosis
anuria
arterial insufficiency
ataxia
chills
cough
diarrhea
dyspnea
earache
epiphora
fatigue
fever
hearing loss
heartburn
hemiplegia
hyperhidrosis
hypersalivation
insomnia
joint enlargement
kyphosis
leg ulcers
loss of vision
muscular weakness
nuchal rigidity
pallor
paresthesia
seizures
splenomegaly
syncope
tremor
urinary frequency
vaginal discharge

CHAPTER 18

Clinical manifestations of diseases

The emphasis in the first section of this book has been on mechanisms of disease and diagnostic methods in certain disease processes. This section of the book is devoted to the clinical manifestations of disease, which are the signs and symptoms that lead the attending physician to make a specific or possible diagnosis. Diagnostic procedures are ordered by the attending physician based on the physical examination of the patient and the clinical manifestations of his illness.

The signs and symptoms of a disease process are the basic parameters of diagnosis, since they are the final expressions of the disease. The significance of the symptoms of a disease and the role they play in medical diagnosis become clear as your knowledge of the mechanisms of a disease process unfolds. This is the basis for the teaching of the disease mechanisms in the first section of the book before studying the clinical manifestations of disease. Symptoms are error signals that warn of threat to the integrity of an organism. They may or may not be specific indicators of a specific disease, but a symptom alone or in combination with others can often point to a specific illness and lead to a correct diagnosis.

We have attempted to establish a profile of common symptoms. Some can be used as a check-off list of symptoms by paramedical personnel when they assume the responsibilities of interviewing a patient and obtaining a clinical history of the patient's complaints. The demand for in-creased knowledge of diseases among paramedical personnel as medical assistants is increasing in modern medicine at a rapid rate. Consequently, paramedical personnel are being trained to assume more and more responsibilities in a doctor's office, clinic, or admitting office of hospitals to free the attending or examining physicians for the more important task of establishing a diagnosis, determining the extent of illness of the patient, and treating him accordingly.

The major symptoms selected for study in this profile are defined in the correct medical terminology. It is important that you learn this technical language, since it enables you to receive and convey information accurately. It is also important that you know which diseases are characterized by certain symptoms. Some of the major diseases for each symptom have been selected for discussion. Other diseases that are more or less common are defined briefly so that it will not be necessary to consult a medical dictionary for further details. All these steps have been taken to increase your medical vocabulary and thereby further your knowledge of diseases. The illustrations increase your knowledge of anatomy and pinpoint the location of diseases.

You will probably note that pain as a symptom is not discussed. This deletion was deliberate, and while it is a universal and outstanding symptom of disease, it is believed that only the physician by careful questioning, observation, and physical examination can interpret the significance of

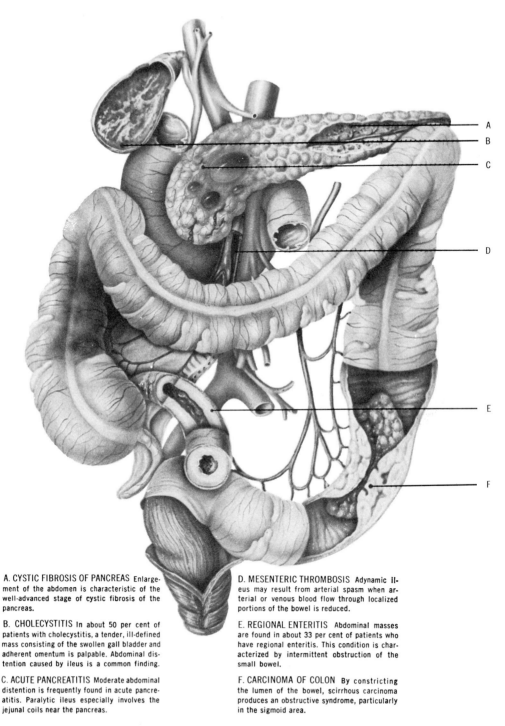

A ——
B ——
C ——
D ——
E ——
F ——

A. CYSTIC FIBROSIS OF PANCREAS Enlargement of the abdomen is characteristic of the well-advanced stage of cystic fibrosis of the pancreas.

B. CHOLECYSTITIS In about 50 per cent of patients with cholecystitis, a tender, ill-defined mass consisting of the swollen gall bladder and adherent omentum is palpable. Abdominal distention caused by ileus is a common finding.

C. ACUTE PANCREATITIS Moderate abdominal distention is frequently found in acute pancreatitis. Paralytic ileus especially involves the jejunal coils near the pancreas.

D. MESENTERIC THROMBOSIS Adynamic Ileus may result from arterial spasm when arterial or venous blood flow through localized portions of the bowel is reduced.

E. REGIONAL ENTERITIS Abdominal masses are found in about 33 per cent of patients who have regional enteritis. This condition is characterized by intermittent obstruction of the small bowel.

F. CARCINOMA OF COLON By constricting the lumen of the bowel, scirrhous carcinoma produces an obstructive syndrome, particularly in the sigmoid area.

Fig. 18-1. Abdominal distention. (From Therap. Notes **70:**10, Jan.-Feb., 1963, Parke, Davis & Co.)

the pain described by the patient. Pain is a personal experience of the patient, and he often has difficulty in communicating the nature, extent, and location of the pain partly because of his inability to put into proper words a true description of his feelings.

ABDOMINAL DISTENTION[83]

Abdominal distention is a localized or generalized swelling of the abdomen. It is usually caused by excessive amounts of gas or fluid in the intestine, but less frequently, it may be the result of free air or gas in the peritoneal cavity after rupture of an air-containing viscus. Abdominal distention occurs in a number of diseases, some of which are illustrated in Fig. 18-1.

The obstructive causes are mechanical and nonmechanical. The mechanical obstructions are intraluminal and are caused by foreign bodies, gallstones, meconium bezoars (concretions), enteroliths (stony hard concretions), or worms. Mechanical obstruction (mural) is caused by compression of the intestinal wall by adhesions, stenosis, hernia (described below), volvulus (twisting of an intestine), intussusception (invagination of a portion of intestine into an adjacent portion), tumors, or atresia (absence or closure of an orifice). Paralytic ileus results from paralysis of the musculature of a portion or all of the intestinal tract. It may occur as a reflex after certain manipulations during surgery, as peritoneal damage from chemical agents, as a reflection of metabolic changes initiated by electrolyte imbalance, or after mechanical hypoactivity.

Ascites[38] (collection of fluid in the peritoneal cavity) may cause pronounced distention of the abdomen. It occurs most often in association with disease processes associated with portal hypertension (increased blood pressure in the portal venous system).[27] These disease processes are cirrhosis of the liver (p. 290), constrictive pericarditis, cardiac decompensation, right heart failure, and sometimes thrombosis of the portal or hepatic vein. Ascites also occurs in malignant diseases and in chronic or tuberculosis peritonitis.

Abdominal distention from a distended bladder may occur with retroversion of the gravid uterus in women and with prostatic hypertrophy in men. Other causes of bladder distention include compression paraplegia, lateral sclerosis, or tabes dorsalis (neurosyphilis).

The abdomen may be distended from abdominal tumor or enlargement of the pancreas, liver, or gallbladder. The abdomen of newborn infants may be distended before the first plug of meconium is passed.

Some specific causes of abdominal distention selected for discussion are as follows.

Cholecystitis[35, 73, 81, 82]

Cholecystitis is an inflammation of the gallbladder. It occurs most often in the fifth and sixth decades, predominantly in women. It is usually caused by partial or complete obstruction to the outflow of bile by stones obstructing the cystic duct. When the outflow of bile is obstructed, the bile becomes progressively concentrated in the gallbladder, causing chemical irritation of its wall. The irritated gallbladder wall is subject to secondary bacterial infection. Pancreatic reflux is sometimes implicated in acute inflammations, with active lipases, amylases, and proteases being identified in the bile. Diagnosis is usually established by cholecystography. Symptoms of chronic inflammation are vague and insidious, usually including an intolerance to fatty foods, belching, pain after eating, nausea, and sometimes vomiting. In acute cholecystitis the pain is usually in the right upper quadrant of the abdomen, radiating to the right shoulder area. There is fever, nausea, vomiting, and rigidity of the abdominal wall, especially in the right upper quadrant, and the gallbladder may be palpable. Jaundice may also occur. Complications are perforation of the gallbladder wall followed by peritonitis, or pericholecystic liver, or sub-diaphragmatic abscess.

Acute pancreatitis[24, 48]

Acute inflammation of the pancreas may be caused by a number of factors, among which are gallstones, alcohol, and idiopathic processes. The underlying mechanism in the production of the inflammation is the escape of activated enzymes into the interstitial tissues of the pancreas. Exactly what triggers the liberation and activation of the proteolytic and lipolytic enzymes normally found in the pancreas is not clearly delineated. The increase of amylase and lipase in the serum is important in establishing a diagnosis. The symptoms are severe epigastric pain, abrupt in onset, which radiates especially to the back; nausea, vomiting, shock, and a peculiar ecchymotic mottling of the skin of the flanks. It is a disease of adults between 40 and 70 years and is more common in females than males. Gross hemorrhage late in the disease occurs in the pancreas from necrosis of arteries and arterioles.

Regional enteritis[3, 38, 51]

Regional enteritis, an inflammatory disease of the small intestine, is a somewhat common disorder, with a peak incidence in middle age. Males are more often affected than females. The etiology is unknown, but lymphatic obstruction is believed to play a primary role. Psychosomatic causes have also been considered but have not been proved. Early in the stage of the disease the bowel walls thicken and later become fibrotic. The distal ileum is usually affected up to the ileocecal valve, but the condition may extend into the cecum and sometimes into the ascending colon. The lumen of the bowel is narrowed. This is clearly seen on x-ray examination because only a thin stream of barium passes through the narrowed passageway. The inflexibility of the bowel wall that occurs in some cases has been compared to that of a lead pipe or a rubber hose. Symptoms are not constant, but are characterized by exacerbations and remissions. Pain at first may be vague in the right lower quadrant, followed by colicky cramps, and constipation and diarrhea may alternate. As the disease progresses symptoms become more pronounced, with loss of appetite, nausea, vomiting, and loss of weight. The severe diarrhea may create a serious disturbance of fluid and electrolyte balance. Melena (passage of dark stools stained with blood pigments or with altered blood) occurs in many cases. After remission, the symptoms may be reactivated by stress, either physical or emotional. Complications are hemorrhage, perforation, and peritonitis.

Cirrhosis[27, 43, 73, 79]

Cirrhosis is a disease of the liver in which the liver cells are damaged or necrotic and are replaced by fibrous connective tissue. The disease derives its name from the Greek word *kirrhos*, meaning yellow or orange, but this is a misnomer, since not all cirrhotic livers are this color. Cirrhosis is classified into a number of types according to etiology, but all cirrhotic livers have certain distinctive changes in common, such as a diffuse, real or apparent increase in fibrous connective tissue, necrosis of liver cells, and either nodular or diffuse regeneration of the liver cells. The symptoms and end results are also similar regardless of etiology.

Laennec's cirrhosis, which is also called alcoholic cirrhosis, fatty nutritional cirrhosis, hobnail liver, portal cirrhosis, and diffuse nodular cirrhosis, is the most common type. In the United States and some foreign countries it is most commonly associated with long-continued use of alcohol. The exact mechanism of the injurious effect of alcohol on the liver is unknown. In some countries like India and Africa where cirrhosis is common, it seems to be related more to malnutrition and hepatitis. One theory is that perhaps it is caused by dietary insufficiency and is preceded by prolonged and excessive fatty infiltration of the liver. Many alcoholics suffer from malnutrition, particularly of protein-containing essential amino acids, since their persistent and excessive drinking interferes with an adequate diet. Experiments in animals have shown that alcohol in excess interferes with fat metabolism. The liver in Laennec's cirrhosis is often large, fatty, and uniformly granular, and the abdomen may be distended.

Laennec's cirrhosis occurs at any age but is more prevalent among those between 40 and 65 years, and it is more frequent in males than in females.

Some symptoms of Laennec's cirrhosis that may also to a certain extent, or in many instances, be found in cirrhosis from other causes are portal hypertension, which results from interference of blood flow through the portal system, splenomegaly, and hemorrhoids. When the portal venous circulation is obstructed, the body attempts to bypass the liver by establishing shunts between the portal circulation and the peripheral venous circulation. A shunt sometimes develops in the lower end of the esophogus and cardia of the stomach. The dilated veins in such instances form varices that connect the veins with the diaphragm and through the diaphragm with the superior vena cava. In these cases esophageal varices occur and have a tendency to rupture, sometimes with fatal hemorrhage. Hematemesis (vomiting of blood) occurs in some cirrhotics and may be the first symptom of the disease. Other clinical manifestations of cirrhosis are telangiectasis or spider vascular lesions on the upper chest and sometimes on the face and neck. Palmar erythema (morbid redness of the skin) is sometimes a symptom. A symptom of obstructive cirrhosis is progressive jaundice associated with intense itching. The stools are clay colored, and the urine is dark brown and contains bile pigments. The liver may or may not be enlarged and may even be decreased in size, depending upon the etiology of the cirrhosis. Not all these symptoms occur in every type of cir-

rhosis, but they are more or less common findings.

Postnecrotic cirrhosis has also been called toxic cirrhosis and posthepatic cirrhosis. In this type of cirrhosis the liver is coarsely nodular with large areas of scarring and subnormal weight. The smallest of the cirrhotic livers is seen in this type. A distended abdomen is not a feature of this form of cirrhosis.

Pigmentary cirrhosis is a type in which an excess of iron is stored in the liver. It is commonly seen in the disease hemochromatosis and in other conditions in which absorption of iron is excessive. The liver is not so large as that in Laennec's cirrhosis. There may be pigmentation of the skin, with deposits of hemosiderin and hemofuscin and increased melanin pigment.

Biliary cirrhosis is caused by obstruction of the biliary tract, either extrahepatic or intrahepatic. The most common cause in adults is obstruction by a tumor or stones. It also occurs in infants with congenital atresia of the extrahepatic bile ducts.

In infectious or cholangitis biliary cirrhosis, the liver is usually large and finely nodular. An infection by colon bacillus is commonly the cause. The infection spreads from the bile ducts into the liver cells on the periphery of the liver nodules. This type may be both obstructive and infectious.

Syphilitic cirrhosis results from syphilitic infection. There is extensive scarring or diffuse fibrosis of the liver.

A parasitic type of cirrhosis is the result of infection by schistosomes or liver flukes.

Hernias[38]

A hernia is protrusion of an organ or part of an organ through the wall that contains it. Hernias are considered to be mechanical disturbances or obstructions. Most hernias are abdominal and consist of extension of a peritoneal pouch or sac through a defect or structural weakness of the abdominal wall. The abdominal hernias may contain any of the mobile viscera, usually the omentum or portions of the intestinal tract or both. In indirect inguinal hernia the abdominal contents herniate through the internal inguinal ring and along the inguinal canal into the scrotum. This type of hernia is caused by persistence of the peritoneal vaginal processus that normally accompanies the testis on its descent into the scrotum and subsequently becomes obliterated. The hernia appears as a soft mass, usually in the groin or scrotum, that may disappear when the patient lies down. In direct inguinal hernia, herniation is through the external ring of the male or through the femoral ring beneath the inguinal ligament. When this occurs in the female, it is called a femoral hernia. Ventral hernias are related to trauma of the abdominal wall, usually from improper healing following surgery.

When a hernia is reducible or uncomplicated, the symptoms are a dull, burning, prickling sensation that becomes worse when walking or standing. Coughing precipitates the same type of sensation.

When a hernia is incarcerated, the intestinal loop is caught in the opening. The walls distend with blood. The trapped hernia may not be pushed back, and the intestinal flow of blood is obstructed. The symptoms include pain, nausea, and vomiting.

If the hernia becomes strangulated, the loop of intestine in the sac becomes twisted, producing constriction. Blood supply is cut off, and necrosis of the intestinal loop occurs. If uncorrected, it will progress to perforation and peritonitis. Symptoms of uncorrected strangulated hernia are acute abdominal pain, nausea, and vomiting. There is blood in the stool. The white blood cell count is high.

ABDOMINAL RIGIDITY[84]

Abdominal rigidity is a sustained reflex contraction of the abdominal wall muscles in response to stimuli arising in the viscera or walls of an organ or cavity. Visceral

stimuli are frequently not strong enough to complete the spinal cord reflex arc, but they do increase enough to produce excitability to near threshold levels. For rigidity to occur, an additional stimulus from the abdominal wall or peritoneum is necessary. The reflex is influenced by the higher nervous system centers; therefore patients who are hypersensitive or who are undergoing anxiety states will have increased excitability. Excitability is lowered in patients in shock or suffering from toxic conditions. Sensory nerves are abundant in the anterior and lateral abdominal walls, but the pelvis and medial portion of the posterior abdominal wall are poorly supplied, and hence, stimuli from these areas are less likely to produce rigidity.

Forceful contraction in weak and thin abdominal muscles and in obese abdomens may not cause rigidity, even if adequate stimuli are present.

The conditions causing abdominal rigidity are illustrated in Fig. 18-2 and are discussed in the accompanying captions. These need not be amplified except to note that rigidity is divided into two types— localized and generalized. Localized rigidity occurs in the abdominal wall overlying an affected organ, such as in appendicitis, cholecystitis, and occasionally pancreatitis. Intestinal obstruction causes localized rigidity if gangrene and localized peritonitis have developed. Transient localized rigidity occurs during paroxysms of pain in patients with colic. Generalized rigidity occurs when peritonitis is generalized from a number of causes.

ABNORMAL UTERINE BLEEDING[64, 69, 85]

Abnormal uterine bleeding is usually divided into three types—menorrhagia (excessive bleeding during normal menstruation), metrorrhagia (bleeding between menstrual periods), and postmenopausal bleeding. The organic lesions and complications of pregnancy are common causes of abnormal uterine bleeding.

Abortion[36] is one of the most common

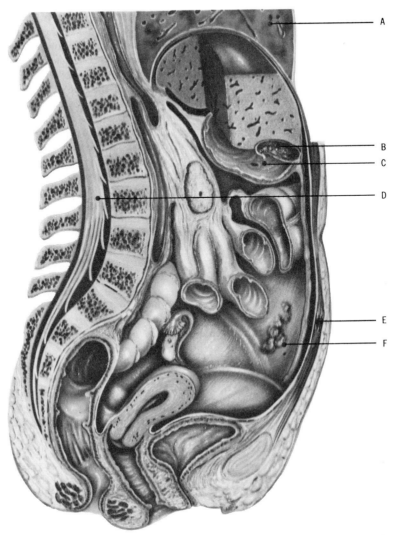

A ———————————

B ———————————
C ———————————
D ———————————

E ———————————
F ———————————

A. INTRATHORACIC CONDITIONS Diaphragmatic pleurisy, which is usually secondary to lower lobe pneumonia, may cause upper abdominal rigidity. Epidemic pleurodynia is a less common cause, while acute pericarditis is a rare cause of abdominal rigidity.

B. INTRA-ABDOMINAL INFECTION Infection of intra-abdominal organs, such as acute cholecystitis or appendicitis, may spread to adjacent peritoneum and cause localized rigidity. Infection which extends from an infected uterus, a pyosalpinx, or a pyonephrosis causes rigidity. Acute pancreatitis is an infrequent cause of localized rigidity. A strangulated loop of intestine or a segment of intestine affected by mesenteric thrombosis or embolism may become devitalized; organisms escape into the peritoneal cavity and cause peritonitis and rigidity. Rupture of an abscess of the liver or spleen causes rigidity.

C. PERFORATED VISCUS Perforation at the site of a gastric or duodenal ulcer, a tuberculous or typhoid ulcer of the intestine, or a carcinoma, stercoral ulcer, or a diverticulum

of the bowel causes generalized rigidity. A gangrenous gall-bladder, appendix, or intestine may rupture and cause generalized rigidity.

D. CENTRAL NERVOUS SYSTEM Anxiety, hypersensitivity, and hysteria condition the reflex arc within the spinal cord and cause rigidity. The gastric crises of tabes dorsalis also cause rigidity.

E. ABDOMINAL WALL Injury to the abdominal wall from direct trauma or, more rarely, from rupture of the rectus abdominis muscle following severe muscle strain causes abdominal rigidity localized to the affected segment. Abdominal wall infection is a rare cause of rigidity.

F. INTRA-ABDOMINAL BLEEDING Bleeding into the peritoneal cavity from a carcinoma of the peritoneum, tuberculous peritonitis, thrombosis of the portal vein, rupture of the liver or spleen, or rupture of vascular adhesions of a cirrhotic liver cause rigidity. Rupture of an ectopic pregnancy may cause rigidity which is not marked and may be absent if shock is severe.

Fig. 18-2. Abdominal rigidity. (From Therap. Notes **70:**143, Sept.-Oct., 1963, Parke, Davis & Co.)

causes of abnormal uterine bleeding. A spontaneous abortion is synonymous with miscarriage and is the premature delivery of a medically nonviable fetus of less than 27 to 28 weeks of age. The legal age of viability is much less, averaging about 20 weeks. About one half of miscarriages occur from the tenth to thirteenth week, irrespective of apparent etiology. Among the most frequent causes of spontaneous abortions are early death and absorption of the embryo; severe abnormality of the embryo and its later death; or, less commonly, abnormal implantation of the embryo. Maternal factors involved in abortion are criminal or elective legal abortions, uterine abnormalities, and inflammatory diseases. Trauma has also been implicated. A number of abortuses have been found to have chromosomal anomalies.[36]

An ectopic pregnancy,[76] another cause of abnormal uterine bleeding, is one in which the embryo has implanted anywhere outside the endometrial cavity. The fallopian tube is the most common site of ectopic pregnancy, which has been attributed to physiologic or mechanical slowing down of the rate of progress of the ovum through the tube or delay in entering the tube. Rupture of the tube occurs because of the extension of the trophoblast and chorionic villi into the tubal muscle rather than into a mass of decidua as in the uterus.

Endocrine disturbances may cause menorrhagia or metrorrhagia. In this type of abnormal bleeding the endometrium is often hyperplastic, usually because of failure of ovulation that results from an imbalance in estrogen-progesterone ratio. Disordered hormonal regulation is one of the most common causes of metrorrhagia. Metrorrhagia may occur throughout the menstrual cycle from puberty to menopause, but it is most common is adolescence and near the menopause. Adolescent metrorrhagia is often self-limited, and normal menstrual cycles are eventually established. Hormonal disturbances may be manifested by functional follicular lutein ovarian cysts or by granulosa or theca cell ovarian tumors. Salpingo-oophoritis (inflammation of the tube and ovary) or pituitary and thyroid disturbances may be associated with hormonal imbalance.

Psychogenic factors may be responsible for functional bleeding, possibly caused by the influence of emotional stimulation of the hypothalamus.

Postmenopausal bleeding is defined as a sanguineous discharge from the genital tract occurring at least 6 months after cessation of menses in women over the age of 45. The incidence of malignant lesions in patients with postmenopausal bleeding is high. In all cases of menorrhagia, metrorrhagia, or postmenopausal bleeding, diagnostic measures for the presence of carcinoma are Papanicolaou smears and dilatation and curettage with a biopsy.

Some of the specific causes, other than those illustrated in Fig. 18-3, are selected for discussion as follows.

Endometriosis[36]

Endometriosis is a disorder principally occurring in the third to fourth decades. In this condition endometrial glands or stroma, or both, are found in abnormal locations. In a type called adenomyosis there is abnormal growth activity of the endometrium into the myometrium, and glands and stroma penetrate between the muscle fibers of the myometrium. Patients frequently have menorrhagia, dysmenorrhea (painful menstruation), dyspareunia (difficult or painful sexual intercourse in women), and drawing pelvic pain, particularly during the premenstrual period.

In external or indirect endometriosis, abnormal nests of endometrium develop in the tubes, ovaries, or peritoneum or any other site in the body outside the uterus, such as the vagina, vulva, appendix, umbilicus, uterine ligaments, rectovaginal septum, and laparotomy scars. Unlike adenomyosis, the foci in this type of endometriosis are prone to undergo cyclic menstrual changes with periodic bleeding. When they

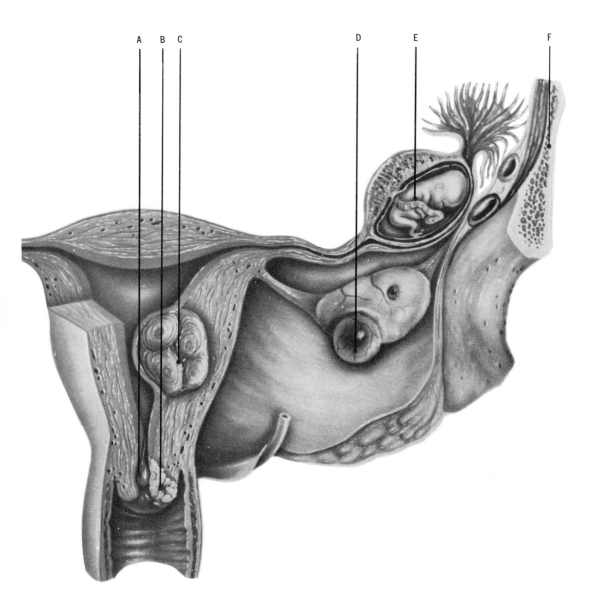

A. POLYPS Endometrial or cervical polyps may cause abnormal bleeding. Multiple endometrial polyps may be related to endometrial hyperplasia. Cervical polyps associated with intermenstrual bleeding or postmenopausal bleeding should prompt thorough investigation to rule out carcinoma.

B. CARCINOMA Cancer of the cervix may cause intermenstrual spotting, often after coitus. In endometrial cancer a watery leukorrhea may progress to a bloody discharge, intermittent spotting, and eventually to gross hemorrhage.

C. FIBROIDS Submucous leiomyomas, or fibroids, are a common cause of uterine bleeding; menstrual bleeding tends to increase with growth of the tumors while the interval between periods remains the same.

D. OVARIAN LESIONS Dysfunctional bleeding may be caused by cysts of the ovary as well as by theca or granulosa cell tumors. These lesions produce excess estrogenic stimulation leading to endometrial hyperplasia and abnormal bleeding.

E. COMPLICATIONS OF PREGNANCY Irregular bleeding after a period of amenorrhea may be caused by ectopic pregnancy or abortion. Hydatidiform mole and chorioepithelioma are other complications of pregnancy associated with uterine bleeding.

F. BLOOD DYSCRASIAS Thrombocytopenic purpura and leukemia may cause uterine bleeding through interference with clotting mechanisms.

Fig. 18-3. Abdominal uterine bleeding. (From Therap. Notes **72:**59, Mar.-Apr., 1965, Parke, Davis & Co.)

are symptomatic, there may be severe dysmenorrhea and pelvic pain caused by intrapelvic bleeding. As the disease advances and affects neighboring structures, pain may result from tension on suspensory ligaments of the uterus. Sterility is a late complication when the tubes and ovaries are involved.

Abnormalities of the placenta[36, 61]

The placenta is the organ by means of which the nutritive, respiratory, and excretory functions of the fetus are carried on from the earliest days of pregnancy until delivery. Consequently, if the placenta is not healthy or intact, this will have an adverse effect on the fetus, perhaps causing death or inflicting permanent damage. The two abnormalities that occur most frequently and are responsible for the majority of maternal hemorrhages and a significant number of fetal anoxias are placenta previa and abruptio placentae. Both of these represent abnormalities of implantation and separation.

Placenta previa.[36, 61, 63] In placenta previa the placenta is implanted and developed in the lower uterine segment instead of normally higher on the uterine wall. This implantation may either cover or adjoin the internal cervical os and is thus in the zone of effacement and dilatation. Effacement of the internal cervical os occurs as pregnancy progresses.

Placenta previa is a relatively infrequent complication of pregnancy. When the placenta is implanted in the lower uterine segment, the uterine cavity during the last half of pregnancy remains spheroid instead of developing into an ovoid structure. The spheroid shape prevents engagement of the fetal head and contributes to the increased incidence of breech and transverse presentations. If the placenta is implanted on the posterior wall of the uterus below the true pelvic brim, the size of the inlet is reduced by the thickness of the placenta. As the lower segment of the uterus enlarges and thins, the lower portion of the placenta is

disrupted, and acute hemorrhage results. Fetal malpositions requiring manual and instrumentation manipulation are also likely to rupture the lower uterine segment during delivery.

Painless genital bleeding is the most significant symptom, but other symptoms may give an indication of placenta previa before hemorrhage occurs. These include fetal malposition, particularly in a nulliparous woman. The location of the placenta can be established by a single lateral soft-tissue roentgenogram or by use of radioisotopes. When the cervical os begins to dilate in the latter weeks of pregnancy and during labor, some placental separation occurs. Maternal blood vessels are torn, causing hemorrhage when the dilated cervix pulls away from the placental implantation. This can cause premature rupture of the membranes, premature labor, and abnormal presentation.

Abruptio placentae.[36, 61] In abruptio placentae the normally implanted placenta is prematurely separated from its uterine attachment. It occurs about once in every 85 to 250 deliveries, and it occurs after the twentieth week of pregnancy. Such separation before this week of pregnancy is considered an abortion. The two dangers of this type of placental detachment are external hemorrhage and concealed hemorrhage.

Initially there is an extravasation of blood into the decidua basalis and the formation of a hematoma that separates and compresses the adjacent placental portions. The bleeding may dissect between the membranes and the uterine wall and be manifested by external hemorrhage. It may also remain hidden in the uterus. If the fetal head is in the lower segment of the uterus, the exit of blood may be blocked externally and may remain as a concealed hemorrhage. The concealed hemorrhage can also result when the placenta is partially separated but the margins remain attached, or if the placenta is completely detached but the membranes remain attached to the

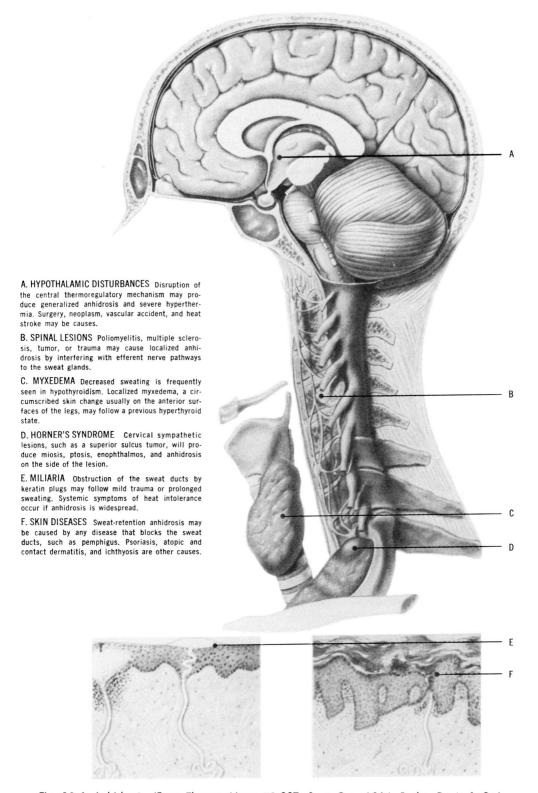

A. HYPOTHALAMIC DISTURBANCES Disruption of the central thermoregulatory mechanism may produce generalized anhidrosis and severe hyperthermia. Surgery, neoplasm, vascular accident, and heat stroke may be causes.

B. SPINAL LESIONS Poliomyelitis, multiple sclerosis, tumor, or trauma may cause localized anhidrosis by interfering with efferent nerve pathways to the sweat glands.

C. MYXEDEMA Decreased sweating is frequently seen in hypothyroidism. Localized myxedema, a circumscribed skin change usually on the anterior surfaces of the legs, may follow a previous hyperthyroid state.

D. HORNER'S SYNDROME Cervical sympathetic lesions, such as a superior sulcus tumor, will produce miosis, ptosis, enophthalmos, and anhidrosis on the side of the lesion.

E. MILIARIA Obstruction of the sweat ducts by keratin plugs may follow mild trauma or prolonged sweating. Systemic symptoms of heat intolerance occur if anhidrosis is widespread.

F. SKIN DISEASES Sweat-retention anhidrosis may be caused by any disease that blocks the sweat ducts, such as pemphigus. Psoriasis, atopic and contact dermatitis, and ichthyosis are other causes.

Fig. 18-4. Anhidrosis. (From Therap. Notes **71:**227, Sept.-Oct., 1964, Parke, Davis & Co.)

uterine wall, or if the blood can break through the membranes and enter the amniotic cavity. External hemorrhage usually follows partial separation. This type of hemorrhage is more common but less severe than the hidden type.

The primary cause of abruptio placentae is unknown, but predisposing factors include eclampsia, preeclampsia, and chronic hypertensive disease. Eclampsia is a serious toxemia of pregnancy and is associated with the symptoms of hypertension, edema, or proteinuria.

Complications of abruptio placentae include shock, since there is excessive blood loss, and occasionally acute renal failure when the condition is severe and accompanied by concealed hemorrhage.

ANHIDROSIS[87]

Anhidrosis is deficiency in sweat, either from inability to sweat or from an inability to deliver sweat to the surface of the skin. It may be limited to certain areas or it may be generalized (Fig. 18-4). If it is generalized over a large area of the body, fatal hyperthermia may occur or there may be a severe intolerance to heat. Neural causes include exhaustion or a damaged hypothalamus (central thermoregulatory control center), leading to breakdown of the sweating mechanism. Heatstroke is an example. It has been described in Chapter 11.

Degeneration of the peripheral sympathetic fibers may occur in diabetes mellitus and gout, resulting in lack of sweating in the lower extremities, with orthostatic hypotension and heat intolerance. Sweating may also be absent in peripheral nerve lesions, such as those in leprosy and in various forms of polyneuritis (multiple peripheral neuritis). Ganglionic blocking agents, local anesthetics, anticholinergic drugs, and sympathectomy are other causes of absence of sweating.

Hormonal disorders that can cause anhidrosis include myxedema, diabetes mellitus, diabetes insipidus, and pituitary and adrenal insufficiency. These disorders have been discussed elsewhere in the text. Absence of sweating is also present in poisoning with thallium, lead, arsenic, or morphine. Sweating may be absent in the diseases of glomerulonephritis, cirrhosis, and in certain malignancies. These have also been discussed elsewhere.

Cutaneous causes include congenital absence of sweat glands and congenital alopecia (deficiency of scalp hair). The sweat glands may atrophy in radiodermatitis (dermatitis caused by exposure to x rays or other radiation), scleroderma (Chapter 13), and in vitamin A deficiency.

The following causes of anhidrosis have been selected for discussion.

Horner's syndrome

Horner's syndrome[52] is caused by paralysis of the cervical sympathetic fibers. In this syndrome there is sinking inward of the eyeball, ptosis (falling) of the upper eyelid, slight elevation of the lower lid, constriction of the pupil, narrowing of the palpebral fissure, and absence of sweating on the ipsilateral side of the face and neck.

Hereditary ectodermal defect[87]

There is an inherited ectodermal defect that causes anhidrosis. It is an uncommon condition in which dysgenesis of the epidermis and its appendages is the main feature. It occurs more often in males and is inherited as a recessive autosomal dominant. The facies of the afflicted persons is characterized by wide, high, scanty eyebrows, prominent frontal bones, saddle nose, thick swollen lips, underdeveloped maxillas and mandibles, and a pointed chin. The skin is likely to be thin, dry, white, and soft. The restricted sweating is caused by an absence of or a decrease in the number of sweat glands, which are often rudimentary. There is also a decrease in the number of sebaceous glands. The nails may be ridged or decreased in thickness. Body hair is scant or absent. There may be absence or decrease in the number of per-

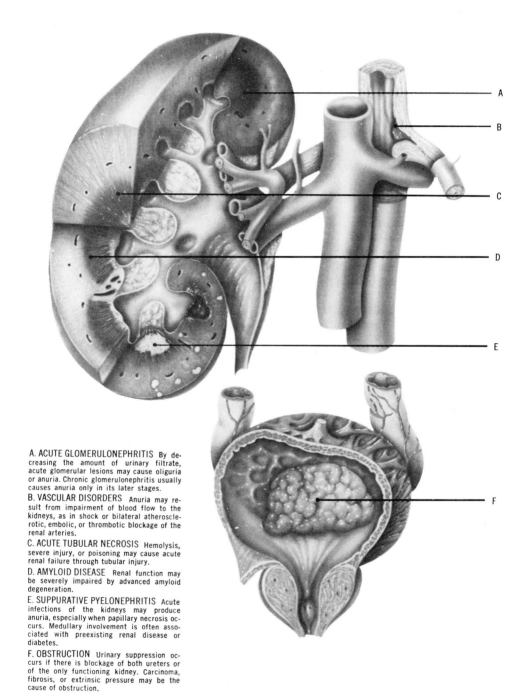

A. ACUTE GLOMERULONEPHRITIS By decreasing the amount of urinary filtrate, acute glomerular lesions may cause oliguria or anuria. Chronic glomerulonephritis usually causes anuria only in its later stages.

B. VASCULAR DISORDERS Anuria may result from impairment of blood flow to the kidneys, as in shock or bilateral atherosclerotic, embolic, or thrombotic blockage of the renal arteries.

C. ACUTE TUBULAR NECROSIS Hemolysis, severe injury, or poisoning may cause acute renal failure through tubular injury.

D. AMYLOID DISEASE Renal function may be severely impaired by advanced amyloid degeneration.

E. SUPPURATIVE PYELONEPHRITIS Acute infections of the kidneys may produce anuria, especially when papillary necrosis occurs. Medullary involvement is often associated with preexisting renal disease or diabetes.

F. OBSTRUCTION Urinary suppression occurs if there is blockage of both ureters or of the only functioning kidney. Carcinoma, fibrosis, or extrinsic pressure may be the cause of obstruction.

Fig. 18-5. Anuria. (From Therap. Notes **71:**127, Mar.-Apr., 1964, Parke, Davis & Co.)

manent and deciduous teeth. The lenses may have cataracts or be absent. This defect may be associated with other congenital anomalies, such as central nervous system defects, cleft palate, and supernumerary fingers or toes.

ANURIA[88]

Anuria is cessation of urinary secretion. Clinically this would be secretion of less than 100 ml. of urine daily. In oliguria (scanty urine), 100 to 400 ml. is formed daily. Hyperkalemia (abnormally high content of potassium in the blood), azotemia (presence of urea or other nitrogenous substances in the blood), and overhydration result from this excretory deficit. Anuria may be caused by prerenal, renal, or postrenal lesions (Fig. 18-5).

The prerenal and postrenal lesions include narrowing of the renal arteries from atherosclerosis, occlusion by embolus or thrombus, and bilateral renal vein thrombosis. A diminished urinary secretion occurs in dehydration from excessive sweating, severe diarrhea or febrile illnesses, decreased cardiac output or shock, or inadequate water intake.

Urinary calculi in the ureters also cause anuria, but the blocking of both ureters is rare, and this type of obstruction leading to anuria is more likely to occur when one kidney is absent or poorly functioning from disease. Other types of obstruction are carcinoma of the bladder, pressure on the ureters by uterine fibroids, cysts of the ovaries, visceral tumors, aberrant vessels, or retroperitoneal hematomas. Precipitation of sulfonamide, oxalic acid, cystine, or calcium crystals may also cause obstruction.

The renal lesions that may produce anuria are acute tubular necrosis, suppurative pyelonephritis, and acute glomerulonephritis. Preeclampsia, purpuric affections, and hypersensitivity reactions can cause partial or complete anuria.

Selected lesions that may produce anuria are discussed in the following section.

Acute renal failure[4, 16, 86]

Acute renal failure, a frequently reversible renal syndrome, is known by a number of names, such as lower nephron nephrosis, renal anoxia, acute tubular necrosis, and hemoglobinuric nephrosis. It is characterized by a severe oliguric or anuric phase followed by a diuretic phase. It starts with progressive reduction in urine formation, which may be reduced to 50 to 200 ml. per day. Complete shutdown or anuria is the exception rather than the rule and is suggestive of postrenal obstruction, acute glomerulonephritis, or renal vascular accident. The oliguric phase lasts about 10 to 12 days and is followed by diuresis, which is potentially dangerous because of the loss of fluid and electrolytes. Uremic symptoms are nausea, vomiting, spontaneous bleeding from the bowel, tachycardia, anemia, and rising blood pressure as the azotemia progresses. There is also central nervous system irritability with muscular twitching and convulsions, hyperkalemia, and pulmonary edema in a large percentage of the patients. Cardiac dysfunction is the most serious complication and is usually the principal cause of death.

A number of prerenal conditions can lead to kidney failure. Decreased cardiac output, hemorrhage, and severe dehydration, especially if the latter is associated with extensive burns, are contributing factors. Severe trauma can cause hemorrhage, shock, and tissue destruction, leading to renal shutdown. The crush syndrome is an example of traumatic injury. Nephrotoxins, such as metals of mercury, uranium, and bismuth, or the chemicals of carbon tetrachloride, diethylene glycol, and DDT, are common causes of acute renal failure.

A number of diseases of the kidney cause acute renal failure. These include acute pyelonephritis with papillary necrosis associated with pregnancy toxemias. Vascular diseases of the kidney that are implicated are renal artery occlusion and renal venous thrombosis. Intravascular hemolysis is another cause. This can occur as a result of mismatched transfusions, infusions of distilled water, and certain infections, such as blackwater fever (a form of malaria), epidemic hemorrhagic fever, and septicemia caused by *Clostridium welchii*. It may be encountered in sickle cell crisis and during transurethral resection and septic abortions. Occasionally acute renal failure occurs following intravenous pyelography, particularly in patients with myeloma, but it can also occur in cholecystography, and it can follow obstetric complications.

Postrenal failure is largely the result of obstructive uropathy, such as ureteral obstruction with calculi, stricture, blood clot, edema following instrumentation, accidental surgical ligation, and tumor.

Dialysis[46, 53] has been instrumental in saving lives by reversing acute renal failure and in prolonging lives of those with chronic kidney disease. The artificial kidney was first developed to give temporary relief to patients with reversible acute renal failure. It is used to supplement the normal kidney in treatment of acute poisoning, such as from barbiturates, bromides, salicylates, and methanol intoxications. In cases of advancing azotemia, uremic syndrome, and hyperkalemia, the use of the artificial kidney may allow time for the renal function to recover.

Dialysis is used to remove nephrotoxins

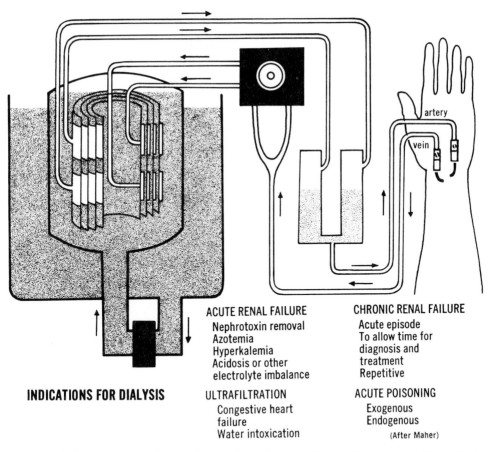

INDICATIONS FOR DIALYSIS

artery
vein

ACUTE RENAL FAILURE
Nephrotoxin removal
Azotemia
Hyperkalemia
Acidosis or other
electrolyte imbalance

ULTRAFILTRATION
Congestive heart
failure
Water intoxication

CHRONIC RENAL FAILURE
Acute episode
To allow time for
diagnosis and
treatment
Repetitive

ACUTE POISONING
Exogenous
Endogenous
(After Maher)

Fig. 18-6. Diagram of artificial kidney. (From Therap. Notes **71**:222, Sept.-Oct., 1964, Parke, Davis & Co.)

before overt uremia ensues. The electrolyte abnormalities, such as acidosis, hypermagnesemia, and hyponatremia, may also be corrected by use of the artificial kidney.

Advances in the methods of dialysis have made it possible to keep patients alive with an artificial kidney for years after kidney function has ceased. For most patients, dialysis will continue to be used until a suitable cadaver kidney can be found for transplantation. In a small group, transplantation is contraindicated for medical or immunologic reasons, and dialysis offers the only hope as a form of treatment at this time.

There are two methods of dialysis: one is peritoneal, in which the dialyzing fluid is introduced into the peritoneal cavity, with the peritoneum acting as a semipermeable membrane across which dialysis occurs. The other method is hemodialysis, in which an artery and vein, for example in the wrist or arm, are connected by cannulas to the dialyzer (Fig. 18-6). The principle is that blood is routed through the dialyzing fluid where nephrotoxins are removed and the purified blood is then routed back to the body.

Glomerulonephritis[4, 73, 115]

Glomerulonephritis is an inflammatory or degenerative condition affecting primarily the glomeruli of the kidney. It may be caused by hypersensitivity, embolization, or bacteria. It occurs in chronic, subacute, and acute forms. It is one of the most common types of kidney disease and is often referred to as Bright's disease. Glomerulonephritis may occur at any time of life, but the majority of patients are in the first and second decades. It appears to occur twice as often in males as in females.

The inflammatory changes in the glomeruli narrow or obliterate the capillaries of the glomerular tufts. This obstructs the flow of blood through the capillaries and thus interferes with the formation of glomerular filtrate and injures the filter itself. The blood supply of the tubules is likewise affected. As the condition progresses, the effect is a gradual hyalinization of glomerular tufts, with many of them disappearing. The corresponding tubules atrophy. Atrophy and disappearance of nephrons result in shrinkage of renal substance. In prolonged chronic cases sclerotic changes are found in the small arteries and arterioles. In the late stages with marked hypertension the arteriosclerotic changes may be severe and may accelerate the fatal ending.

Acute glomerulonephritis seems to be more clearly related to infection than are the other stages. Streptococcus predominates among the causative bacterial agents. The infectious diseases that may precede the attack are upper respiratory infection, tonsillitis, scarlet fever, rheumatic fever, or bacterial endocarditis. The acute stages of glomerulonephritis occur mainly in children and young adults. The initial symptoms are fever, malaise, weakness, loss of appetite, and chills. Edema may be slight to marked, and although its mechanism is not easily explained, it may be caused by low plasma proteins as a result of albuminuria or because of associated cardiac decompensation. The blood pressure may be elevated. Hematuria is a classic sign, usually associated with pyuria (pus in the urine), albuminuria, and casts. The urine output may progressively fall to anuric level. The acute forms may cause death, or they may progress to subacute or chronic forms.

Subacute glomerulonephritis may be an extension of a typical acute diffuse glomerulonephritis that is prolonged, or it may be a less severe type of inflammation from its onset. The evidence of renal functional deficiency is progressive, and death is usually from uremia.

Chronic glomerulonephritis may be present over many years. There may be periods of clinical latency, or it may be punctuated by mild acute flare-ups. The chronic form, however, does not subside completely, but usually relentlessly progresses to renal functional failure terminating in uremia.

Pyelonephritis[4, 73, 115]

Many different types of bacteria cause kidney infection. They may also follow a bladder infection or may be carried to the kidneys by the bloodstream. *Escherichia coli* are the most frequent cause, but others include staphylococcus and streptococcus. Tuberculosis may also attack the kidneys as a bloodborne infection. In pyelonephritis both the parenchyma of the kidney and the renal pelvis are involved by interstitial inflammation. It is the most common single type of renal disease. In many cases there is an associated obstruction somewhere in the urinary tract, since obstructions predispose to infection by organisms carried in the bloodstream. This type is called descending pyelonephritis. When the infection is spread from the lower urinary tract, the bacteria ascend to involve the kidney, and this is called ascending pyelonephritis.

In the acute type there is a sudden pain in the back that radiates to the region of the gallbladder, to the abdomen over the appendix, to the loin, and along the course of the ureters. Chills, fever, nausea, and vomiting may be present. Burning urination is frequent, and there is dysuria (painful urination). Anuria may develop, especially when papillary necrosis occurs.

ARTERIAL INSUFFICIENCY[40, 89]

In arterial insufficiency, peripheral arterial circulation is impaired, producing ischemia of the affected tissues. Manifestations of arterial insufficiency vary with the intensity of the ischemia and the tissues affected. Pain is a manifestation of cutaneous ischemia. The skin changes in color, reflecting the color and amount of blood circulating to the affected parts, as in frostbite (Chapter 11). Skin temperature is also affected. Ulceration and gangrene are manifestations of severe ischemia of the skin and underlying tissues, such as occurs in diabetic gangrene.

Acute arterial insufficiency may be spastic or thromboembolic. Raynaud's phenomenon is an example of spastic arterial insufficiency. Paroxysmal digital cyanosis is a symptom of this phenomenon. The shoulder-girdle compression syndrome, cervical rib syndrome (supernumerary first rib), ergotism (chronic poisoning from prolonged use of ergot drugs or ingestion of ergotized rye or wheat), scleroderma and disseminated lupus erythematosus (Chapter 13), and occlusive arterial disease are associated with Raynaud's phenomenon. Sudden occlusion of an artery by an embolus causes severe, rapidly progressive arterial insufficiency. Sudden arterial thrombosis may occur in patients with debilitating diseases such as ulcerative colitis, septicemia, pneumonia, and peritonitis, as well as with a number of infections.

Leriche syndrome[40] is a gradual thrombosis of the terminal portion of the abdominal aorta. It differs from sudden occlusion of the aorta and is more common. Discomfort develops in the thighs, hip region, or buttocks and represents intermittent claudication at a high level. Arterial pulses are absent or decreased in the lower extremities. Bruits may be heard over the abdominal aorta and over the iliac and femoral arteries. Atrophy of leg muscles occurs in time.

Chronic arterial insufficiency is far more frequent in the lower extremities than acute arterial insufficiency. The most common cause is occlusive atherosclerosis. In nondiabetic patients it tends to be segmental and more proximal in distribution.

Pulseless disease or Takayasu's disease[40] is rare, and the diagnosis is usually made during the third decade of life. Most of the patients are females. It was once thought to be confined to Japan, but this is no longer true. The clinical symptoms are vertigo, syncope (temporary loss of consciousness), convulsions, aphasia, headache, transient cerebral ischemia resulting in hemiplegia or hemiparesis, nonpalpable carotid arteries on one or both sides, transient episodes of blindness, amblyopia (dimness of vision), rapidly developing cataracts, retinal atrophy, photophobia, optic atrophy, and

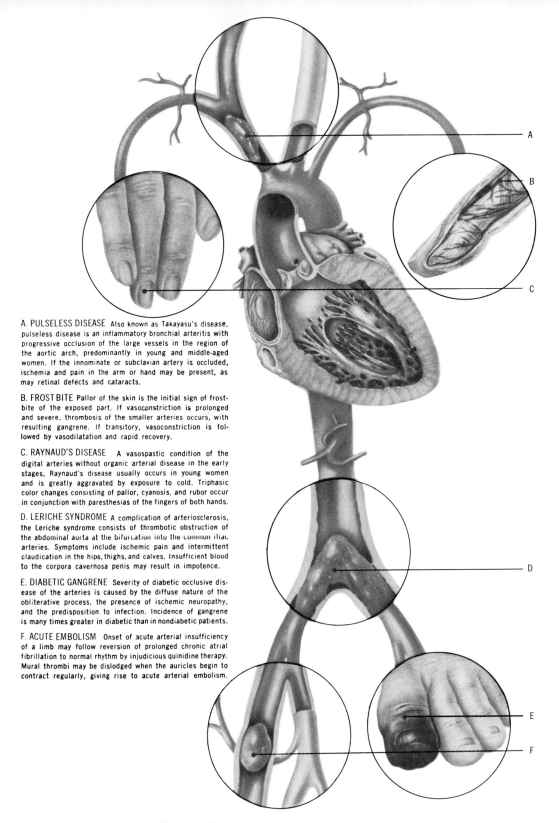

A. PULSELESS DISEASE Also known as Takayasu's disease, pulseless disease is an inflammatory bronchial arteritis with progressive occlusion of the large vessels in the region of the aortic arch, predominantly in young and middle-aged women. If the innominate or subclavian artery is occluded, ischemia and pain in the arm or hand may be present, as may retinal defects and cataracts.

B. FROSTBITE Pallor of the skin is the initial sign of frost-bite of the exposed part. If vasoconstriction is prolonged and severe, thrombosis of the smaller arteries occurs, with resulting gangrene. If transitory, vasoconstriction is fol-lowed by vasodilatation and rapid recovery.

C. RAYNAUD'S DISEASE A vasospastic condition of the digital arteries without organic arterial disease in the early stages, Raynaud's disease usually occurs in young women and is greatly aggravated by exposure to cold. Triphasic color changes consisting of pallor, cyanosis, and rubor occur in conjunction with paresthesias of the fingers of both hands.

D. LERICHE SYNDROME A complication of arteriosclerosis, the Leriche syndrome consists of thrombotic obstruction of the abdominal aorta at the bifurcation into the common iliac arteries. Symptoms include ischemic pain and intermittent claudication in the hips, thighs, and calves. Insufficient blood to the corpora cavernosa penis may result in impotence.

E. DIABETIC GANGRENE Severity of diabetic occlusive dis-ease of the arteries is caused by the diffuse nature of the obliterative process, the presence of ischemic neuropathy, and the predisposition to infection. Incidence of gangrene is many times greater in diabetic than in nondiabetic patients.

F. ACUTE EMBOLISM Onset of acute arterial insufficiency of a limb may follow reversion of prolonged chronic atrial fibrillation to normal rhythm by injudicious quinidine therapy. Mural thrombi may be dislodged when the auricles begin to contract regularly, giving rise to acute arterial embolism.

Fig. 18-7. Arterial insufficiency. (From Therap. Notes **69**:6, July-Aug., 1962, Parke, Davis & Co.)

atrophy of the iris. The facial skin is thin and pigmented. The nose and palate may be ulcerated. Blood pressure is decreased or absent in the upper extremities and increased in the lower extremities. The patients usually die of cerebral ischemia or heart disease.

Causes of arterial insufficiency, other than those illustrated in Fig. 18-7 or described above, are disseminated arteritis, hypertensive ischemic ulceration, erythema induratum, and thromboangiitis obliterans or Buerger's disease.

ATAXIA[18, 90]

Incoordination of muscular movement, ataxia, is of two types—sensory and cerebellar. In sensory ataxia, sensory impulses involved in conscious proprioception are lost because the sensory cortex is deprived of proprioceptive information necessary for regulation of voluntary motor acts. The gait is staggering and broadbased. Eyes are fixed on the ground to compensate for dysfunction. Movements are awkward and clumsy. When the eyes are closed, postural stability is lost. Dysarthria (imperfect articulation in speech) may be present, as well as loss of tendon reflexes, sense of joint position, and vibratory sense. Polyneuritis in such deficiency states as pellagra, beriberi, chronic malnutrition, and alcoholism may cause sensory ataxia. Many chemical substances, such as mercury, lead, arsenic, thallium, organic solvents and insecticides, have been implicated, as well as diphtheria toxins and various drugs. Sensory ataxia may also occur in leprosy, porphyria, the collagen diseases, and subacute combined degeneration of the spinal cord. Acute intermittent porphyria is familial or inherited as a mendelian dominant. It is characterized by neuromuscular disturbances, muscle spasms, foot- and wrist-drop, flaccid quadriplegia or paraplegia, psychotic behavior, and intense abdominal colic. Another familial type is caused by an inborn error of porphyrin metabolism. There is photosensitization, with skin blisters from exposure to light, and later the fingers and portions of the nose and ears may be lost. Another type called porphyria cutanea tarda may also be familial and follows exposure to sunlight, trauma, or use of hepatotoxic drugs. Symptoms are photosensitivity, a brown pigmentation of the skin, which may become violaceous or purplish, and changes in the color of the hair.

In lesions of the cerebellar system the ataxia is more marked on the side of the lesion. Closing the eyes does not worsen the condition. Common signs and symptoms are staggering gait, reeling toward the side of the lesion, intention tremor, nystagmus (involuntary rapid movement of the eyeballs), vertigo, dysmetria (disturbance of power to control range of muscular acts), hypotonia, and impaired speech. Cerebellar symptoms of ataxia may occur with encephalitis and other infections of the brain. Acute intoxications with alcohol, barbiturates, bromides, and carbon monoxide often produce ataxia.

Hysterical ataxia may be primarily psychogenic or it may be a reaction to true organic disease. In hysterical ataxia there are inconsistencies in the neurologic picture and obvious psychologic disturbances that suggest the diagnosis to the examining physician.

The causes of ataxia are illustrated in Fig. 18-8.

Multiple sclerosis[18, 73, 124, 125]

Multiple sclerosis (M.S.) is also known as disseminated sclerosis, particularly in England and Canada. It is a major disorder of the central nervous system, principally affecting the white matter. It is one of the most frequent nonvascular disorders of neurologic disabilities. It generally begins in adult life between the ages of 20 and 40, although it may affect children and even some adults in the later years. It is more common in the temperate zones than in hot climates, but the reason for this is unknown. The exact number of persons with M.S. is not known; the National

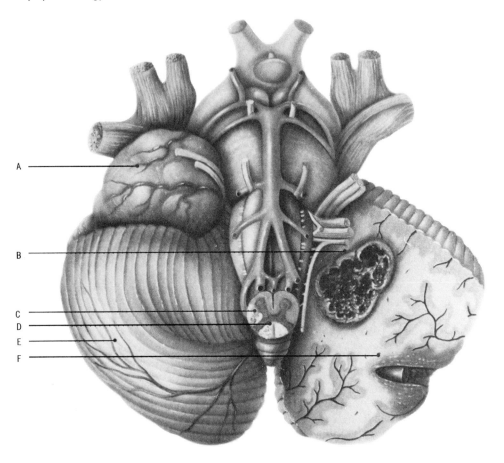

A

B

C
D
E
F

A. ACOUSTIC NEUROMA Cerebellar ataxia is produced by this tumor, which arises from the neurilemma of the eighth nerve and expands to fill the cerebellopontine angle. Deafness, headache, tinnitus, diplopia, and vertigo are frequent symptoms.

B. ABSCESS Usually secondary to middle-ear or mastoid infections, abscesses of the cerebellum may cause ataxia. Staphylococci, pneumococci, and streptococci are the most common organisms involved.

C. DISSEMINATED SCLEROSIS Patchy areas of demyelinization are found in multiple sclerosis, producing protean and varying symptoms. Lesions of the dorsal columns and spinocerebellar tracts may produce both sensory and cerebellar ataxia.

D. TABES DORSALIS A late manifestation of syphilis, tabes dorsalis is characterized by degeneration of the dorsal columns of the cord secondary to infiltration of the posterior roots.

E. THROMBOSIS Infarction of the cerebellum may be caused by thrombosis of the cerebellar arteries. Horner's syndrome, facial analgesia, ataxia, and palatal weakness are present on the side of the lesion, whereas analgesia and paresis may be found on the opposite side of the body when the posterior inferior cerebellar artery is affected.

F. TRAUMA Direct injury to the cerebellum from gunshot or knife wounds as well as closed head injuries, which lead to contusion or hematoma of the cerebellum, may cause ataxia.

Fig. 18-8. Ataxia. (From Therap. Notes **71**:95, Mar.-Apr., 1964, Parke, Davis & Co.)

Multiple Sclerosis Society estimates that about 500,000 Americans have the disease or closely related neurologic ailments.[125]

Multiple sclerosis is a disease of patchy areas of demyelinization or breaking up of the myelin sheath, a protective fatty covering of the nerves. (A recent finding is that myelin is laid down around the nerves by glial cells or neuroglial cells.) The disease derives its name from the multiple areas of sclerosis or hardened scars or plaques that appear along the course of nerves of the central nervous system. The lesions have a predilection for the optical nerves, areas around the anterior and posterior parts of the lateral ventricles, the brainstem, the cerebellar peduncles, and the dorsal half of the spinal cord. They may spread to involve the gray matter of the brain. In spite of remissions that are hallmarks of the disease, it is progressive.

The onset may be insidious, and sometimes there is a 6-year lag between the first symptoms, which may be vague, and the establishment of a definite diagnosis. Some early signs are slurring speech and tingling and numbing sensations, which are followed later by shaking or tremor, extreme weakness, and progressive paralysis. Some patients may experience nystagmus and diplopia. Cerebellar incoordination is reflected in difficulty in walking. The end stage is often characterized by dementia caused by cerebral white matter lesions and blindness from bilateral retrobulbar neuritis; lesions of the dorsal columns and spinocerebellar tracts may produce both sensory and cerebellar ataxia. Not all these symptoms will occur in a patient, and some of them are also symptoms of other central nervous system diseases that must be distinguished in the final diagnosis. Multiple sclerosis is difficult to diagnose in the early stages, and a physician bases the diagnosis on the patient's history and clinical symptoms and signs. The first attack may arouse suspicion of multiple sclerosis, but quite frequently an additional attack or attacks must follow for the diagnosis to be conclusive.[124]

The etiology is unknown, but many theories have been investigated and many others are still under investigation. These include familial tendency, trauma, vascular ischemia and anoxia, bacteria, viruses, disorders of carbohydrate and fat metabolism, intoxication by zinc and other substances, nutritional defects, and allergies.

CHILLS[91]

A chill is an involuntary contraction of voluntary muscles accompanied by a feeling of cold and by pallor of the skin, that is, shivering or shaking; chills are also known as rigors. Chills occur in many febrile illnesses (illnesses characterized by a rise in temperature). Whether chills occur as a single episode or as repeated episodes has diagnostic significance. The single chill occurs typically at the onset of an acute infection and is common in lobar pneumonia, smallpox, influenza, severe colds, septicemia, pyemia, pneumonic tuberculosis, typhus, and relapsing fever. Other diseases in which a single attack of chills may occur initially are cerebrospinal fever, acute poliomyelitis, malaria, yellow fever, Weil's disease, trench fever, and erysipelas. A chill may also occur after catheterization, certain injections, and blood transfusions.

In lobar pneumonia (Fig. 18-9) the initial single attack of chills is often severe and prolonged. There is a sudden shaking chill in the majority of patients, accompanied by a rapid rise in temperature and tachycardia. More than a single rigor or chill is unusual in pneumonia. Second at-

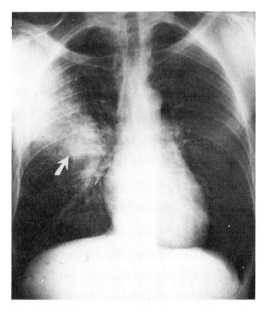

Fig. 18-9. Lobar pneumonia. Arrow points to increased density of lung, typical of lobar pneumonia. (From Young, C. G., and Likos, J. J.: Medical specialty terminology, x-ray and nuclear medicine, St. Louis, 1972, The C. V. Mosby Co.)

tacks of chills in this condition may indicate complications. If a second chill occurs in typhoid fever or in paratyphoid fever, it may be a warning of complications such as perforation of the intestine, acute peritonitis, pleurisy, pneumonia, middle ear infection, periostitis, or cholecystitis.

Multiple or recurring chills occur in several conditions. The best example of which is malaria. (See Figs. 18-15, *F*, and 18-17, *E*.) Malaria is characterized by chills recurring at regular intervals of 48 to 70 hours in the benign tertian and quartan infections, and at shorter intervals if the infection is mixed.

Malaria is a protozoan infection.[55, 126] It is spread from person to person by the bite of the female *Anopheles* mosquito. When this mosquito bites an individual with malaria, the blood she sucks may contain malaria parasites. The parasites develop in her body over a 2-week period, and after this time if she bites a healthy person she will inject the infective parasites into the blood. The incubation period in humans lasts about 10 days to 2 weeks after the mosquito bite. In addition to symptoms of a cycle of fever and periodic chills, sweating, headaches, and nausea also occur. In chronic cases, anemia and splenomegaly develop. Carriers among apparently healthy natives in endemic malarial regions are common.

Relapsing fever[34] starts with a chill or series of chills. The chills recur about 2 weeks after the patient begins convalescing. A second relapse may occur at the end of the third week, and in some there is even a third relapse. Relapsing fever[34] is an acute arthropod-borne infection characterized by toxemia and febrile episodes that subside and recur over a period of weeks. Under natural conditions, relapsing fever is transmitted by body lice and ticks. Louse-borne relapsing fever is typically epidemic under conditions in which overcrowded poor populations live under unhygienic conditions that facilitate wide dissemination of body lice. At one time louse-borne relapsing fever was the scourge of armies. Tick-borne relapsing fever is endemic. In both types the initial attack begins with chills, nausea, vomiting, joint and muscle pain, photophobia, and fever. A macular or petechial rash notably develops in louse-borne relapsing fever. It involves the neck, shoulders, chest, and abdomen. Symptoms include abdominal pains, splenomegaly, hepatomegaly, and sometimes jaundice. Epistaxis, hemoptysis, hematuria, and hematemesis also occur. Uterine hemorrhage and abortion are frequent. In tick-borne fever, ophthalmic and neurologic manifestations are special features, including iritis, iridocyclitis, retinitis, choroiditis, and temporary blindness. Cerebral involvement is manifested by coma, focal hemiplegia, meningitis, aphasia, and cranial nerve palsies. Delirium is a symptom of meningeal irritation. Except during epidemics, diagnosis depends on demonstration of borreliae (causative agent) in the peripheral blood, usually in the early stages. Borreliae can sometimes be found in lesions of the rash.

Multiple chills are common in puerperal fever (a bacterial infection of the uterus following childbirth) and malignant endocarditis. Acute infective osteomyelitis and portal pyemia are also commonly characterized by chills. Other conditions are acute leukemia, pyelitis, pyelonephritis, cystitis, cholecystitis, empyema, infective sinus thrombosis, advanced pulmonary tuberculosis complicated by pyogenic infections of tuberculous cavities, and bronchiectasis.

COUGH

A cough is a sudden and noisy expulsion of air from the lungs, usually in an attempt to rid the lungs of foreign or offending material—a response to irritation.

Three mechanisms are involved in the expulsion of foreign material: (1) the action of the cilia (fine hairlike projections lining the respiratory tract), (2) the peristaltic motion of the bronchioles, and (3) the cough reflex. The cough reflex is most commonly initiated by stimulation of the afferent nerve endings in the mucosa of the larynx, but it may result from excitation of vagal afferents in the lungs or of the nerve endings in the pleura. A cough consists of a short inspiration followed immediately by the closing of the glottis and a forcible expiratory effort, resulting in considerable pressure within the lungs. The glottis then opens suddenly, and the offending material may be swept away from the air passages.

A number of diseases affecting the respiratory tract are characterized by cough, such as the common cold, bronchitis, tracheobronchitis, bronchiectasis, pneumonia, and pulmonary tuberculosis. Irritation of the air passages also causes what is termed as a "smoker's cough" in cigarette smokers. A dry spasmodic cough occurs in patients with influenza. The catarrhal inflammation of the respiratory tract that occurs in measles is manifested by cough, sneezing, and nasal discharge. Cough is generally a prominent symptom in psittacosis[74] (a specific infection transmitted to humans by birds, such as the parrot or canary). The cough is productive with small amounts of mucoid material, occasionally streaked with blood.

The cough in mycoplasmal pneumonia[20] is usually not prominent until 2 or 3 days after the onset of the illness. It may be paroxysmal and productive or nonproductive. When productive, there are small amounts of mucoid material, which may be streaked with blood. Mycoplasmal pneumonia is discussed on p. 323. A prominent symptom during the course of pneumococcal pneumonia (p. 323) is a productive cough with bloody sputum.[132] Stimulation of the cough reflex in this disease is caused by irritation of the lower respiratory tract and by mucus and exudate within the bronchial tree.

Cough and a productive sputum are predictable symptoms in pulmonary tuberculosis caused by bronchial involvement.[31] Their presence is indicative of an advanced stage of the disease. The cough may be mild, or there may be severe paroxysms. The sputum may be scant and mucoid or copious and purulent, depending upon the degree of bronchial involvement and cavitation.

Cough is an early symptom of sarcoidosis,[80] a systemic granulomatous disease of undetermined etiology. This disease often undergoes spontaneous remission, but it may progress and involve almost any organ, particularly the lungs, with deposits of granulomas.

In heart failure a productive cough is a frequent symptom.[29] The cough is produced by reflexes from the bronchi and congested lungs. With pulmonary congestion the cough may be severe and interfere with sleep, and paroxysmal coughing will frequently trigger severe nocturnal dyspnea. In mitral valvular disease, enlargement of the left atrium may produce cough by pressing on the bronchi. With pulmonary infarction the cough may produce a bloody sputum. Severe pulmonary edema caused by left ventricular failure produces a frothy, blood-tinged fluid from the bronchial tree.

In esophageal carcinoma (Chapter 6), severe bouts of coughing may occur because of obstruction of the lumen of the esophagus. The bronchial manifestation of neoplasms of the lung (Chapter 6) is a change in a chronic cough caused by irritation of bronchial mucosa by the tumor.[28] A cough with hemoptysis is one of the main reasons patients seek medical attention.

Cough and sputum are associated with emphysema[62] (p. 313). A productive cough with copious amounts of purulent sputum is a classic symptom of bronchiectasis.[39] Asthma is characterized by cough, dyspnea, and wheezing. Coughing and wheezing are also symptoms of pneumoconioses, such as asbestosis, silicosis, chronic beryllium disease, farmer's lung, and byssinosis.

Bronchiectasis[39, 56, 73]

Bronchiectasis is an abnormal dilatation of the bronchi and bronchioles resulting from inflammatory damage to their walls. All ages and both sexes are affected, and it is quite common in childhood.

The etiology is in dispute. Some believe that infections are the predisposing factors. These infections include pulmonary diseases, such as asthma, bronchitis, bronchiolitis, pneumonia, or bronchopneumonia. About one half of the patients give a history of pneumonia or bronchopneumonia, occurring particularly during childhood diseases or infections. Infections occurring in tuberculosis and fibrocystic disease of the pancreas are also implicated. Others believe that deranged pulmonary function causing abnormal dilatation of the bronchi and bronchioles creates the setting for the development of infections because of the destruction of the normal support and function of the bronchi and bronchioles. Antecedent inflammations or infections

with consequent scarring lead to persistent traction on the walls of the air passages, causing them to abnormally dilate. Regardless of which theory is acceptable, for the purposes of our discussion we are interested only in the end results of bronchiectasis. Previous infections or obstructions injure the elastic tissues and musculature of the walls of the bronchi and bronchioles. There is hypersecretion of mucus, which becomes infected, and the infection advances into the walls of the air passages, with subsequent necrosis and dilatation (Fig. 18-10). With total obstruction of the airways, atelectasis develops in surrounding lung parenchyma. Bronchiectasis usually develops in the lower lobes but may be found in an upper lobe, where it is likely to be secondary to tuberculous lesions.

The obstructive ventilatory insufficiency causes marked dyspnea and cyanosis. Clubbing of fingers may also occur. The complications are pleurisy, empyema, lung abscess, pneumonia, cerebral abscess, meningitis, and hypertrophy of the right ventricle.

DIARRHEA[1, 38]

Diarrhea, the passage of excessively liquid or frequent stools, is a symptom of many disorders of intestinal motility. It may be caused by functional disorders, such as allergy to food or drugs, defective absorption, defective digestion in the stomach or pancreas, vitamin deficiencies, and abuse of cathartics.

Diarrhea is present in adult celiac disease and tropical sprue—diseases of malabsorption.[81] In these diseases the intestinal mucosa is incapable of hydrolyzing a peptide or group of peptides because of deficiency or absence of necessary peptidases. About one fourth of the adult patients have a history of childhood diarrhea or steatorrhea.

Diarrhea may be prevalent in pancreatic insufficiency as in cystic fibrosis of the pancreas (Chapter 16). In this disease the diarrhea occurs either alone or in combination with respiratory disease.

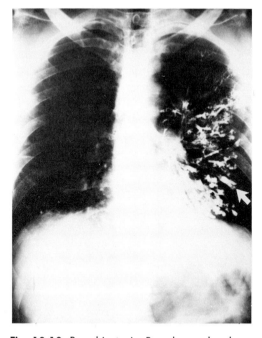

Fig. 18-10. Bronchiectasis. Bronchography showing cystic dilatation (arrow) in lower lobe, left lung. (From Young, C. G., and Likos, J. J.: Medical specialty terminology, x-ray and nuclear medicine, St. Louis, 1972, The C. V. Mosby Co.)

A well-defined functional disorder occurring in patients with diabetes is referred to as diabetic diarrhea.[129] The diarrhea may be persistent or occur in episodes, and it is watery. The attacks are usually severe and explosive and last up to a few days, after which they subside, but they may also be continuous. Fecal incontinence may develop.

Diarrhea of varying severity may occur with urgency and tenesmus in irritable colon.[1, 38] The term irritable colon covers a variety of disturbances of the colon that are accompanied by emotional tension. It ranks with the common cold as a recurrent minor disability. The stools in this type of diarrhea are small and often contain mucus. The diarrhea commonly occurs in the morning, and the accompanying pain is usually relieved with passage of feces and gas.

Diarrhea is also a symptom of intrinsic diseases of the intestines caused by specific viral, bacterial, fungal, and protozoan or metazoan parasites. Amebiasis is an example of protozoal infection (Chapter 14). Bacterial infections include cholera, typhoid, and bacillary dysentery. Common bacterial infections of the gastrointestinal tract are caused by salmonella, *Entamoeba histolytica*, and shigella. Measles, a viral infection, may be complicated by diarrhea, which may appear before the typical rash. Enteroviruses also cause infections of the gastrointestinal tract. Helminthic diseases in which diarrhea occurs are chronic schistosomiasis, roundworm infestation, strongyloidiasis, and trichuriasis (whipworm infection).

Diarrhea is a factor in regional enteritis[3] (p. 290), ulcerative colitis (described in the following section), benign or malignant tumors of the gastrointestinal tract, fistula, and blind loops in the bowels.

Nonbacterial gastroenteritis occurs as an epidemic diarrhea.[9] The onset is abrupt, usually with vomiting and fever, followed shortly by diarrhea. The illness subsides within 24 hours as a rule. The illness has been attributed to the colonization of the bowel by strains of normal intestinal flora. It is prone to occur in school children and among travelers. A similar but more serious diarrhea occurs in infants.

Identifying the cause of diarrhea depends upon determining the location and nature of the responsible disease process. Location is suggested by the character and consistency of the stools and the area involved in pain. When the stool is large in volume, the site of the disorder may be the proximal colon or small intestine, and the referred pain is in the periumbilical area or right lower quadrant of the abdomen. When stools are small, the seat of the disorder may be in the distal colon. The stools in this type of diarrhea may contain mucus or flecks of blood. Pain is in the lower abdomen or sacral region. The nature of the disease may be determined from a history of allergies to food or drugs or exposure to toxic or infectious agents and from the emotional makeup and environment of the patient.

Diagnostic studies include sigmoidoscopy, gross and microscopic examination of feces, culture of stools for pathogens, and barium enema studies.

Ulcerative colitis[38, 51]

Ulcerative colitis is an inflamed condition of the colon and rectum. It is usually a disease of young to middle-aged adults, although its onset may be at any age. It has a long and protracted course and is one of the most serious and common disorders of the colon, except malignant tumors.

Ulcerative colitis is confined to the colon in the majority of cases but may also extend to the ileum. Early lesions tend to occur as crypt abscesses in the rectosigmoid but may be found at higher levels and even in the cecum. As the disease progresses, larger areas are involved with small ulcers, and this may extend throughout the entire colon. The ulcers usually penetrate only to the muscularis, but in severe cases they may penetrate the bowel wall, causing pericolic abscesses or peritonitis. In chronic cases, adhesions may develop to adjacent viscera with the occurrence of fistulous tracts. The appearance of the colon has been likened to that of a garden hose, since the wall becomes thickened and rigid. This appearance will be evident at some stages, but at others the colon is extremely friable with a tendency to bleed freely. Scarring and fibrosis occur in later stages. The disease is noted for remissions and exacerbations.

The symptoms during periods of exacerbation are pain, cramps, and severe diarrhea and melena. Many of the exacerbations are believed to be triggered by emotional disturbances and stress. During exacerbations fluid loss is excessive, along with loss of electrolytes. The persistence of ulcerative lesions in chronic cases creates

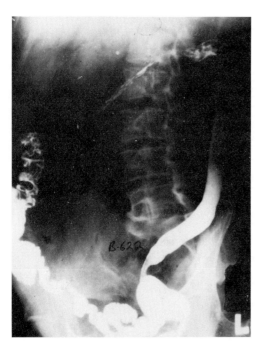

Fig. 18-11. Ulcerative colitis with carcinoma. The incidence of carcinoma of colon in association with long-standing ulcerative colitis is relatively high. (From Young, C. G., and Likos, J. J.: Medical specialty terminology, x-ray and nuclear medicine, St. Louis, 1972, The C. V. Mosby Co.)

severe debilitation, particularly in older people. Anemia is a common finding.

In addition to pericolic abscesses, fistula, and perforation, a serious complication is malignancy (Fig. 18-11).

Diagnostic procedures are sigmoidoscopy and roentgenologic studies.

DYSPNEA

Dyspnea is difficult or labored breathing; it is sometimes referred to by laymen as "shortness of breath." Dyspnea occurs when respirations cannot be carried out with ease and there is a conscious necessity for increased respiratory effort. Respiratory and circulatory functions are concerned with acquiring oxygen and eliminating carbon dioxide. Dyspnea occurs if either of these functions is disturbed to the extent that normal gaseous exchange cannot take place. Dyspnea also occurs when the oxygen requirement and the carbon dioxide production are so great that normal respiratory and circulatory mechanisms have difficulty meeting the demands of the moment. Also the oxygen supply itself may be inadequate, as at high altitudes, resulting in dyspnea.

A prominent cause of dyspnea is prevention of adequate oxygenation of the blood in the lungs. This can result from pulmonary disease, laryngeal or tracheal obstruction, or low oxygen tension in inspired air. Among the pulmonary diseases in which dyspnea is a feature are asthma (Chapter 13), bronchopneumonia, pulmonary edema and congestion; inflammation and fibrosis of the lungs, emphysema (discussed on the following pages), intrathoracic sarcoidosis, and obstructive neoplasms.

A major symptom of interstitial lung disease is exertional dyspnea.[26] In these patients eventually the performance of ordinary activities is hampered by shortness of breath. In advanced form the dyspnea may occur when the patient is at rest. A suffocating and intense dyspnea occurs during the development of interstitial edema. Breathing is rapid and shallow; also, severe attacks of paroxysmal nocturnal dyspnea result from left ventricular failure. Exertional dyspnea is a characteristic of pneumoconioses,[8] such as silicosis and asbestosis. The dyspnea at first is brought on by moderate exercise, but progressively even less activity will result in dyspnea until it is present at rest.

Dyspnea is a manifestation of heart failure.[29] The patient becomes aware of his breathing and describes it as breathlessness. The sensation may appear at rest or during mild exercise. In left heart failure, dyspnea is characteristic of pulmonary congestion and edema. The patient with congested lungs in left heart failure experiences paroxysmal nocturnal dyspnea, especially if he also suffers from orthopnea. Patients with paroxysmal nocturnal dyspnea are pale and in a cold sweat as they struggle to breathe. Tachycardia and gallop rhythm are common. Orthopnea is a type of dyspnea that appears when the subject is lying down; he is unable to breathe except in an upright or nearly upright position. Dyspnea occurs with exertion in certain chronic heart lesions, such as mitral stenosis. Dyspnea is the most common symptom in diseases of the myocardium, with orthopnea and nocturnal asthma being common. It is a feature in acute pericarditis. In aortic stenosis, exertional dyspnea is one of the cardinal symptoms.

Other causes of dyspnea are increased metabolism during muscular exertion, acidosis, nervous condition, emotional disturbances, neurasthenia, and hysteria. Dyspnea may also result from direct stimulation of the respiratory center by cerebral tumor, hemorrhage, edema, or encephalitis.

Emphysema[8, 39, 56, 62, 77, 122]

Emphysema has been included with other pulmonary obstructive diseases such as chronic bronchitis in a common term "chronic obstructive pulmonary diseases or COPD."[122] Emphysema and chronic bronchitis frequently go hand in hand and rank among the fastest growing causes of death in the United States. Bronchitis has been discussed in the chapter on infectious diseases, p. 212. The term emphysema comes from a Greek word meaning inflation. This is an apt description for this disease since in emphysema the ultrathin walls of the alveoli (air sacs in lungs) lose their elasticity and tear, with groups of ruptured sacs combining into larger sacs, which trap used or stale air (Fig. 18-12). This trapped air may give the patient a "barrel chest" appearance. As more air is inhaled and trapped in the alveoli and there is a reduction in the free exchange of oxygen and carbon dioxide, the body is under stress to work harder to get sufficient oxygen. The greatest problem of the patient is to exhale enough stale air so that an adequate replacement of fresh air can be supplied. Instead of the normal fifteen or so breaths a minute, the patient must breathe twice as fast, only to find that he is still short of breath. An adequate supply of oxygen is necessary for efficient functioning of the chest and heart muscles. As the blood levels decrease, there is an accumulation of the toxic waste product, carbon dioxide. The result may be death from heart failure, since oxygen needs cannot be met, or death may be caused by suffocation resulting from a crisis precipitated by cold or other respiratory infection. As the lungs become less efficient, the heart enlarges under the strain (Fig. 18-12).

The basic cause of emphysema is not known, but it is believed by many to be a late effect of chronic infection or irritation of the bronchial tubes, for example, chronic bronchitis. There is proof that tobacco smoking is related to emphysema. Extensive studies conducted by the U.S. Public Health Service and other organizations overwhelmingly show that cigarette smokers are more likely to be victims of emphysema than nonsmokers, and further once emphysema develops it is more progressive in smokers. Repeated exposure to air pollutants and other irritants is implicated in development of emphysema. It is hypothesized that these irritants initially break

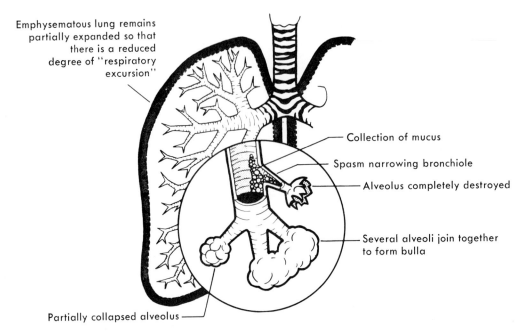

Emphysematous lung remains partially expanded so that there is a reduced degree of "respiratory excursion"

Collection of mucus

Spasm narrowing bronchiole

Alveolus completely destroyed

Several alveoli join together to form bulla

Partially collapsed alveolus

Fig. 18-12. Emphysematous lung. (From Obley, F. A.: You and your emphysema, Philadelphia, 1968, J. B. Lippincott Co.)

down the millions of tiny hairlike cilia that line the bronchial tubes and protect them from inhaled dust, debris, bacteria, and other foreign matter, by sweeping foreign matter out toward the throat where it can be eliminated. When a breakdown of the protective lining occurs, the noxious materials accumulate and block the flow of air by hardening and destruction of the tissues. Repeated attacks of colds, influenza, asthma, bronchitis, and other respiratory infections and ailments also contribute to the development of emphysema and its progress into a debilitating disease.

Of the estimated 1.3 million Americans who have emphysema, over half are under 65 years of age.[122] Emphysema is a leading cause of disability. Emphysema and chronic bronchitis are currently increasing as causes of death in the United States, with over 30,000 fatalities yearly.[122]

Early diagnosis of emphysema and bronchitis is imperative. Both creep up on their victims so slowly and stealthily that they are often ignored until serious damage has occurred. Shortness of breath, cough, or fatigue should be reported to a physician as soon as these symptoms are evident and seem to recur. Many useful tests have been developed to detect and assess deterioration in lung function. These include simple, rapid, single-breath tests of lung volume and gas exchange, which make it possible to screen large numbers of people.

EARACHE[59, 92]

Earache (otalgia) is a pain arising from certain pathologic processes in the external or middle ear or a referred pain from more remote regions. External earache is pain in the auricle and external canal from local lesions. The pain may be severe because of the close adherence of the skin to the underlying cartilage. Numerous dermatitides affect the external ear, many of which produce edema and redness. These lesions include eczema, sunburn, reactions to insect bites, chilblain, and dermatitis venenata (contact dermatitis or acute allergic inflammation caused by cantact with certain

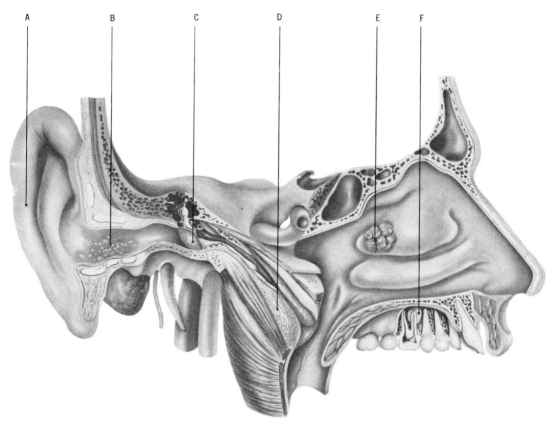

A. FROSTBITE OF PINNA Because pain is absent at onset, frostbite may lead to serious damage of the tissues. As vasoconstriction gives way to vasodilatation, pain may become intolerable.

B. HERPES OF EXTERNAL CANAL Herpes simplex, herpes zoster, and geniculate ganglion herpes may cause pain in the canal or severe neuralgic pain.

C. ACUTE PURULENT OTITIS MEDIA Severity of pain increases as pressure mounts in the middle ear. Drainage via the eustachian tube is usually blocked as a result of concomitant eustachian salpingitis.

D. EUSTACHIAN SALPINGITIS Acute inflammation of the pharyngeal orifice of the eustachian tube may prevent drainage of the middle ear and cause pain even in the absence of middle ear infection.

E. MALIGNANT NEOPLASMS Pressure on the middle turbinate from malignant neoplasms may produce pain referred to the external meatus, behind the pinna, and mastoid area.

F. APICAL ABSCESS An abscessed tooth may be the cause of pain referred to the middle ear. The neural pathway is via the dental branches of the trigeminal nerve to the tympanic plexus.

Fig. 18-13. Earache. (From Therap. Notes **69**:161, May-June, 1962, Parke, Davis & Co.)

substances, which may be chemical, animal, or vegetable). Impaction of the auditory canal with cerumen (wax) or a foreign body causes aural discomfort and may cause pain.

Middle ear pain is caused as a rule by acute purulent otitis media, malignant disease, or acute eustachian salpingitis (Fig. 18-13), Acute inflammatory lesions of the temporal bone or labyrinth may extend into the middle ear.

Aural neuralgia of local origin may be caused by inflammatory changes or otic barotrauma or blast injury. If the aural neuralgia is referred pain, which is more common, it may be from sinus infections (sphenoiditis, ethmoiditis), pressure on the middle turbinate, or from diseases of the upper nasopharynx. Diseases of the tonsils, larynx, pharynx, and tongue may produce pain in the region of the eardrum, in the eustachian tube, and in the external auditory canal. Malocclusion of the jaws, infected or abscessed teeth, tumors of the

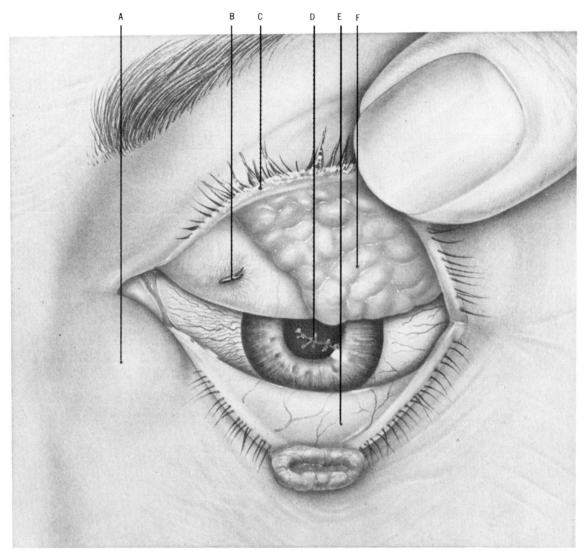

A. DACRYOCYSTITIS Acute inflammation of the lacrimal sac may result from nasolacrimal stenosis, of which epiphora is a characteristic feature.

B. FOREIGN BODY Irritation from a foreign body is a common cause of excessive lacrimation.

C. BLEPHARITIS Hypertrophy of the eyelid edge and conjunctiva from chronic marginal blepharitis results in eversion so that the puncta lacrimalia of the lower lid are no longer in apposition to the eye, and epiphora follows.

D. CORNEAL ULCER Dendritic corneal ulcers are characteristic of herpes simplex. Excessive lacrimation is a major manifestation.

E. ECTROPION Ectropion, by removing the puncta lacrimalia from close apposition to the globe, is a cause of epiphora.

F. VERNAL CONJUNCTIVITIS Conjunctivitis and other inflammatory conditions of the eye result in excessive lacrimation.

Fig. 18-14. Epiphora. (From Therap. Notes **69**:12, July-Aug., 1962, Parke, Davis & Co.)

gums, and inflammation or calculous disease of the parotid, submaxillary, and sublingual glands may cause pain in the drum and middle ear. Osteomyelitis of the mastoid is a source of pain in and behind the ear. Pain in this region also is present with acoustic neuroma.

Traumatic rupture of the eardrum and fracture of the anterior wall of the bony canal cause pain in the ear. Pain in the ear is also associated with vascular headaches. Facial neuralgia, as well as herpes zoster of the fifth and seventh cranial nerves, may cause pain in the ear.

Sudden changes in atmospheric pressure or water pressure in case of submersion may produce severe damage to the tympanic membrane and cause sudden excruciating earache. The most common cause of acute optic barotrauma, or aerotitis media, is rapidly decreasing pressure in the eardrum with rapidly increasing external air density from too quick descent in aircraft or hasty increase in cabin pressure when landing. This condition occurs more frequently in people with nasopharyngitis when patency of the eustachian orifice is impaired.

EPIPHORA[93]

Epiphora is an abnormal overflow of tears, usually caused by stricture or obstruction of lacrimal passages (nasolacrimal ducts). The nasolacrimal ducts open into the inferior meatus beneath the inferior turbinate bone (nasal bone), which is closed before birth by a mucous membrane. Occasionally the membrane does not disappear shortly after birth, and in these infants, tears spill over the cheeks instead of draining into the nose. Any nasal disease that causes obstruction of the canaliculus causes epiphora. Obstructions in the canaliculus sometimes form from concretions produced by infections. Permanent epiphora can occur from injury to the duct or canal.

The most common cause of excessive lacrimation is emotionally induced weeping. Increased lacrimation is common in all ocular diseases in which the fifth nerve is irritated. Senile epiphora is caused by relaxation of the skin of the lower lid. In this condition the blinking of the eyes does not contract the orbicularis muscle and tears do not drain into the nose. In facial paralysis, failure of the orbicularis palpebrarum muscle causes the lower lid to droop away from the globe, causing epiphora.

The conditions or diseases that cause epiphora or excessive lacrimation are illustrated in Fig. 18-14. In addition, chronic inflammation of the lacrimal sac in granulomatous diseases, such as syphilis, tuberculosis, and sarcoidosis, causes epiphora. Head cold and acute catarrhal conditions of the mucous membranes of the nose, as well as hayfever, are responsible for excessive lacrimation.

FATIGUE[94]

Fatigue is a sense of weariness or tiredness or lack of feeling of well-being. It is also referred to as listlessness, loss of energy, weakness, and lassitude. It is the most frequent presenting complaint of patients.

Fatigue may have a psychogenic basis or an organic basis, but it may be a normal response to prolonged activity. The physician must always discern between fatigue from some underlying physical abnormality and that of a psychogenic basis. The majority of patients complaining of fatigue have no organic basis for their complaint, as established by physical examination and diagnostic procedures. These patients describe their fatigue as being present when they arise in the mornings. They also claim that usually it is accompanied by nervousness, irritability, insomnia, restlessness, depression, loss of appetite, or sexual disturbances. They generally have a lack of motivation. The examining physician may discover that the basis of their fatigue is an emotional conflict at home or work. These patients are usually classified as having acute tension or anxiety neuroses.

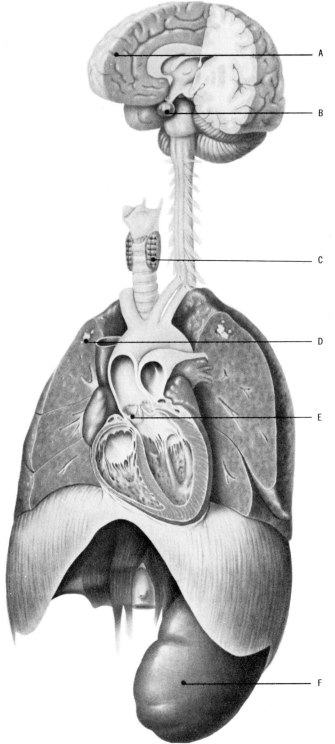

A. PSYCHOGENIC Emotional conflict with home or employment situations may manifest itself as fatigue. The anxiety neuroses are the most frequent causes, but the reactive depressions and phobic and hysterical states also produce fatigue.

B. PITUITARY DISEASE Hypopituitarism may cause fatigue principally by the secondary effects on other glands, as in adrenal cortical insufficiency and pituitary myxedema. In the late stages of acromegaly and gigantism, there may be hypopituitarism with fatigue.

C. HYPOTHYROIDISM Weakness and fatigue, associated with muscular pains and cramps, and pseudomyotonia with muscle enlargement may be the presenting signs and symptoms in myxedema.

D. TUBERCULOSIS Tiredness, particularly at the end of a day, associated with malaise, is often the initial complaint in both the pulmonary and extrapulmonary forms of the disease.

E. BACTERIAL ENDOCARDITIS The subacute variety may begin insidiously, with weakness and fatigue noticed first. Associated symptoms of malaise, fever, and weight loss appear slowly.

F. MALARIA Progressive debilitation with fatigue is frequently seen. In the estivo-autumnal form, the illness may be constant; in the tertian variety, a prodromal state with fatigue, myalgia, and fever may herald the onset of the paroxysm.

Fig. 18-15. Fatigue. (From Therap. Notes **72**:87, May-June, 1965, Parke, Davis & Co.)

Chronic infectious disease is the most frequent organic cause of fatigue. Tuberculosis and subacute endocarditis (discussed below) are characterized by afternoon fatigue. Other infectious processes in which fatigue is often a major symptom are infectious hepatitis, chronic pyelonephritis, brucellosis, malaria, and hookworm infestation. In the convalescent stages of influenza and other acute infectious diseases, fatigue is often a complaint. Severe anemic states are another cause of fatigue. There is a feeling of fatigue in Addison's disease and Cushing's disease. Fatigue may be an initial complaint in diabetes mellitus (Chapter 7). Toxic causes of fatigue include alcoholism, brominism, barbiturate, morphine, and heroin addiction, and uremic states.

In addition to the causes of fatigue illustrated in Fig. 18-15, the following diseases have been selected for discussion.

Bacterial endocarditis[5, 9, 66, 78]

Bacterial endocarditis is an acute or subacute, febrile systemic disease (Fig. 18-17, B). It is characterized by focal infection of the heart valves, with formation of bacteria-laden vegetations. These foci of infection enter the bloodstream and lead to bacteremia or septicemia, with metastatic dissemination of organisms to distant organs.

Acute bacterial endocarditis is caused by pyogenic cocci (*Streptococcus viridans*, *Staphylococcus aureus*, or pneumococcus). The least virulent form is the most common, affecting those in the third, fourth, and fifth decades most often. It is caused by a variety of organisms, *Escherichia coli*, *Proteus*, *Brucella*, alpha hemolytic and beta hemolytic streptococci, meningococci, gonococci, and *Haemophilus influenzae*.

Vegetative endocarditis tends to involve heart valves previously damaged by rheumatic fever, congenital anomalies, or arteriosclerosis. The more virulent forms attack normal heart valves, following focal infections in other tissue and organs. In infections of the less virulent type no extracardiac focus of infection can be found in a number of cases, except for relatively innocuous low-grade infections in the oral cavity, sinuses, or upper respiratory tract. Gonococcic endocarditis is predominantly a disease of the right side of the heart.

The vegetations of the heart valves are bulky, friable, granular thrombotic masses attached to the leaflets of the mitral valve as a rule, but the aortic valve may also be involved.

The onset in most cases is subtle, with malaise, low-grade fever, fatigue, weight loss, and anorexia. Heart murmur is present in most patients. It may be loud when the disease is acute. Symptoms include cutaneous petechial hemorrhages, enlarged spleen, and nail bed splinter hemorrhages. In time, clubbing of the fingers and signs of renal functional impairment may develop. The complications are septicemia, embolism, valvular stenosis or insufficiency, focal embolic glomerulonephritis, and cardiac failure.

Tuberculosis[23, 31, 56, 120]

Tuberculosis is an infectious disease caused by two species of *Mycobacterium*—*M. tuberculosis* and *M. bovis*. Tuberculosis is usually contracted by inhalation of infectious material as in infection with *M. tuberculosis*, but it may be ingested, as in infection with *M. bovis*. The tubercle bacilli is transmitted from one person to another, almost always through the air. A person with active tuberculosis coughs or sneezes and releases into the air tiny, moist droplets, each containing one or two tubercle bacilli. These droplets dry out and float about in the air, but if the germs float out into the sunlight they are quickly killed. In a closed room with poor ventilation, a person can breathe in these tiny droplet nuclei, but in order to cause infection they must penetrate the air deep into the lungs without being stopped. If this happens they can become imbedded and the germs begin to grow and multiply very slowly. The body sets up a defense even in this very early stage, and as a rule it is strong enough to stop the growth of the germ. This is a primary infection and most infections are arrested in this stage. There is no explanation as to why dormant germs from a primary infection of earlier years suddenly erupt into action and active tuberculosis develops.

Tuberculosis is not rare. In 1969 there were over 38,000 new cases of active tuberculosis reported, and more than 5,000 patients died.[120]

The initial constitutional or general symptoms of pulmonary tuberculosis are fatigue; anorexia; weight loss; fever, characteristically in the afternoon; night sweats; and malaise. Fatigue and weight loss are usually the symptoms that lead the patient to seek medical aid. Chest pain and a productive cough, often with hemoptysis, follow the initial symptoms. Cough and sputum usually do not occur until there is cavitation of the lung parenchyma. The hemoptysis may indicate rapid sloughing of a caseous lesion or ulceration in a draining bronchus.

Tuberculosis is traditionally described as being primary or childhood type, and secondary or adult or reinfection type (Figs. 18-16 and 18-17, C). Hilar adenopathy is often a feature in childhood tuberculosis; tuberculosis of the adult is predominantly a disease of the parenchyma of the lung. Regardless of how pulmonary tuberculosis is classified, almost all clinical tuberculosis is the result of evolution of the initial infection.

Tuberculosis is one of the oldest diseases, having existed for at least 6,500 years. Although it is not a common disease today, there is a mass of knowledge about it, and the general public is fairly well informed, at least in the United States. Through the public health services and the National Tuberculosis Association, mass x-ray examinations are made for detection of the disease. Also chest x-ray examinations are a prerequisite for employment in many

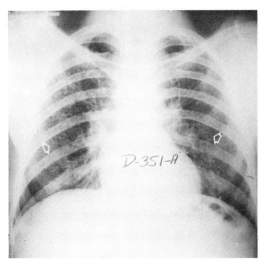

Fig. 18-16. Miliary tuberculosis. Arrows point to areas of fine nodules in both lung fields. (From Young, C. G., and Likos, J. J.: Medical specialty terminology, x-ray and nuclear medicine, St. Louis, 1972, The C. V. Mosby Co.)

businesses, hospitals, and industries. Chest x-ray examinations are also a part of the physical examination for induction into the armed forces and for qualification for health and life insurance in many insurance companies. Further, most patients presenting symptoms related to the respiratory system (lungs) are given x-ray examinations. Any individual whose x-ray films show suspicious shadows on the lungs is advised to undergo further and intensive investigation. In addition to detection of tuberculosis by x-ray examination, a simple skin test called the Mantoux tuberculin test is one of the best of a number of tests.[120] If the test shows that a person has been infected, chest x rays are taken. If the chest x ray indicates possible involvement, a sputum sample is then taken and examined in the laboratory for presence of tubercle bacilli germs. When tuberculous patients are discovered, all persons who come in contact with them, if known, are given x-ray or other examinations for possible infection. Today, with careful diagnosis and conscientious drug therapy and

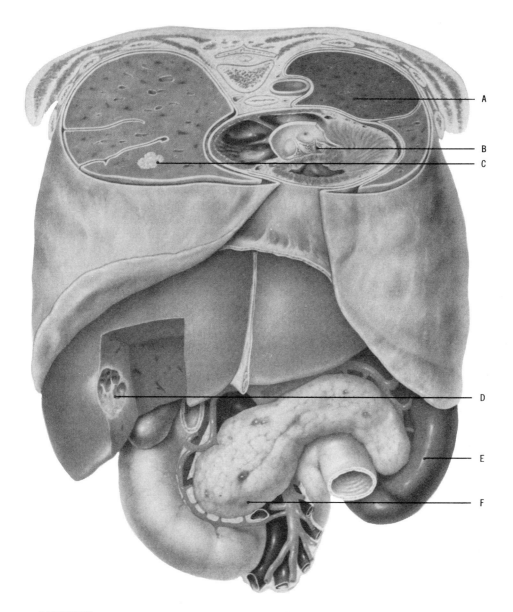

A. PNEUMONIA Diagnosis of bronchopneumonia is made from abnormal physical signs in the chest. Pyrexia may last for two or more weeks and may recur.

B. BACTERIAL ENDOCARDITIS Undiagnosed pyrexia accompanied by focal embolic lesions should always suggest subacute bacterial endocarditis.

C. TUBERCULOSIS Occurrence of some degree of fever without an apparent cause may be the only evidence of tuberculosis.

D. PYOGENIS ABSCESS Localized pus characteristic of pyogenic abscess may be the cause of continued pyrexia.

E. MALARIA Characteristic of malaria are febrile paroxysms, which recur at varying intervals, depending on the form of the disease.

F. PANCREATITIS Fever without the typical pain associated with chronic pancreatitis may be the initial symptom of chronic relapsing pancreatitis.

Fig. 18-17. Fever. (From Therap. Notes **71**:61, Jan.-Feb., 1964, Parke, Davis & Co.)

surgery, if indicated, the chances of curing or arresting tuberculosis are good, regardless of the stage the disease has reached when it is discovered. The tubercle bacillus takes about 18 to 24 hours to reproduce itself just once, and it grows slowly and dies slowly, so there is always the danger that once the germ has entered the lungs, actual disease will result.

FEVER[95]

Fever, also called pyrexia, is an abnormal elevation of body temperature. Fever may have a normal physiologic basis, as that which occurs during menstruation, or it may be an indication of evaporation of moisture on the skin, as occurs during periods of high humidity of the air. Psychic and hypothalamic disturbances and excessive fatigue may be causes of fever. Fever referred to as "surgical" apparently is the result of toxic substances liberated by injured tissues. Injuries to nerves cause neurogenic fever, especially when the lesions are in the neighborhood of the third ventricle, internal capsule, or medulla. Dehydration in young children may cause fever.

Persistent or prolonged fever occurs in a number of diseases, and it is characteristic of typhoid and paratyphoid fevers, typhus, Mediterranean or Malta fever, secondary syphilis, brucellosis, tularemia, psittacosis, influenza, tetanus, and Weil's disease (an infection caused by leptospires). A persistent fever is often a symptom of localized collections of pus, as in abscesses of the tonsils, pharynx, teeth, parotids, mastoid, breast, liver, kidneys, appendix, and prostate. Persistent fever occurs in diseases in which there are localized purulent infections without pus collection, as in cholecystitis, phlebitis, pancreatitis, bronchitis, dental caries, and tonsillitis. Prolonged fever is characteristic of pleurisy with serous effusion, bacterial endocarditis, septicemia, cirrhosis and secondary carcinoma of the liver, gout, rheumatoid arthritis, blood diseases, meningeal hemorrhages, and certain collagen diseases. Malaria, trypano-somiasis, dysentery, cholera, plague, relapsing fever, and sprue are among the tropical diseases of which prolonged fever is characteristic.

In acute leukemia,[54] fever may be an abrupt symptom. Fever is a late manifestation of chronic leukemia, and usually it is caused by an infection, since immunity to bacteria and viruses is reduced. In acute liver disease, fever is a common symptom, usually from infection, tissue necrosis, or drug hypersensitivity. Chronic relapsing pancreatitis may begin with fever when there is no pain or other diagnostic manifestation.

Aseptic fever results when there is destruction of body tissues, as in cardiac and pulmonary infarction, hemolytic anemias, and in pernicious anemia in young adults. Periodic fever occurs in Pel-Ebstein or Hodgkin's disease, a disease of lymphatic tissue, usually regarded as neoplastic.

The cause of fever may be obscure, and it is considered to be of unknown origin if it lasts at least 10 days without a diagnostic basis. Occult neoplasms cause low-grade fever.

Some of the diseases illustrated in Fig. 18-17 have been discussed elsewhere. Pneumonia is selected for discussion to follow.

Pneumonia[26, 56, 75, 132]

Pneumonia is a diffuse inflammation of the lungs. It can occur as a primary infection as with pneumococcus, staphylococcus, streptococcus, *Klebsiella pneumoniae*, *Haemophilus influenzae*, or a viral agent. It can also be secondary to or a complication of viral infections such as influenza, rickettsial diseases, congestive heart failure, bronchiectasis, bronchitis, bronchial obstruction with tumor, or the pulmonary mycoses.

Lobar pneumonia[56, 132] is initiated by pneumococci that reach the alveoli by inhalation or through bacteremia. (See Fig. 18-9.) It is likely to be much more serious in older people who are debilitated or chronically ill from other diseases, in syphilitic patients, and in people who suffer from chronic alcoholism. It is rarely seen today except in those who lie ill and unattended at home, in alcoholics exposed to cold temperatures, in those with chest injuries causing pulmonary congestion and edema, or in patients who recently have undergone general anesthesia. The clinical effects may be toxic psychosis, cardiovascular collapse and shock, empyema, lung abscess, meningitis, cardiac infections, acute otitis media, mastoiditis, and paralytic ileus.

Friedländer's pneumonia[75] is caused by *Klebsiella pneumoniae* or Friedländer's bacillus. It is a particularly destructive type, with the infected lobules creating consolidated nodules, which on confluence become lobar. Abscesses may be extensive. This form affects older men, especially those who are alcoholics, diabetics or have severe oral sepsis.

Staphylococcal pneumonia comprises up to 5% of bacterial pneumonias, except during influenza epidemics. This type of pneumonia is most often seen in infants, in children with cystic fibrosis of the pancreas, leukemia, or measles, and in adults with influenza or who have debilitating diseases. It is characterized by a high-spiking fever, multiple chills, cyanosis, dyspnea, chest pain, and a thick, creamy yellow or reddish-yellow sputum. In infants, empyema or pneumothorax may suddenly develop. The leukocyte count is elevated, even up to 25,000 per cubic millimeter. The mortality rate is high in this type of pneumonia. Recovery is gradual, and bronchiectasis may be a consequence of the disease.

Mycoplasmal pneumonia[20] is a severe respiratory infection caused by *Mycoplasma pneumoniae*. It has an insidious onset, with malaise and headache as prominent symptoms. Later there is fever, myalgias, and pharyngitis. Cough is delayed in appearing, but it later becomes the dominant symptom. The fever is variable in duration, lasting 3 days to about 2 weeks. Relapses can occur after clinical recovery. Compli-

cations are bronchiectasis, pericarditis, myocarditis, and thrombocytopenic purpura. Mortality rates are low.

Streptococcic pneumonia is caused by beta hemolytic *Streptococcus pyogenes* in most cases and is secondary to influenza, measles, or other childhood viral infections. This organism was the principal cause of death during the pandemic of influenza in 1918 to 1919. It is rare today.

Bronchopneumonia is an infection that originates in the terminal and respiratory bronchioles and spreads into the surrounding peribronchiolar alveoli.[56] The elastic walls of the bronchioles are readily destroyed, allowing the inflammatory changes to spread into the peribronchiolar tissues and adjacent alveoli. The organisms commonly responsible are *Staphylococcus aureus*, *Streptococcus*, *Klebsiella*, *Haemophilus*, and pneumococcus, but there is also a tuberculous type. The onset is more likely to be severe if the patient is an infant, is over 50 years of age, is debilitated, is suffering from chronic diseases, or has had a prior viral infection. Causes other than bacterial infections are inhalation of noxious gases and dusts and aspiration of fluid and solid contents of the alimentary tract. Bronchopneumonia also occurs with rickettsial diseases, congestive heart failure, bronchiectasis, lung tumors, and pulmonary mycotic diseases. There is a tendency for bronchopneumonia to inflict permanent damage on the lung, leading to bronchiolar fibrosis and narrowing or bronchiectasis.

Inhalation or aspiration pneumonia may occur from a variety of causes. It results from the inhaling of food, gastric contents, or foreign bodies into the lungs, which may occur when anesthesia has been induced on a full stomach during pregnancy or emergency surgery. Such inhalation of foreign material may also occur in drunkenness, in epileptic attacks, during coma or neurologic disorders that interfere with breathing, in swallowing, or in coughing. Feeble infants may also inhale regurgitated materials.

Lipid or lipoid pneumonia[26] is from aspiration of oil. The exogenous type is caused by long-continued use of oily nose-drops or sprays, mineral oils, oily medications and vitamins forcibly given to infants and young children, and from instillation of oily radiopaque contrast media. This type of pneumonia tends to be symptomless, unless a bacterial infection is superimposed. The lung structure in severe lipoid pneumonia may be almost completely replaced by fat and fibrous tissue. An endogenous variety of lipoid pneumonia results from metabolic, allergic, neoplastic, or inflammatory processes that release lipoid by causing tissue breakdown.

Pneumocystis carinii pneumonia[25, 44] (*P. carinii* pneumonia) is caused by the opportunist organism, *Pneumocystis carinii,* and is an important cause of pulmonary infection in immunosuppressed patients. The organism is presumed to be a protozoan but it has never been cultivated for positive identification. The pneumonia occurs in endemic and epidemic forms in many parts of the world, particularly in Southeast Asia.[70] The disease mainly affects the very young poorly nourished or debilitated children, premature infants, and patients who have been treated with corticosteroids, antimetabolites, or antibiotics. It has been found in Vietnamese infants, and a recent case of a diffuse fulminant disease with recovery has been reported in an adopted infant from Vietnam.[70] It has recently been diagnosed by the use of bronchopulmonary lavage.

HEARING LOSS[41, 59, 60, 96, 131]

Hearing loss or deafness is of two types —conduction deafness and nerve deafness. Deafness is one of the most emotionally disabling conditions from which people suffer. Children who are born deaf learn to speak only with intensive study, and regardless of the amount of education and training given to them, they remain behind other children in school achievement. If these afflicted children are not discovered, they are often termed feebleminded. Those who later become deaf and are forced to live in a world of silence are prone to withdraw and live within themselves, since they are deprived of their primary means of communication.

Infantile deafness may be familial or the result of developmental defects. It may be caused by damage in utero or during the passage through the birth canal, or it may result from erythroblastosis fetalis from Rh incompatibility. Other causes are given below under nerve deafness.

Deafness after birth arises from a variety of causes, such as infections, like meningitis, viral infections (particularly measles or mumps), nonspecific high fevers, diabetes, syphilis, and myxedema, as well as ototoxic drugs (streptomycin, kanamycin, salicylates, and quinine). The ototoxic drugs affect the cochlea. Traumatic injuries like skull fracture, injury to the drum when diving, and exposure to sudden loud noise account for some deafness. Constant exposure to a noisy environment may also affect the hearing. Advancing age causes hearing to become less acute, usually beginning with high frequencies and progressing downward.

Conduction deafness is caused by any condition in the middle ear or external ear that interferes with or prevents the conduction of air-borne sound waves to the inner ear. Chronic infections of the ear are a common cause of this type of deafness, as in tonsillitis and adenoiditis. In these conditions the tonsils and adenoids become swollen and obstructive, preventing proper aeration of the middle ear. Serous otitis media is one of the most important causes of acquired deafness or conduction deafness. It is insidiously progressive. Mucoid, purulent, or clear fluid develops in the middle ear, and if untreated, it produces metaplasia of the mucosa, scar tissue forms, and a chronic adhesive type of deafness occurs. Usually serous otitis media follows a respiratory infection, but it may also be on an allergic basis. Irreversible changes can occur in the middle ear, and the hearing loss may be abrupt.

Nerve deafness or sensory neural hearing loss results from any condition that interferes with the analysis of the transformed sound waves in the inner ear or transmission of nerve impulses to the brainstem. Nerve deafness is also called perceptive deafness and sensorineural deafness. The partial or complete loss of hearing of the sensory neural type may be caused by congenital abnormalities of the inner ear inherited through defective genes, dominant or recessive. Congenital nerve deafness may also be acquired in utero. The inner ear of the embryo is especially susceptible to trauma, toxins, viral infections, and anoxia, which is particularly true in the first and last trimesters of pregnancy. Nerve deafness may also be caused by lesions involving the terminals of the cochlear nerve in the internal ear. Chronic otitis interna is a cause of deafness, and it may follow an infection of the middle ear secondary to blockage of the eustachian canal or acute labryinthitis. The infection may also follow acute purulent otitis media, meningococcal meningitis, or mumps. Some drugs cause deafness by damaging the auditory nerve or the auditory centers in the pons. Other causes include damage to the eighth cranial nerve by tumor or by meningovascular syphilis.

Vascular spasms or a clot in one of the vessels supplying the inner ear produce deafness. The hearing loss usually is sudden and is accompanied by tinnitus (ringing in the ears) and vertigo (a form of dizziness).[41]

Otosclerosis is an important cause of hearing impairment in adults. It has a relatively high incidence in the population. This disease of the bone is unique to the human otic capsule. It may begin at any time in life but appears most frequently after puberty, during pregnancy, the puerperium, or menopause. The initial process is resorption of bone, progressing until the entire capsule may be involved, including the walls of the semicircular canals and both labyrinthine windows. Hearing acuity is reduced. In the early stages the bone conduction by which we hear our own voices remains relatively unaffected, but later to the person with advanced otosclerosis, his own voice sounds loud and he attempts to compensate by pitching his voice low, sometimes to the point that he cannot be understood. Otosclerotic victims can usually hear fairly well on the telephone, which provides an amplified signal, provided the disease is not too far advanced. They can also hear better in noisy places, such as a train or subway, or in any place where people have to talk above the surrounding noises.

Meniere's syndrome[59, 60] causes perceptive deafness, as well as vertigo. For some unknown reason, endolymph is formed in excessive amounts and produces increased pressure through the cochlear duct and the vestibular system. This results in progressive atrophy of the hair cells. Low tones are affected to a greater degree than high tones in the early stages. Tinnitus is usually the first complaint. It is a chronic disease that may be mild or quite severe, lasting a few minutes to several days. The head noises are hissing, roaring or ringing. These auditory symptoms are usually bilateral. The attacks of vertigo are characterized by a turning, swaying, or rocking sensation. Rarely, however, does the vertigo cause the victim to fall. The attacks are frequently accompanied by nausea and vomiting. Nystagmus may also be present during an attack.

Tuning fork tests frequently confirm the presence of unilateral nerve type deafness. Audiologic studies furnish characteristic findings, showing a flat or low-tone sensorineural hearing loss.

Prominent causes of hearing loss are illustrated in Fig. 18-18.

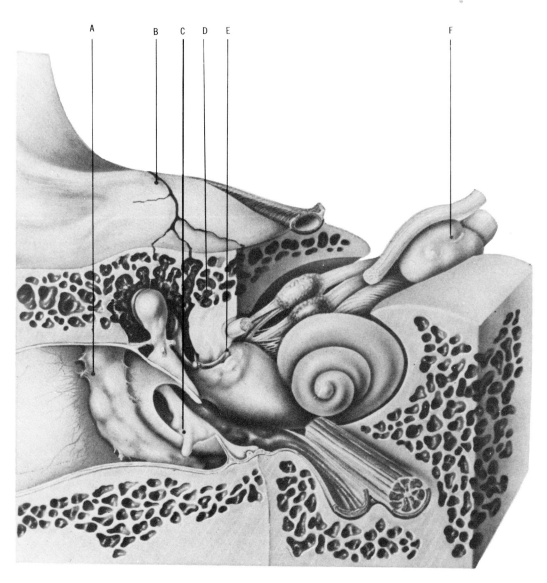

A. CERUMEN Wax and foreign bodies within the external auditory canal should be carefully removed. Method of choice is introduction of warm water by syringe.

B. SKULL FRACTURE When damage to the eighth nerve caused by fracture through the petrous portion of the temporal bone involves the cochlear or vestibular portion, complete deafness of the perceptive type ensues.

C. CHRONIC OTITIS MEDIA Chronic suppurative otitis media is characterized by tympanic inflammation which is accompanied by perforation of the eardrum and persistent discharge of pus.

D. HEMORRHAGE Spontaneous hemorrhage into the inner ear, although rare, sometimes occurs in blood dyscrasias, such as leukemia, pernicious anemia, hemophilia, or hemorrhagic conditions associated with purpura.

E. OTOSCLEROSIS Extent of otosclerosis ranges from small, inactive areas to involvement of the entire cochlear capsule. Progressive loss of hearing is the most characteristic symptom of this condition.

F. ACOUSTIC TUMOR Tumor of the eighth nerve (acoustic neuroma), whether unilateral or bilateral, usually causes symptoms during the fifth decade of life.

Fig. 18-18. Hearing loss. (From Therap. Notes **70:**9, Jan.-Feb., 1963, Parke, Davis & Co.)

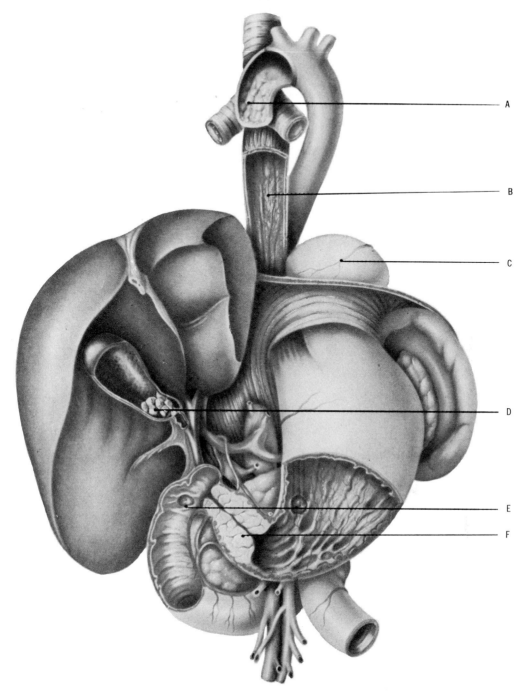

A ———————————————— A

B ———————————————— B

C ———————————————— C

D ———————————————— D

E ———————————————— E

F ———————————————— F

A. SYPHILITIC AORTITIS   Aortitis is a frequent visceral manifestation of acquired syphilis. Atypical angina resulting from syphilitic aortitis may take the form of heartburn.

B. ACUTE ESOPHAGITIS   Substernal distress may be caused by acute esophagitis, which may complicate upper respiratory infections; occur after operation, especially in the presence of severe vomiting or prolonged gastric intubation; or result from ingestion of corrosive agents.

C. ESOPHAGEAL HIATUS HERNIA   In esophageal hiatus hernia, the most common kind of acquired hernia, part of the stomach herniates through the esophageal hiatus of the diaphragm. Heartburn is a specific symptom of hiatus hernia.

D. GALLSTONES   Stones in the gall bladder can cause heartburn. Distress often is more pronounced after ingestion of certain foods, such as pork, cabbage, or fried foods.

E. PEPTIC ULCER   About one quarter of patients with peptic ulcer complain of heartburn. Although usually single, ulcers may be multiple. They may be present in both stomach and duodenum or as multiple lesions in the same organ.

F. PYLORIC STENOSIS   When pyloric stenosis results from healed ulcer or from gastric carcinoma, it may cause persistent heartburn. Because symptoms of cancer of the stomach are indefinite, indigestion in a person of cancer age is suspect.

Fig. 18-19. Heartburn. (From Therap. Notes **69:**8, Nov.-Dec., 1962, Parke, Davis & Co.)

HEARTBURN[97]

Heartburn (pyrosis) is a painful burning sensation in the chest, located behind the sternum in the midline between the xiphoid process (tip of sternum) and the manubrium (uppermost part of the sternum). Practically every form of anterior chest pain or discomfort is referred to as heartburn, and this includes angina pectoris. Pain may occur spontaneously and have no relation to activity, eating, or other phenomena, or it may accompany belching.

The physiologic causes of heartburn include irritation of a sensitive esophagus when gastric contents are regurgitated, structural and functional derangements of the esophagus, burning retrosternal pain following rapid swallowing of water or dilute bicarbonate of soda, and overdistention of the stomach caused by eating rapidly or drinking excessive amounts of water or carbonated drinks with meals.

Heartburn is primarily a symptom of esophageal disorders, such as cancer, peptic esophagitis, acute or chronic esophagitis, and stricture of the esophagus. Chronic esophagitis causes heartburn when injury to the esophagus is so severe that it prevents healing of the damaged structures. It may also occur as a result of irradiation damage, tuberculosis, actinomycosis, or syphilis. Esophageal hiatal hernia (discussed in the following section) is a common cause of heartburn.

Among other causes of heartburn are nervous tension causing increased irritability of the esophageal motor system, and faulty eating habits. Pregnant and obese people or those with large intra-abdominal tumors often complain of heartburn. Heartburn is not a symptom of organic heart disease as a rule, unless the heart condition is severe enough to initiate secondary gastric disturbances.

Fig. 18-19 gives a number of causes of heartburn; some have been selected for discussion as follows.

Esophageal hiatal hernia[21, 38]

Esophageal hiatal hernia is one in which the proximal segments of the stomach herniate through a weakened esophageal hiatus of the diaphragm into the thoracic cavity. It is called a sliding hernia. The loss of the acute angle of entry of the esophagus into the stomach interferes with the mechanism of the cardiac sphincter and permits reflux of gastric juice into the esophagus. The complications are esophagitis and possibly erosion and ulceration of the esophageal wall. The esophagus is commonly shorter than normal, either as a congenital defect or as the result of inflammation and scarring.

The cardinal symptoms and signs of sliding hiatal hernia are epigastric and substernal pain or distress, heartburn, regurgitation, dysphagia, and hematemesis or melena. Substernal pain may mimic coronary artery disease except that it is usually related to meals and posture. Patients often experience regurgitation or a reflux of the sour gastric liquid into the mouth when they bend forward, lie down, or engage in strenuous activity that raises intra-abdominal pressure. Dysphagia may occur during a meal and then disappear. The patient has the sensation of a bolus of food sticking in the esophagus. The symptomatic hiatal hernia usually occurs in obese, middle-aged individuals.

Peptic ulcer[38, 116]

Peptic ulcers are craterlike lesions or sores in the lining of the walls of the stomach or duodenum. (See Figs. 18-2, 18-21, and 18-29.) The ulcers erode through the inner mucous membrane lining of these organs and into the deeper muscular wall. Peptic ulcers occur only in the environment of acid gastric secretions. The acid gastric secretion is hydrochloric acid, which is usually limited to the fundus of the stomach. The stomach also secretes a protein-digesting enzyme called pepsin, from which the peptic ulcer derives its name. The secretion of hydrochloric acid and pepsin brings about the digestion of meat and other proteins as they reach the stomach. Ordinarily they are not secreted in the absence of food. The oversecretion of hydrochloric acid and pepsin is the important factor in the production of ulcers. The other factor is the inability of the intestinal wall to resist erosion by this mixture. There are a number of theories on why the stomach will oversecrete hydrochloric acid and pepsin. In some people the stomach will secrete acid not only in the presence of food but also on and off between meals when the lining of the stomach and duodenum are unprotected by food against the corrosive action of the gastric juices. Factors that are believed to stimulate the increase in the amount of acid secretion and also to irritate the stomach and duodenal wall are certain foods or medications, such as alcohol, coffee, and aspirin. In the normal person the mucous membrane lining of the stomach and duodenal wall is resistant to the secretions of hydrochloric acid and pepsin, and no ulcer will develop. In others, however, this resistance breaks down, and an ulcer develops. Anxiety and stress are believed to contribute to hyperacidity. In this connection, there is a theory that the hypothalamus–anterior pituitary–adrenal cortex stress mechanism is of significance in the production of an ulcer, possibly through the vagus nerve, which stimulates the stomach to produce its secretions. The vagus nerve is sometimes severed in the stomach as a surgical procedure in ulcer therapy.

Duodenal ulcers are much more common than gastric ulcers, and they occur much more often in young adults and middle-aged males. Gastric ulcers occur more frequently in women and in older people. Gastric ulcers occur in the antrum of the stomach and infrequently in the cardia. They are usually on or near the lesser curvature of the stomach, but a few are in close proximity to the pylorus on the anterior or posterior wall. Some gastric ulcers are large, but the duodenal ulcer is typically small. Duodenal ulcers usually occur 1 or 2 cm. distal to the pylorus on the anterior or posterior wall.

The almost universal symptom of ulcers is pain. It is usually steady, with a gnawing or burning character. It generally appears from 30 minutes to 2 hours after a meal and is relieved by eating or taking antacid medications. The pain is usually located in the small area of the abdomen somewhere between the umbilicus and the lower end of the sternum. As the stomach empties, the continued secretion of the undiluted acid comes in contact with the ulcer causing the pain.

The complications of ulcers are narrowing or obstruction of the intestinal opening into the stomach, hemorrhage, and perforation. The duodenal ulcers or those in the pylorus may become inflamed and swollen or scarred, and the intestinal opening may be narrowed or even closed. A symptom of obstruction is vomiting of meals and regurgitation of the stomach secretions. As the ulcer erodes into the muscular portion of the wall of the stomach or duodenum, the blood vessels are damaged. The small blood vessels may leak slowly over a period of time causing anemia. If the ulcer has damaged a large blood vessel, the hemorrhage is more rapid and potentially dangerous. The symptoms of hemorrhage are a feeling of faintness or even collapse. The internal hemorrhage may cause death. In cases of bleeding the stools become a tarry black from the digested blood. The danger of perforation is peritonitis, since the erosion all the way through the wall of the stomach or duodenum allows partially digested food and bacteria to pass into the peritoneal cavity. The symptom of a sudden perforation is acute pain throughout the abdomen.

The diagnostic procedure for confirming the presence of an ulcer is the x-ray procedure in which the patient swallows a barium meal. In the x-ray films taken from the various angles of the stomach and duodenum, ulcer craters are revealed to be filled with the barium. Many ulcers heal with epithelium growing over the defect, but permanent scars are the rule. Steroid administration may activate an existing ulcer, which may have become quiescent through healing.

HEMIPLEGIA[18, 98]

Hemiplegia is spastic paralysis of one side of the body; it is usually the result of a lesion involving the corticospinal tract. The paralysis at first is flaccid from spinal shock and gradually becomes spastic, which characterizes it as a lesion of the upper motor neuron.

Hemiplegia of sudden onset is commonly the result of a vascular lesion involving the internal capsule, with thrombosis the most frequent cerebrovascular lesion. This is usually found in conjunction with a previously formed atherosclerotic plaque. Cerebral hemorrhage and sometimes embolism are commonly the cause of hemiplegia, and both may initiate a state of apoplexy. Embolism is nearly always of cardiac origin and may be from thrombi in large arteries or from pulmonary vein thrombosis. Cerebral hemorrhages occur in patients with essential hypertension, in whom the intracerebral bleeding is caused by rupture of an atheromatous artery. Cerebral hemorrhage from rupture of a cerebral aneurysm is another important cause.

Patients with hypertensive encephalopathy may experience a transient hemiplegia during periods of high blood pressure. General paresis is another cause of transient hemiplegia.

Head injuries such as cerebral contusion, cerebral laceration, and epidural hemorrhage with fracture of the skull and tearing of branches of the middle meningeal artery are traumatic causes of hemiplegia. Injury of the spinal cord at a high cervical level may occasionally result in hemiplegia. When hemiplegia is of gradual onset, it is often caused by intracranial space-occupying lesions, such as brain tumors (especially gliomas), brain metastases, and brain abscesses (Fig. 18-8, B). Tuberculoma occurs infrequently, and gummas and parasitic cysts rarely develop, but all may cause hemiplegia. Cervical cord neoplasms, congenital malformation (platybasia[18]—upward invagination of the first two cervical vertebrae into the posterior fossa), and multiple sclerosis (p. 305) may also give rise to hemiplegia.

The major causes of hemiplegia are illustrated in Fig. 18-20, some of which are discussed in Chapter 9.

HYPERHIDROSIS[99]

Hyperhidrosis is excessive production of sweat; it can be generalized or localized. Generalized sweating normally follows exercise or occurs during excessively hot weather. Hyperhidrosis is a classic sign of fever and occurs in such illnesses as malaria, tuberculosis, brucellosis, and pneumonia. Hyperhidrosis may result from disturbances in the central heat regulatory mechanism in fevers of unknown origin. Tumor, trauma, or inflammatory diseases of the brain affecting the hypothalamus or its tracts may cause generalized hyperhidrosis in an occasional patient. In certain hormonal disorders, such as hyperthyroidism and occasionally hyperpituitarism, there may be generalized hyperhidrosis. It may also occur regularly in diabetes and during pregnancy and menopause. Excessive sweating may be associated with pathologic obesity, gout, alcoholic intoxication, and drug reactions. Profuse generalized sweating occurs in children with acrodynia, a condition occurring in infants in which there is edema, bluish red color of hands, disordered digestion, multiple arthritis, and muscular weakness. Excessive perspiration is a characteristic feature in familial dysautonomia, an inherited disease transmitted by a simple recessive autosomal gene, in which there is defective lacrimation, skin

A. SUBDURAL HEMATOMA A chronic subdural hematoma should be suspected in patients in whom hemiplegia develops soon after a head injury and who manifest fluctuations of consciousness and varying degrees of mental disturbance.

B. GLIOBLASTOMA MULTIFORME This malignant neoplasm invariably proves fatal regardless of treatment or location in the brain. Hemiplegia may result from hemorrhage into the tumor.

C. CEREBRAL THROMBOSIS Cerebral ischemia caused by thrombosis of a cerebral artery frequently impinges on the corticospinal tracts, resulting in hemiplegia.

D. CEREBRAL ANEURYSM Localized dilatation of an intracranial arterial aneurysm may cause pressure on neighboring upper motor neurons or may rupture, leading to subarachnoid hemorrhage with resultant hemiplegia.

E. CEREBRAL LACERATION Hemiplegia may result from a head injury in which a cerebral laceration, with bruising and hemorrhage into brain substance, occurs.

F. CEREBRAL ABSCESS Hemiplegia accompanied by a focal brain lesion, intracranial infection such as sinusitis, mastoiditis, or osteomyelitis, elevated intracranial pressure, and pleocytosis suggests a diagnosis of cerebral abscess.

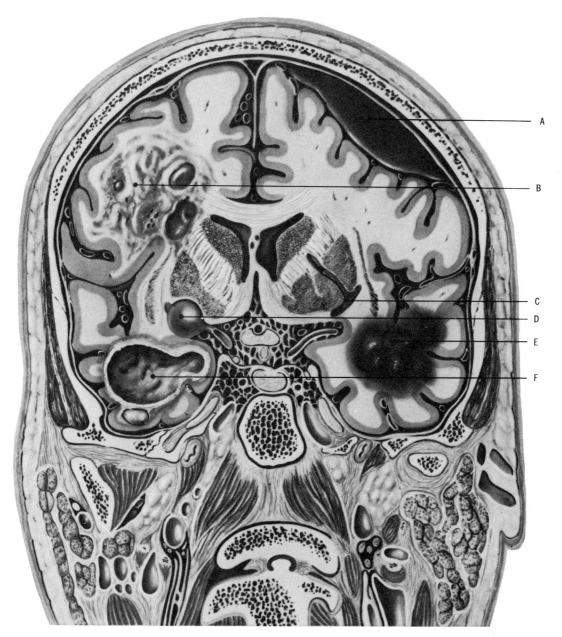

Fig. 18-20. Hemiplegia. From Therap. Notes **69**:4, Mar.-Apr., 1962, Parke, Davis & Co.)

blotching, emotional instability, motor incoordination, and hyporeflexia.

Localized hyperhidrosis occurs as a result of emotional stimuli. The usual locations are the axillae, palms, soles, forehead, eyebrows, tip of nose, sternal area, antecubital fossa, and perianal areas. Localized excessive perspiration may occur in the areas surrounding frostbite, trench foot, thrombophlebitis, and scleroderma. Organic lesions that may be characterized by localized hyperhidrosis are brain tumor, spinal cord injury, or peripheral nerve injury. Postencephalitic parkinsonism is characterized by localized areas of continuous sweating. Excessive perspiration may occur in paralyzed parts of the body. In the auriculotemporal syndrome in which there is injury in the region of the parotid gland, excessive sweating and flushing characteristically occur.

A type of sweating known as gustatory reflex sweating occurs on the face in some persons during eating, particularly of spicy foods.

HYPERSALIVATION[100]

Hypersalivation (ptyalism) is flow of saliva in excess of 1,200 to 1,500 ml. a day. Normally salivation is stimulated by the psychic response to the sight, smell, taste, or thought of food; it may occur as a conditioned reflex response.

True hypersalivation occurs following ingestion of iodides, bromides, arsenic, antimony, bismuth, mercury, lead, phosphorus, and copper salts. In botulism, a form of food poisoning caused by the toxin produced by *Clostridium botulinum* in improperly canned or preserved foods, there may be an initial increase of hypersecretion of the salivary glands followed by a decrease. Cholinergic drugs may also cause hypersalivation.

Various forms of stomatitis produce hypersalivation, as seen in the oral lesions of diphtheria, syphilis, tuberculosis, pyogenic infections, and Ludwig's and Vincent's angina. Stomatitis associated with foot and mouth disease, sprue, scurvy, and pernicious anemia may also cause hypersalivation. Painful swallowing in some of these conditions may cause the saliva to drool from the mouth.

A jagged tooth or filling, salivary gland calculus, dental caries, ill-fitting dentures, and oral tumors may cause excess salivation from reflex irritation of the trigeminal nerve. Neuralgia of the fifth nerve is another cause of hypersalivation. A self-limited type of excessive salivation may occur during pregnancy, usually ending during the second trimester. In this condition, there is almost constant expectoration. A number of gastrointestinal disorders cause increased salivation, but the most frequent one is an ulcer on the posterior wall of the duodenum.

Pseudoptyalism is drooling of saliva from the mouth, simulating hypersalivation. It is attributable to difficulty in swallowing. Swallowing of saliva may be interfered with in acute tonsillitis, mumps, abscesses, and tumors and granulomas of the palate, pharynx, larynx, or esophagus. Inability to swallow may be caused by paralysis of the pharyngeal or facial muscles as in bulbar paralysis, facial paralysis, myasthenia gravis, and paralysis agitans.

Some of the most prominent causes of hypersalivation are illustrated in Fig. 18-21. Epilepsy and rabies have been selected for further discussion.

Rabies (hydrophobia)[67, 127]

Rabies is an infectious disease that affects the nervous system, including the brain and spinal cord. It is caused by a neurotropic virus present in the saliva of infected animals and transmitted usually through a bite; however, infected saliva may occasionally contaminate a wound, but this is rare. It is a disease of all warm-blooded animals, including humans, but principally of such biting animals as dogs, cats, skunks, wildcats, foxes, wolves, and coyotes. Cattle, sheep, horses, and hogs may also contract the disease. During the last

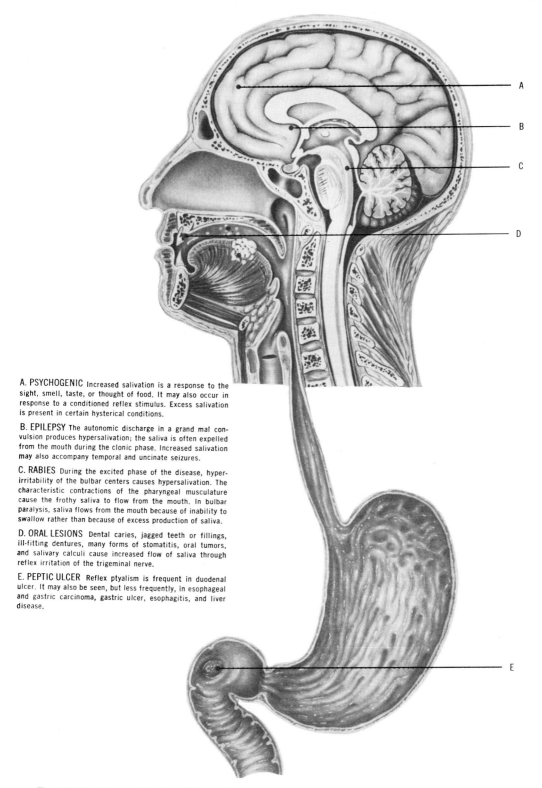

A. PSYCHOGENIC Increased salivation is a response to the sight, smell, taste, or thought of food. It may also occur in response to a conditioned reflex stimulus. Excess salivation is present in certain hysterical conditions.

B. EPILEPSY The autonomic discharge in a grand mal convulsion produces hypersalivation; the saliva is often expelled from the mouth during the clonic phase. Increased salivation may also accompany temporal and uncinate seizures.

C. RABIES During the excited phase of the disease, hyperirritability of the bulbar centers causes hypersalivation. The characteristic contractions of the pharyngeal musculature cause the frothy saliva to flow from the mouth. In bulbar paralysis, saliva flows from the mouth because of inability to swallow rather than because of excess production of saliva.

D. ORAL LESIONS Dental caries, jagged teeth or fillings, ill-fitting dentures, many forms of stomatitis, oral tumors, and salivary calculi cause increased flow of saliva through reflex irritation of the trigeminal nerve.

E. PEPTIC ULCER Reflex ptyalism is frequent in duodenal ulcer. It may also be seen, but less frequently, in esophageal and gastric carcinoma, gastric ulcer, esophagitis, and liver disease.

Fig. 18-21. Hypersalivation. (From Therap. Notes **71**:259, Oct.-Nov., 1964, Parke, Davis & Co.)

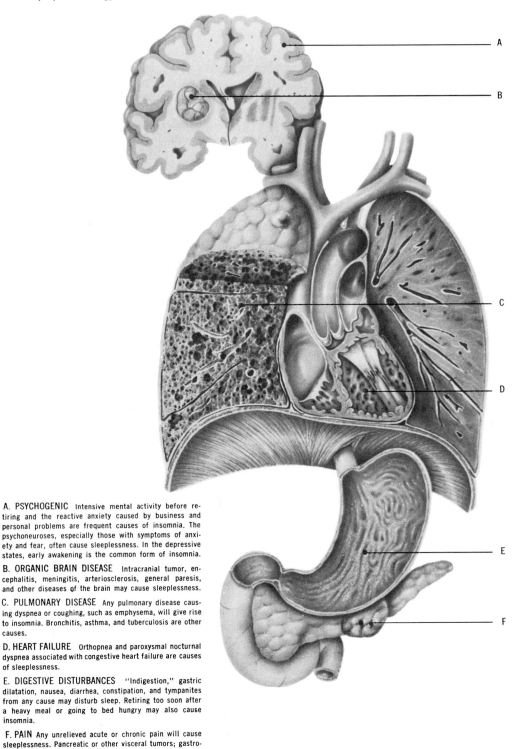

A

B

C

D

E

F

A. PSYCHOGENIC Intensive mental activity before retiring and the reactive anxiety caused by business and
personal problems are frequent causes of insomnia. The
psychoneuroses, especially those with symptoms of anxiety and fear, often cause sleeplessness. In the depressive
states, early awakening is the common form of insomnia.

B. ORGANIC BRAIN DISEASE Intracranial tumor, encephalitis, meningitis, arteriosclerosis, general paresis,
and other diseases of the brain may cause sleeplessness.

C. PULMONARY DISEASE Any pulmonary disease causing dyspnea or coughing, such as emphysema, will give rise
to insomnia. Bronchitis, asthma, and tuberculosis are other
causes.

D. HEART FAILURE Orthopnea and paroxysmal nocturnal
dyspnea associated with congestive heart failure are causes
of sleeplessness.

E. DIGESTIVE DISTURBANCES "Indigestion," gastric
dilatation, nausea, diarrhea, constipation, and tympanites
from any cause may disturb sleep. Retiring too soon after
a heavy meal or going to bed hungry may also cause
insomnia.

F. PAIN Any unrelieved acute or chronic pain will cause
sleeplessness. Pancreatic or other visceral tumors; gastrointestinal disease, such as peptic ulcer or gastritis; and
spinal root or peripheral nerve disease may produce pain
with resulting insomnia.

Fig. 18-22. Insomnia. (From Therap. Notes **71**:293, Nov.-Dec., 1964, Parke, Davis & Co.)

few years a high incidence of rabies has been reported in bats. Rabies is one of the most widespread diseases known, being found all over the world and present in animals during any season of the year.

The virus enters the body usually through the bite of an infected animal and travels along nerves or perineural lymphatics until it reaches the brain and spinal cord, causing an acute encephalomyelitis. The incubation period in humans is from 14 days to a year, with an average of 20 to 60 days. The length of the incubation period is influenced by the location of the bite as well as by the severity of the wound. Bites on the hands, neck, and head are likely to produce symptoms most rapidly.

The characteristic symptoms range from restlessness, irritation, and nervousness in the beginning to delirium and paralysis. Swallowing is difficult and painful. (The disease was originally named hydrophobia because it was observed that rabid dogs feared swallowing water.) Death results from exhaustion and paralysis. Victims of bites by wild or domestic animals should receive immediate medical attention, and Pasteur treatment should be given if it is not known whether the animal was rabid, and if there is reason to believe it was ill with hydrophobia.

Diagnosis is based on presence of Negri bodies (inclusions) in the brain.

INSOMNIA[101]

Insomnia is abnormal wakefulness, either from inability to sleep or from interference with depth and duration of sleep. It may be a symptom of many diseases (Fig. 18-22).

Insomnia is most often the result of functional disturbances that result from faulty habits or hygiene. Conditions that may interfere with sleep are a lighted, noisy, airless, or overheated bedroom; a mattress that is too hard or too soft; insufficient or too many bedclothes; sudden change in daily routine or insufficient daytime activities; overfatigue; stimulating drinks, such as coffee or tea, or drugs ingested before retiring; excessive smoking; sleeping during the day; and stimulating mental work late at night.

Disorders of the nervous system that interfere with sleep are manic depressive illness and involutional depression, often causing insomnia because of early morning awakening and inability to fall asleep again. The sleep rhythm is disturbed in mania, delirium, and in acute confusional states. Schizophrenic hallucinations may also prevent sleep. Children as well as some adults are often awakened by nightmares, which may be triggered by emotional disturbances.

Organic causes of insomnia other than those given in Fig. 18-22, are chronic renal disease, cirrhosis, hypertension, anemia, polycythemia, febrile illnesses and hyperthyroidism. Such symptoms of organic disease as muscular cramps, dysuria, polyuria, polydipsia, urinary retention or frequency, and pain will usually interfere with sleep.

JOINT ENLARGEMENT[12, 102]

Joint enlargement or swelling of a joint may result from a number of conditions, such as accumulation of fluid within the joint space, synovial or capsular thickening, localized periarticular effusion in a tendon sheath or bursa, subcutaneous edema around the joint, bony enlargement, or tumor growths.

Arthritis is a common cause of joint enlargement. It can be produced by any number of infectious agents. In arthritis caused by tuberculosis, usually only one joint is involved, and it occurs most frequently in children. In congenital syphilis a chronic effusion into the knee joint may appear around puberty. In secondary syphilis, transient swelling of joints may occur, and in tertiary syphilis, gummas of the synovial membranes may be a feature. Purulent infections of the joints are commonly caused by hemolytic streptococcus, *Staphylococcus aureus*, pneumococcus, and meningococcus. Gonococcic infections may

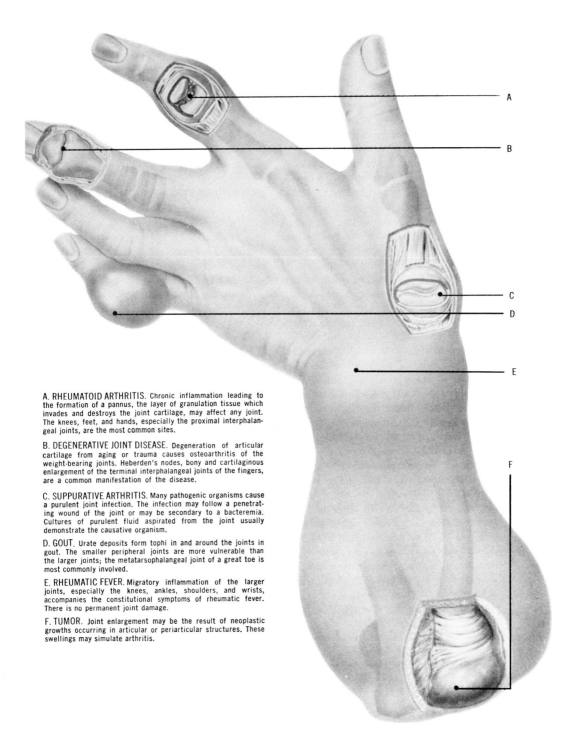

A. RHEUMATOID ARTHRITIS. Chronic inflammation leading to the formation of a pannus, the layer of granulation tissue which invades and destroys the joint cartilage, may affect any joint. The knees, feet, and hands, especially the proximal interphalangeal joints, are the most common sites.

B. DEGENERATIVE JOINT DISEASE. Degeneration of articular cartilage from aging or trauma causes osteoarthritis of the weight-bearing joints. Heberden's nodes, bony and cartilaginous enlargement of the terminal interphalangeal joints of the fingers, are a common manifestation of the disease.

C. SUPPURATIVE ARTHRITIS. Many pathogenic organisms cause a purulent joint infection. The infection may follow a penetrating wound of the joint or may be secondary to a bacteremia. Cultures of purulent fluid aspirated from the joint usually demonstrate the causative organism.

D. GOUT. Urate deposits form tophi in and around the joints in gout. The smaller peripheral joints are more vulnerable than the larger joints; the metatarsophalangeal joint of a great toe is most commonly involved.

E. RHEUMATIC FEVER. Migratory inflammation of the larger joints, especially the knees, ankles, shoulders, and wrists, accompanies the constitutional symptoms of rheumatic fever. There is no permanent joint damage.

F. TUMOR. Joint enlargement may be the result of neoplastic growths occurring in articular or periarticular structures. These swellings may simulate arthritis.

Fig. 18-23. Joint enlargement. (From Therap. Notes **72**:27, Jan.-Feb., 1965, Parke, Davis & Co.)

also involve the joints. Swelling and pain of the joints may occur in brucellosis, mycotic diseases, typhoid fever, rubella, and bacillary dysentery. In rheumatic fever, which often involves the joints of the knee, ankle, shoulder, and wrist, there may be inflammation of the joints. The joint cavities are distended with a turbid yellowish fluid, but there is no permanent joint damage.

The benign neoplasms that cause joint enlargement are the chondromas, chondromyxomas, and xanthomatous giant-cell-tumors. A malignant synovioma may arise from an articular synovial membrane or bursa and cause joint enlargement. Multiple exostoses may also arise from pre-cartilaginous tissue near the joints.

Some of the causes of joint enlargement, such as rheumatoid arthritis, degenerative joint disease, gout, and rheumatic fever, have been selected for discussion as follows. These are illustrated in Fig. 18-23.

Rheumatic fever[2, 57, 66, 78]

The cause of rheumatic fever is unknown, but the attacks are preceded by hemolytic streptococcic infection. This may be in the form of a streptococcic pharyngitis, scarlet fever, otitis media, or some other streptococcic infection without symptoms. Not every person who has a streptococcic infection will develop rheumatic fever, but if it does develop, the symptoms are apparent 2 to 4 weeks after the onset of the infection. Rheumatic heart disease is the result of rheumatic fever, which usually occurs in children between the ages of 5 and 15 years, but it is not limited to this age group. Rheumatic fever is hard to recognize; it mimics many other diseases. It may last for several weeks or many months, and even after it has become inactive, there may be recurrence after another streptococcic infection. The heart can be damaged with each attack. If the heart is affected, its pumping action is weakened, and it becomes enlarged. The inflammation may leave no permanent damage to the child's

heart or one so slight that the child can lead a normal life.

When injury is permanent, the valves of the left side of the heart have been involved in inflammation that after healing left a scar, preventing the proper opening or closing of the valve. Thus there is interference with the normal blood flow.

The symptoms of rheumatic fever are usually joint pains and joint enlargement. There may be failure to gain weight, pallor, poor appetite, fatigue, frequent colds, and pharyngitis or tonsilitis. The joint pains are in the arms and legs and are more likely to occur during the night. There is unusual restlessness, irritability, chorea, St. Vitus dance, and behavior and personality changes. Not all of these symptoms, of course, signify an attack of rheumatic fever, but they could, and, if unrecognized, damage to the heart could result. Rheumatic fever is not a contagious disease, but the streptococci infection that causes it is contagious. Prevention of streptococcic infections is the key to control of rheumatic heart disease.

Arthritis[12, 113]

Arthritis has plagued mankind through the ages. Signs of this bone disease have been found in the bones of the Java Ape Man and the mummies of Egypt. The forms of arthritis are rheumatoid arthritis, osteoarthritis, and fibrositis. No cause for rheumatoid arthritis has been found as yet, but the disease has followed sprains, infections, and joint injury in some cases. Some suspect that the cause is a virus or bacteria; others suspect an allergy. Some believe the nervous system or hormones are involved, and still others think it might be a disorder of the metabolic system. Also there is support for arthritis being an autoimmune disease. Some evidence exists that rheumatoid and gouty arthritis have a familial basis.

Arthritis is the number one crippler at present in the United States, despite new and improved forms of therapy. To date no cure has been found. The disease affects both sexes, young and old.

Rheumatoid arthritis.[12, 113] (See Fig. 18-28, *E*.) Rheumatoid arthritis is known as atrophic arthritis and proliferative arthritis. In the young it is called juvenile rheumatoid arthritis. When the spine is solely or predominantly involved, it is called rheumatoid spondylitis or Strümpell-Marie spondylitis.

Rheumatoid arthritis is a systemic disease characterized by a chronic and progressive inflammatory involvement of the joints and by atrophy of the muscles. About one third of arthritic people have the rheumatoid type; it occurs most frequently in the early decades of adult life. About 80% of the cases begin between the ages of 20 and 50 years, with women being affected three times as often as men.

The onset may be insidious or abrupt and violent. Prodromal symptoms include slight fever, loss of weight, fatigue, and increased sweating of the hands and feet, but these are not always present. Most patients have polyarticular joint involvement that tends to be bilateral and somewhat symmetric in distribution. Early symptoms are pain and stiffness of joints. The joints may also be swollen and the covering skin red with increased warmth. The lining of the joints is inflamed and thickened. The lining may grow into the joint space and fill it, and the cartilage of the bones may become eroded. Swelling in combination with atrophy of muscles gives rise to fusiform or spindle-shaped digits. Small bony spurs may form. The bones may also grow together, and the joint become permanently fused. Probably the most characteristic lesion associated with rheumatoid arthritis is the subcutaneous nodule. These nodules range from pea size to walnut size and appear under the skin covering bony prominences, especially the olecranon process (elbow). A striking feature of the disease is its tendency for exacerbations and remissions. Remissions may occur irregularly and last for months or years at a time.

Osteoarthritis.[12, 113] Osteoarthritis is a degenerative joint disease (Fig. 18-24, *D*). It is far more common than rheumatoid arthritis but, as a rule, less damaging. It seems to result from a combination of aging, irritation of the joints, and normal wear and tear. Joint changes in this disease are found to some degree in all persons beyond the third or fourth decade of life. Chronic irritation of the joints is the main contributing factor, possibly caused by overweight, poor posture, or injury or strain from occupation or recreation.

In osteoarthritis, degeneration is mainly of the joint cartilage. It becomes soft and wears away, often completely, exposing the underlying bone. Thickening of the ends of the bones may also occur. Except when the disease involves the hip joints or knees, serious deformity or crippling does not occur.

The common symptoms include pain, aches, and stiffness of joints. The joints of the fingers and the weight-bearing joints, such as the hips, knees, and feet are mostly affected. Enlargement of the fingers at the last joint often occurs. Nodes, referred to as Heberden's nodes, are permanent but seldom lead to disability.

Gout.[12, 113] Gout, sometimes called gouty arthritis, affects the joints of the feet, especially the big toe. It is regarded as a familial disease of unknown etiology that is associated with altered uric acid metabolism. About 2% to 5% of chronic joint diseases have a gouty component. It occurs predominantly in males at any age and in most instances is characterized by acute recurrent arthritis.

The onset is usually sudden, often with no apparent provocation. Some attacks may follow minor injury, excessive eating or drinking, heavy exercise, or surgical operations. The attacks may last days or weeks, during which time joint inflammation is acute. Between attacks the patient is free from symptoms. The affected joint, usually metatarsal phalangeal, becomes swollen, tender, and red. In some instances it may

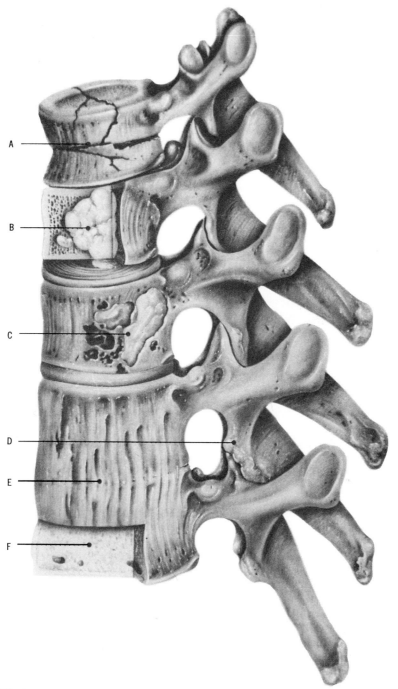

A. CRUSH FRACTURE OF VERTEBRAL BODY If a vertebral fracture is not recognized and treated at time of injury, the cancellous tissue yields to the weight of the trunk, and the injured vertebral body is compressed into a wedge shape, causing eventual appearance of angular kyphosis.

B. SPINAL TUMOR Spinal tumors may be primary or metastatic. Tumors of the breast, prostate, lungs, thyroid, and kidneys especially tend to metastasize to the vertebrae.

C. SPINAL CARIES In caries, the most common cause of angular kyphosis, tenderness of the spine at the level of the deformity may be elicited by percussing the affected vertebrae.

D. OSTEOARTHRITIS Characteristic of advancing age is a diffuse kyphosis caused by osteoarthritic changes taking place in the vertebral bodies.

E. SPONDYLITIS DEFORMANS An inflammatory condition primarily affecting the ligaments and joints of the spine, spondylitis deformans culminates in an ossifying periostitis that immobilizes adjacent vertebrae.

F. PAGET'S DISEASE Kyphosis caused by Paget's disease appears as a uniform curve developing after middle age, usually accompanied by additional evidence of the disease in other parts of the body.

Fig. 18-24. Kyphosis. (From Therap. Notes **71**:29, Jan.-Feb., 1964, Parke, Davis & Co.)

shift from one joint to another, particularly in the young. Uric acid concentrations in the blood are increased and excretion in the urine reduced. Chalky deposits of compounds of uric acid (urates) are found in the soft tissues, such as the lobes of the ears or around the joints. These deposits are called tophi. Eventually, because of the urate deposits, the arthritis becomes chronic. The articular tissues are progressively destroyed by the increasing amounts of urate deposits and by the inflammation that accompanies them. In late stages the tophi may completely destroy the articulation, and the subcutaneous deposits of sodium urate may eat through the covering tissues to permit the extrusion of chalky white, crystalline material from an ulcerated lesion.

Fibrositis.[113] Fibrositis is a common rheumatic condition that does not affect the joints directly. When it occurs within the muscles, it is called myositis, and when it is in the lumbar region and low back, it is referred to as lumbago. There is pain and stiffness or soreness of fibrous tissue, especially in the muscle coverings or sheaths. It is not a progressive or destructive disease, but it may persist for years, or it may disappear spontaneously. The attacks may follow an injury, repeated muscular strain, or prolonged muscular tension.

KYPHOSIS[11, 12, 103]

Kyphosis, a posterior angulation of the spine, is generally associated with severe spinal protrusion and loss of stature. It is also usually associated with scoliosis (lateral curvature of the spine). Kyphosis, in which a limited small portion of the spine is involved, is called angular; when a large portion of the spine or the entire spine is affected, it is called diffuse.

Angular kyphosis is caused by collapse of one or more vertebral bodies, resulting from tuberculosis of vertebral bodies, abnormal spinal growths (primary sarcoma or metastatic carcinoma), crush fracture, or hydatid (cystlike structures) disease of the spine. Caries is a common cause of angular kyphosis. It usually appears in children under 10 years. In healthy adults, angular curvature is usually caused by crush fracture. Angular kyphosis in persons over 50 years is usually the result of malignancy. The metastatic lesions as a rule are from carcinoma of the breast, prostate, lungs, or kidneys.

A primary cause of diffuse kyphosis is weakness of the muscles supporting the trunk, but it may also be caused by diseases of the bones or joints of the spine. These diseases include muscular dystrophy, paralytic poliomyelitis, congenital spastic paralysis, syringomyelia, Friedreich's ataxia, and neurofibromatosis.[71] Neurofibromatosis, also called von Recklinghausen's disease, is an ectodermal congenital defect. It is characterized by multiple tumors of the spinal and cranial nerves and skin and by cutaneous pigmentation. Poor postural tone of spinal muscles in adolescence, if not corrected, causes secondary changes in bones and joints leading to a fixed curve of the spine.

Other causes of diffuse kyphosis include rickets, osteitis deformans or Paget's disease, spondylitis deformans, and osteoarthritis.[11] Spondylitis deformans is an inflammatory condition of the joints and ligaments of the spinal column, usually the result of gonococcal infection, septic foci, and rheumatoid arthritis. Paget's disease of bone[11] is a chronic progressive disease of the bones of unknown etiology, characterized by increased destruction of bone and replacement with abnormal bone, resulting in enlargement and deformity of skeletal bones. The onset is between 50 and 55 years of age, and it is twice as common in males as in females.

In the aged, kyphosis may be caused by osteoarthritis. Kyphoscoliosis is often associated with thoracic diseases such as empyema and pleural retraction, or it may be a congenital malformation.

The major causes of kyphosis are illustrated in Fig. 18-24.

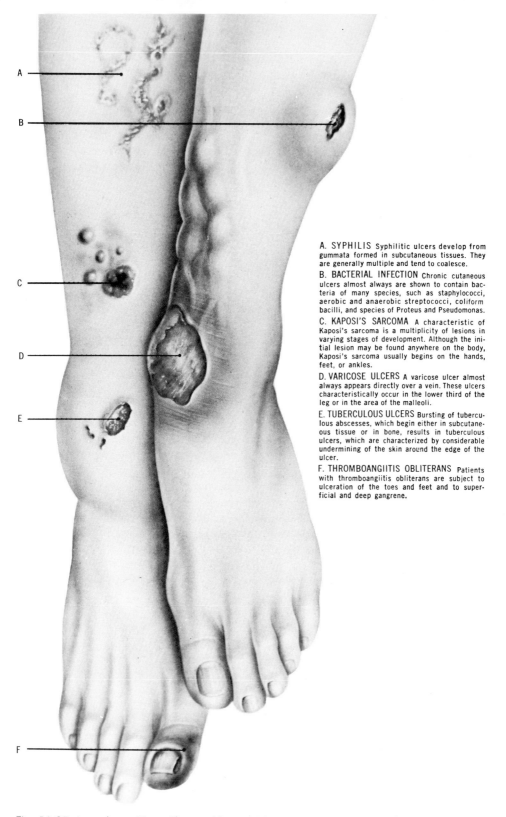

A. SYPHILIS Syphilitic ulcers develop from gummata formed in subcutaneous tissues. They are generally multiple and tend to coalesce.

B. BACTERIAL INFECTION Chronic cutaneous ulcers almost always are shown to contain bacteria of many species, such as staphylococci, aerobic and anaerobic streptococci, coliform bacilli, and species of Proteus and Pseudomonas.

C. KAPOSI'S SARCOMA A characteristic of Kaposi's sarcoma is a multiplicity of lesions in varying stages of development. Although the initial lesion may be found anywhere on the body, Kaposi's sarcoma usually begins on the hands, feet, or ankles.

D. VARICOSE ULCERS A varicose ulcer almost always appears directly over a vein. These ulcers characteristically occur in the lower third of the leg or in the area of the malleoli.

E. TUBERCULOUS ULCERS Bursting of tuberculous abscesses, which begin either in subcutaneous tissue or in bone, results in tuberculous ulcers, which are characterized by considerable undermining of the skin around the edge of the ulcer.

F. THROMBOANGIITIS OBLITERANS Patients with thromboangiitis obliterans are subject to ulceration of the toes and feet and to superficial and deep gangrene.

Fig. 18-25. Leg ulcers. (From Therap. Notes **70**:11, Mar.-Apr., 1963, Parke, Davis & Co.)

LEG ULCERS[104]

Leg ulcers are of four types—noninfective, infective, ulcerating tumors, and ulcers associated with blood disorders (Fig. 18-25).

Noninfective ulcers are those that result from interference with the vitality of the part by injury or circulatory disturbances. Senile ulcers are of this type. They occur on the extremities of persons over 70 years of age from injuries to thin, atrophic skin, or by arteriosclerosis of vessels supplying blood to the skin. Chronic venous insufficiency may result in stasis ulcers. These ulcers are commonly located in the lower extremity on the medial surface of the leg. Ischemic ulcers associated with hypertension are usually low on the lateral or posterior surface of the leg or ankle. Ulcers, usually on the toes, may be caused by arteriosclerosis obliterans, a disease in which there is arteriosclerotic narrowing and obstruction of large and small arteries supplying the lower extremities. Gangrene may develop and necessitate amputation of the affected limb. These ulcers may also develop over the anterior and lateral lower calf. Varicose ulcers usually occur over the affected veins. Ulcers of the toes and feet may be the result of thromboangiitis obliterans (Buerger's disease), an obliterative vascular disease affecting chiefly the peripheral arteries and veins. Ischemic leg ulcers occur in chronic pernio (erythrocyanosis) of the lower part of the leg. These indolent lesions are dull red or violaceous with bleb formation. Perino is seen only in cold, damp climates. Ulcers from frosbite are from freezing of tissue that damages the skin, muscle, blood vessels, and nerves.

Cutaneous ulcers on the lower extremities may result from spirochetal, mycotic, and tuberculosis infections. *Corynebacterium diphtheriae* may gain entrance to the deeper skin structures when the integrity of the epithelium has been destroyed, as in burns and wounds, and cause ulcerative lesions.

Slowly healing, nonvaricose superficial ulcers on the legs of Negroes may indicate sickle cell anemia. Similar ulcers may also be observed in congenital hemolytic jaundice or Cooley's anemia.

Drug eruptions on the lower extremities may develop into ulcerative lesions.

In Kaposi's sarcoma[32] affecting the lower extremities the initial lesions are red to purple skin nodules. They usually affect elderly men, many of whom are of Italian or Jewish descent. Gradually over a prolonged period, nodules develop in internal viscera. The causes of death are intestinal hemorrhage from sarcomatous foci or intercurrent disease.

LOSS OF VISION[32, 134]

There are a number of eye lesions that lead to permanent or partial loss of vision; others may lead to temporary blindness.

Intraocular injuries

Intraocular injuries[32] from blunt instruments or agents, acids and alkalies thrown into the eyes, and deep penetrating foreign bodies may impair vision. Acid burns of the eyes tend to cause an immediate, usually localized and nonprogressive tissue necrosis. Alkalies, such as plaster and lime, cause progressive tissue necrosis. Later, adhesions may form between the areas denuded by the burn. Foreign bodies on the cornea may not cause pain until an ulcer is produced. If they are not over the pupil, there may be no impairment of vision. Foreign bodies, such as metallic objects (iron or steel), may leave a scar when deeply embedded. If located over the pupil, the scar will interfere with vision, the degree of interference depending on the scar's density and breadith.

Corneal scars[32, 134] cause trouble only if they are over the pupil and especially over its center. A *corneal ulcer*[32] is a localized necrosis of corneal epithelium, usually caused by an infection following trauma to the cornea or by spread of infection from the conjunctiva or an infected lacrimal sac.

In severe progressive corneal ulcers, known as serpent ulcers, pus collects in the bottom of the anterior chamber (hypopyon). Complications of a corneal ulcer are iritis, cyclitis, purulent iridocyclitis, and loss of the eye. The defect left by the ulcer fills with fibrous tissue devoid of transparency. In erythema multiforme, an acute inflammatory systemic disease characterized by skin or mucous membrane lesions, scarring of the cornea may cause partial or complete loss of vision.

When corneal diseases or injuries are not treated promptly, impaired vision or blindness may result from the cornea becoming scarred or opaque, blocking the passage of light.[119] In many cases the sight lost by corneal disease or damage is restored by a corneal transplantation. The corneal transplants are the most successful of all organ transplant surgery. Until recently, fresh tissue was necessary for about one half of corneal transplants. Now, however, corneas can be frozen and preserved for indefinite periods of time.[119] Despite the high rate of successful corneal transplants, the body still rejects some grafts. In diseases where blood vessels infiltrate the cornea and circulating antibodies are introduced, transplants are usually rejected.[119] Donor corneas are obtained posthumously from people who have willed their eyes for this purpose.

Inflammation

Inflammation of the eye is one of the most frequent causes of disability, and the most common lesions are *iridocyclitis* with hypopyon and *iritis*.[32, 134] Inflammation of the iris (iritis) may be acute or recurrent or chronic. When the ciliary body is involved, it is usually known as iridocyclitis. The principal symptoms are pain and blurring of vision. The pain is localized in the temporal area of the affected eye. The blurring of vision may be caused by inability to focus because of spasm of the ciliary body, edema of the cornea, edema of the retina if the posterior

eye becomes involved, and fibrin in the anterior chamber. Secondary glaucoma can occur. When the aqueous humor cannot pass into the anterior chamber, the iris balloons forward like a doughnut around the pupil. Vision is destroyed unless an artificial pupil is created to allow free flow of aqueous humor from the posterior chamber to the anterior chamber.[32]

Complications of inflammatory ocular lesions may lead to blindness. In the acute suppurative and granulomatous forms of inflammation, necrosis of the retina and choroid may occur, leading to permanent scarring and loss of function of these tissues. If the macula or all of the retina is involved, severe impairment of vision will occur. Acute inflammations follow penetrating or perforating wounds of the globe. Bacteria and fungi may be introduced into the eye and cause endophthalmitis (inflammation within the eye) or panophthalmitis (inflammation of all ocular structures).[134] Fungi may be introduced into the eye from vegetation or soil through a scratch in the cornea or penetration of the vitreous body.[134] Endogenous suppurative inflammations may occur through spread by the bloodstream of primary bacterial or mycotic infections elsewhere in the body or through extension by way of the optic nerve or subarachnoid fluid of an intracranial infection. In destruction of intraocular tissues, there is severe scarring and gliosis, and disorganization of the internal architecture of the globe. With marked depletion of aqueous humor the eye becomes soft, atrophic, and shrunken. This advanced degeneration and disorganization of the entire eyeball is called *phthisis bulbi*.[134] Malignant melanomas sometimes occur in phthisical eyes.

Trachoma and *inclusion conjunctivitis*[42] are chronic infections of the eye and genital tract, caused by agents of the psittacosis-lymphogranuloma venereum-trachoma group. They were formerly considered to be viruses, but are now called *chlamydiae* (parasites). The infection may be mild and self-limited, but it may also be severe and cause blindness. Trachoma in children and adults begins as a follicular conjunctivitis but progresses to evolve into a dense fibrovascular pannus that extends over part or all of the cornea, impairing vision. Inclusion conjunctivitis of the newborn begins as an acute purulent conjunctivitis with little involvement of the cornea, and it eventually heals without corneal scars and with minimal, if any, pannus. In adults, inclusion conjunctivitis may progress to a limited pannus and a few scars of the conjunctiva and cornea. Trachoma infection is prevalent in Africa and Asia and occurs mainly where there is a shortage of water and poor hygienic conditions. There is widespread blindness in these countries. In parts of the United States, particularly Indian reservations of the Southwest, endemic trachomatous infection is relatively common, but it rarely leads to major visual impairment.

Optic neuritis and *retrobulbar neuritis* may be responsible for sudden loss of vision.[32] This condition is caused by infection or hyperemia or by trauma. Vision is decreased, and a complication may be central vision loss.

Keratitis may be syphilitic or caused by tuberculosis and possibly by influenza or herpes zoster. There is local pain, lacrimation, and photophobia, and vision may be permanently impaired. Congenital infection of the fetus occurs with maternal infection with German measles, and the eye stigmas of the infection in the newborn are cataracts, glaucoma, and microphthalmia.

Chronic nongranulomatous inflammatory processes[134] may cause a leakage of plasma proteins, accumulation of inflammatory cells in the aqueous or vitreous humor, opacification of the cornea, adherence of the iris to the lens or cornea, formation of cataracts, chorioretinal degeneration, and optic atrophy. Glaucoma may develop.

Glaucoma

In glaucoma[6, 32, 47, 114, 134] the aqueous humor accumulates within the eye, creating intraocular pressure. Glaucoma may be acute, subacute, or chronic, primary, or

A   B

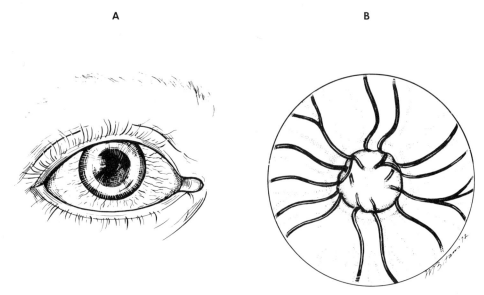

Fig. 18-26. A, Acute glaucoma, showing pupillary dilatation, ciliary injection, and a steamy cornea. **B,** Glaucomatous changes in the optic cup. Note the temporal retinal vessels bend sharply into the cup.

secondary to another condition such as intraocular tumor, iritis, or choroiditis. Most cases of glaucoma are of the chronic type.

Acute glaucoma is caused by an acute obstruction of the anterior chamber angle of the eye or angle between the root of the iris and cornea through which the aqueous humor drains back into the circulation. If the obstruction is unrelieved, vision will be lost. The initial symptoms and signs are excruciating pain, nausea, vomiting, and the seeing of halos around lights. On examination the affected eye may have a stony hardness as compared with a normal eye. There is also dilatation of the pupil, congestion of the globe, and haziness and steaminess of the cornea (Fig. 18-26). Tonometry is used to determine the intraocular pressure. Gonioscopy is used to look directly into the angle of the anterior chamber to determine whether the angle is normally open or if it is closed.

Chronic forms of glaucoma are divided into those with an open or wide anterior chamber angle and those in which the angle is closed or narrow. Open angle glaucoma is caused by some failure in the facility of outflow of aqueous humor, which may be the result of some defect in the trabeculae of the anterior chamber. It is rarely associated with acute attacks or with definitive symptoms, but it is a chronic, slowly progressive disease. The patient may complain of vague headaches, and his glasses may require changing. Since there are no danger signals at all, the eyes may go unchecked until the disease has caused much loss of vision, which prompts the victim to consult an ophthalmologist. The eye chart is not helpful in establishing the diagnosis, since central vision is preserved until late in the disease. The elevation of the intraocular pressure is measured by a tonometer. Eventually if this type of glaucoma is untreated, and possibly even when treated, excavation of the optic nerve occurs with loss of visual field and vision.

Closed angle glaucoma (narrow angle) occurs in intermittent attacks during which the angle is closed. The attacks may be brief and clear spontaneously. But each attack tends to produce adhesions in the anterior chamber angle. Eventually the angle will be either partially or completely closed.

About 20% of glaucoma cases are of the secondary type. These are the result of trauma, tumor, inflammation, or hemorrhage.

Cataracts

A cataract[32, 134] is opacification of the lens. Those present at birth are the result of rubella (German measles) acquired in utero or are associated with other malformations caused by chromosomal abnormalities. After birth, cataracts may be acquired as the result of ocular trauma, malignant melanoma of the uvea, diabetes, or as a complication of some other primary ocular or systemic disease, such as ocular inflammation. Senile cataracts are manifestations of aging. Chemical intoxication from some drugs may also cause cataracts. A morgagnian cataract is a hypermature senile cataract. In these cataracts the lens epithelium is necrotic and the lens shrinks.

The gradually progressive opacities can occur in the cortex, subcapsular area, and in the nucleus. At one time operations were not performed for removal of the cataract or cataracts until the breakdown of cortical material was complete, causing the area to appear white. Surgery is now performed when the patient no longer has useful vision.

Retinopathy

One of the leading causes of new cases of blindness in the United States among adults is *diabetic retinopathy*.[134] It is the most dreaded of all vascular complications in diabetics. It tends to develop in diabetics who have had diabetes for a period of 15 to 20 years, and those who have had diabetes in childhood are more vulnerable. It is characterized by retinal ischemia, hemorrhages, and exudation in the retina.

There are microinfarcts, proliferation of new vessels and connective tissue on the retinal surface, and occasionally retinal detachment.

In chronic renal failure the important eye change is *hypertensive retinopathy.*[32, 134] If papilledema is present, visual acuity is impaired and scotomas corresponding to large hemorrhages may be noted. Ocular manifestations usually clear when the hypertension is controlled. Vision usually returns to normal, but in some patients there may be permanent loss of visual acuity and also optic atrophy.

Sudden loss of vision[32] unaccompanied by pain is nearly always caused by an occlusion of the central retinal artery or occlusion of the central retinal vein. In arterial occlusion the retina is usually edematous and nonhemorrhagic. In venous occlusion involving the central retinal vein, a hemorrhagic retinitis is produced with blood and transudate covering the entire retina.

Another cause of sudden loss of vision is *retinal detachment.*[32, 134] However, the loss of vision usually requires several hours to a few days to develop. There may or may not be a history of injury. Retinal detachment occurs as a result of pathologic conditions in the vitreous or in the anterior segment of the eye, such as abscesses and hemorrhages in the vitreous, accidental trauma, complications of intraocular surgery, inflammations or tumors of the choroid, and passage of liquefied vitreous or aqueous humor, or both, through a hole in the retina. In retinal detachment the sensory retina is separated from its normal position adjacent to the retinal pigment epithelium. The first symptoms are the seeing of scintillating flashes or stars out of one corner of the eye, followed later by a curtain moving across the eye and still later by a progressive and marked loss of vision.

In *retinal* and *vitreous hemorrhage,* blood will soak into the vitreous from a huge retinal hemorrhage, completely obscuring retinal details.[126] Vision is destroyed until the hemorrhage is absorbed or removed.

In *syphilitic retinitis* secondary to congenital or acquired syphilis, central vision may be defective.

MUSCULAR WEAKNESS[18, 105]

Muscular weakness or loss of muscular strength can be mild and generalized, as occurs in patients who have been bedridden for some time, or can be severe and involve a group of muscles, as is seen in palsy or paralysis. It can also be persistent or episodic.

The term "asthenia" is applied to generalized muscular weakness, usually occurring in the elderly or in those confined to bed because of surgical procedures, chronic diseases, or psychiatric disorders. It is less common but more serious than malaise or lassitude. It is never psychogenic as in fatigue or weariness. Generalized weakness may be caused by severe anemia, nutritional deficiencies, chronic infection, endocrine disorders, or diffuse disorders of the motor system. Episodic or recurrent generalized muscular weakness is associated with a number of conditions, including hypoglycemia, orthostatic hypotension, anxiety attacks with hyperventilation, cerebral ischemia, hyperaldosteronism, and familial periodic paralysis.

Motor paralysis restricted to a part or parts of the body is caused by organic disease of muscle or nerve tissue.[18] Muscular weakness from motor paralysis may be the result of disease of the upper motor neuron, the lower motor neuron, or the muscle itself. Hemiplegia (p. 330) is an example of a lesion in the upper motor neuron, commonly in the internal capsule.

A group of biochemical disturbances often produce profound weakness in certain muscle groups rather than generalized loss of motor power. Myotonia congenita, myasthenia gravis, tetanus, tetany, botulism, thyrotoxic myopathy, and disorders of potassium, sodium, calcium, and magnesium metabolism are representative diseases of biochemical disturbances.

Lower motor neuron lesions include pro-

A. HEMIPLEGIA Hemiplegia, or loss of strength on one side of the body, is the most common distribution of paralysis. Hemiplegia is a sign of an upper motor neuron lesion and is caused by damage to the corticospinal tract.

B. MUSCULAR DYSTROPHIES Muscular atrophy caused by primary changes in the muscles themselves is known as muscular dystrophy. Muscular dystrophies are familial and usually appear in childhood. Enlarged calf muscles may be the first sign of the pseudohypertrophic type.

C. SYRINGOMYELIA Weakness, muscle wasting, and sensory abnormalities are among the typical findings in syringomyelia. The condition is characterized by cavity formation in the spinal cord or medulla, and is considered to be a developmental disorder.

D. AMYOTROPHIC LATERAL SCLEROSIS The most common form is one of wasting of the small muscles of the hands, causing weakness and deformities such as clawhand. Lesions are found in both upper and lower motor neurons.

E. MYASTHENIA GRAVIS Weakness and fatigability of facial, oculomotor, laryngeal, pharyngeal, and respiratory muscles that improve with rest are characteristic of myasthenia gravis. In this disease, there is a specific functional abnormality at the myoneural junction. Relief of symptoms by administration of neostigmine is diagnostic.

F. POLIOMYELITIS Acute anterior poliomyelitis is one of the most frequently found types of acute spinal muscular atrophy in a limb. The lesion occurs in the ventral-horn cell of the lower motor neuron and is of viral origin.

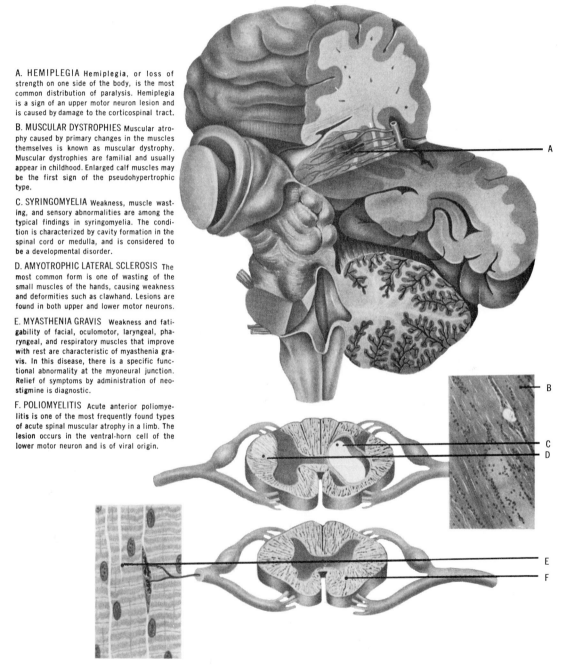

Fig. 18-27. Muscular weakness. (From Therap. Notes **69**:259, Sept.-Oct., 1962, Parke, Davis & Co.)

gressive muscular dystrophy (Chapter 16), poliomyelitis (discussed below), and peripheral neuropathies. These lesions produce severe atrophy of the muscles supplied by the involved nerve, resulting in flaccid muscles and at times fascicular twitching.

The major lesions that produce muscular weakness are illustrated in Fig. 18-27. Myasthenia gravis (MG) and poliomyelitis have been selected for discussion.

Myasthenia gravis (MG)[117]

Myasthenia gravis or MG is a neuromuscular disease affecting the voluntary muscles with weakness and abnormal fatigue. Any muscle may be affected but those most frequently involved are muscles of the eyes, face, lips, tongue, throat, and neck.

MG is a relatively common disease, affecting about 30,000 people in the United States at the present time. It rarely occurs before the age of 10 or after 60 years, being most common between 10 and 40 years of age.[117]

The cause of myasthenia gravis is still unknown, but a metabolic, endocrine, or an immunologic disorder is suspected. A defect in the transmission of the nerve impulse at the point where the nerve ends in the muscle is thought to be the cause. The muscles and nerves in most cases are normal, the only trouble being at their junction. Normally, nerve impulses liberate a chemical—acetylcholine—at the junction, which stimulates the muscle to contract. There is either an insufficient amount of this element or some substance blocks the action, resulting in muscle weakness. Abnormalities in the thymus gland are often found associated with MG, but the direct relationship between the disorder and this finding is still unknown. There is no evidence that the disease is inherited but offspring of a myasthenic mother may have the disease. This condition in the infant may persist a few weeks but responds to treatment or spontaneously disappears. The symptoms of MG may be sudden with extensive paralysis, but often they are slight in early stages and progress gradually. Weakness is the most frequent symptom. It is greatest after exercise or at the end of the day. Weakness of the eye muscles causes ptosis (drooping eyelids), and double vision (diplopia) in one or both eyes is often the first sign. This condition improves in the morning after rest and is worse in the afternoon or evening. The muscles involved in the early stages, other than eye muscles, are those that are used in talking, swallowing, and chewing. The voice may become nasal and tends to fade until almost inaudible during a conversation. Proper chewing is difficult because of weakened muscles. Liquids may get into nasal passages, and food may stick in the throat. Arms and legs may weaken and tire abnormally as the disease progresses. In a crisis or during an attack even the muscles of respiration may fail to function. The normal course of the disease is punctuated with a number of remissions and recurrences. Some mild cases may recover completely.

Diagnostic drugs, electromyography, x-ray studies, and immunologic studies are used to identify the disorder and chart the proper treatment. Over half of the patients today can lead normal and useful lives because of the proper administration of drugs.[117]

Poliomyelitis[17, 67, 128]

Poliomyelitis is also called infantile paralysis, chiefly because it occurs most often in young children. It has been attributed to the enterovirus class. Adults are relatively immune, which is believed to be because of a mild or atypical and unrecognized infection in earlier life. Infants under 1 year rarely contract the infection. Poliomyelitis occurs in endemic or epidemic form in the late summer and autumn, but sporadic cases occur throughout the year. Convalescents and healthy individuals may be carriers. The mode of transmission is believed to be the gastrointestinal tract, as in typhoid fever. In monkeys given intranasal injections the virus reached the brain by the olfactory nerves. This route of infection in humans apparently is rarely if ever followed. The gastrointestinal tract has been found to contain a high concentration of the virus, and it has been isolated from sewage and flies.

Clinical symptoms vary. In the first 1 to 3 days in most cases there is fever, headache, sore throat, drowsiness, irritability, gastrointestinal disturbances, and a stiff neck. Paralysis may or may not occur as a result of damage to the anterior horn cells. In bulbar poliomyelitis the cranial nerves are involved, and respiratory and circulatory distress occur. Respiratory paralysis is the usual cause of death. Involvement of the cerebrum and cerebellum is also occasionally seen. Nonparalytic types are called abortive, and these are more common than the paralytic type. They simulate gastrointestinal or respiratory infections from other causes. Some residual paralyses respond to physiotherapy, but others are apt to be crippling. One attack usually confers immunity; second attacks are rare. The incidence of this disease has decreased markedly since the advent of vaccines for prevention.

NUCHAL RIGIDITY[106]

The principal causes of nuchal rigidity or stiffness of the neck are meningitis, subarachnoid hemorrhage, meningeal carcinomatosis, pressure cones created by space-occupying intracranial lesions, and diseases of the cervical spine or paraspinal tissue.

The intracranial causes include meningism, meningitis, poliomyelitis, subarachnoid hemorrhage, and pressure cones at the tentorial hiatus and foramen magnum, arising as a result of space-occupying lesions. These lesions include tumor, abscess, hematoma, internal hydrocephalus, and cerebral edema caused by vascular lesions. The meninges may also be invaded by carcinomatosis or sarcoidosis, causing a stiff neck.

There are a number of cervical or para-spinal causes of a stiff neck. The most common one is a whiplash injury produced by a sudden snapping of the head and neck, usually occurring in a rear-end automobile collision. A fracture or dislocation of the cervical spinous process may occur. In such accidents, there are ligamentous or capsular sprains, subluxations, anterioposterior narrowing of the intervertebral canals, and subsequent irritation of nerve roots. Neck pain and stiffness may also be the result of spasm of the anterior scalenus muscle, with or without associated cervical rib. A persistent acute stiff neck after a minor sprain, especially in elderly people, may be from vertebral lipping or a degenerative disc lesion. Enlarged cervical nodes following tonsillitis or severe nasopharyngitis, especially in children, may be associated with an acute stiff neck.

Spasm of the neck muscles may occur from muscular fatigue, ligamentous strain, postural defects, anomalies of development, and ruptured disc, and any of these conditions may develop into chronic stiffness of the neck. Degenerative arthritis of the lateral articulations and osteophytic changes of the vertebral ligaments are other causes of nuchal rigidity.[12]

The principal causes of nuchal rigidity are illustrated in Fig. 18-28, and most of these have been described elsewhere.

PALLOR[54, 107]

Although pallor, a pale color of the skin and mucous membranes, is usually associated with anemic states, it can also be seen in a variety of other conditions and in healthy persons as well.

Pallor is a symptom of anemia. The red blood cells are responsible for imparting color to the skin, and consequently any disorder of disease that interferes with the production of red blood cells is likely to cause pallor. Acute blood loss, as in hemorrhage, causes pallor through compensatory vasoconstriction. Pallor may be caused by chronic blood loss from pelvic organs in women or from the gastrointestinal tract in

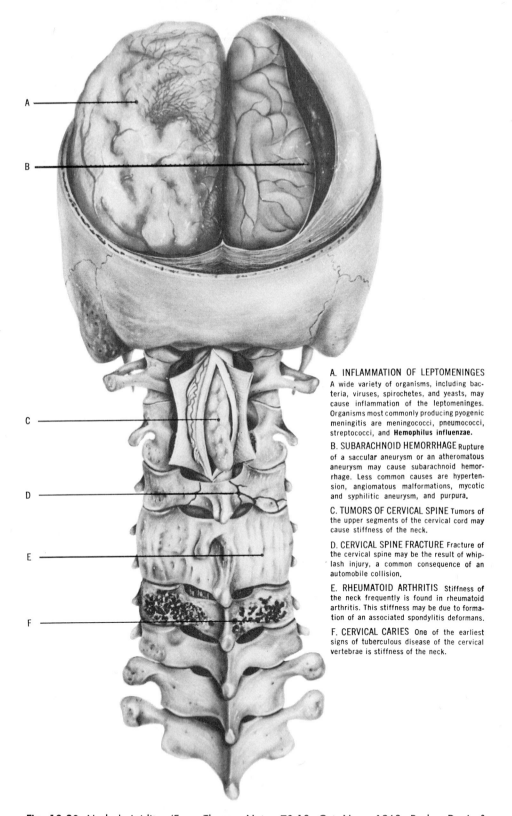

A. INFLAMMATION OF LEPTOMENINGES
A wide variety of organisms, including bacteria, viruses, spirochetes, and yeasts, may cause inflammation of the leptomeninges. Organisms most commonly producing pyogenic meningitis are meningococci, pneumococci, streptococci, and **Hemophilus influenzae.**

B. SUBARACHNOID HEMORRHAGE Rupture of a saccular aneurysm or an atheromatous aneurysm may cause subarachnoid hemorrhage. Less common causes are hypertension, angiomatous malformations, mycotic and syphilitic aneurysm, and purpura.

C. TUMORS OF CERVICAL SPINE Tumors of the upper segments of the cervical cord may cause stiffness of the neck.

D. CERVICAL SPINE FRACTURE Fracture of the cervical spine may be the result of whiplash injury, a common consequence of an automobile collision.

E. RHEUMATOID ARTHRITIS Stiffness of the neck frequently is found in rheumatoid arthritis. This stiffness may be due to formation of an associated spondylitis deformans.

F. CERVICAL CARIES One of the earliest signs of tuberculous disease of the cervical vertebrae is stiffness of the neck.

Fig. 18-28. Nuchal rigidity. (From Therap. Notes **70:**13, Oct.-Nov., 1963, Parke, Davis & Co.)

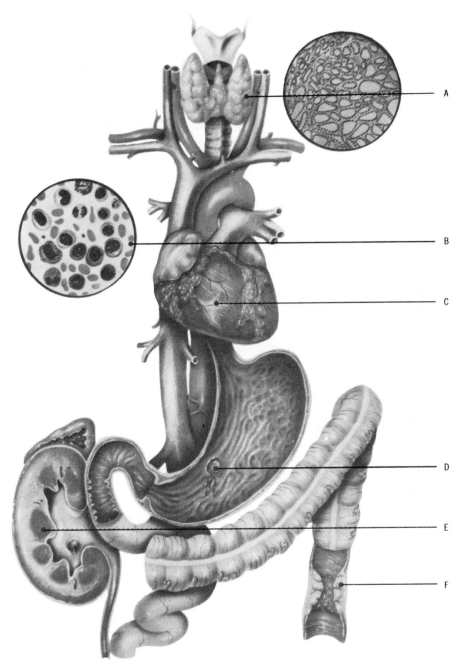

A. HYPOTHYROIDISM A pallid, often yellowish complexion is seen in myxedema. Pallor may be intensified by anemia, which frequently complicates the disease.

B. ANEMIA Insufficient quality or quantity of hemoglobin causes pallor. Decreased production (bone marrow smear, above) or increased destruction of red blood cells may be the cause.

C. CARDIOVASCULAR DISORDERS Vasoconstriction following the lowered blood pressure of an anginal attack or myocardial infarction produces blanching of the skin.

D. ACUTE HEMORRHAGE Profound pallor and symptoms of shock are seen in response to an episode of massive bleeding. The most common cause of massive gastrointestinal hemorrhage is peptic ulcer.

E. RENAL DISEASE Pallor may be apparent in the nephrotic states before the development of anemia.

F. CHRONIC BLOOD LOSS Carcinoma, parasitic infestations, diverticuli, and granulomatous lesions may lead to a hypochromic microcytic type of anemia.

Fig. 18-29. Pallor. (From Therap. Notes **71:**161, May-June, 1964, Parke, Davis & Co.)

both sexes. Most of the infections and systemic diseases produce anemias of the normochromic normocytic type, and pallor is a feature. Anemias resulting from a combination of decreased erythropoiesis (production of red blood cells) and increased destruction of red blood cells by extracorpuscular hemolysis are present in hepatic disease, malnutrition, rheumatoid arthritis, endocrine deficiencies, renal disease, malignancy, and some infections. Icterus, however, is not usually present, since the hemolysis is not generally severe. The anemias associated with severe red blood cell destruction include congenital hemolytic anemia, sickle cell anemia, thalassemia, and acquired hemolytic anemia. Jaundice in these conditions may mask the pallor. Pallor with icterus occurs in some infections, in severe burns, and after ingestion of various drugs and chemicals. In these conditions, destruction of red blood cells is extensive. Pallor in pernicious anemia has a characteristic lemon yellow color.

Pallor also occurs in a number of nonanemic states. The urban dweller may have a pale sallow complexion. A markedly pale complexion may be seen in elderly persons who have occlusion of superficial capillaries in arteriosclerosis. A pallid appearance of the skin is present in such skin diseases as scleroderma. An ashen gray pallor occurs in lead poisoning.

Anxiety states may produce a pallor that is mistaken for anemia. Blanching of the skin occurs in lowered blood pressure in anginal attacks or myocardial infarction. Peripheral vascular disease is characterized by a localized pallor.

Causes of pallor are illustrated in Fig. 18-29. Some of these have been discussed elsewhere.

PARESTHESIA[108]

Paresthesias are abnormal and inappropriate sensations evoked by a normal stimulus, as in tingling of the skin when it is touched lightly, or sensations of tingling described as "pins and needles" or numbness, coldness, or a feeling like small insects are crawling over the skin. Either the central or peripheral sensory system is involved when there is paresthesia (Fig. 18-30).

Psychoneurotics may complain of a variety of sensory disturbances, such as creeping sensations in the skin or bursting sensations.

Central sensory causes of paresthesia include disease of the brainstem, the lateral nucleus of the thalamus, and the sensory cortex.[18] In sensory jacksonian seizure (see epilepsy) the tingling is followed by numbness, proceeding rapidly from the fingers to the shoulders, then to the face, and finally to the leg on the affected side. The aura of migraine headaches is sometimes described as an unpleasant tickling or tingling sensation progressing slowly from hand to face. In multiple sclerosis (p. 305), paresthesias in the extremities may be a presenting symptom, and in tabes dorsalis (neurosyphilis) they may be an early symptom. In pernicious anemia the paresthesia is described as a sensation of "pins and needles" in the hands and feet, and it may be accompanied by signs and symptoms of extensive peripheral nerve and spinal cord degeneration. As pernicious anemia progresses, the paresthesias extend upward to symmetrically involve the distal two thirds of the extremities. Paresthesia may also accompany microcytic hypochromic anemia. In tumors of the cauda equina there may be tingling of the feet or the saddle area of the buttocks. In pressure on the spinal cord the sensations appear early and are described as intense cold, deadness, and numbness of the legs. About one half of the patients with amyotrophic lateral sclerosis have pain and paresthesia in the extremities.[71] In this disease, which is a chronic progressive disease of the nervous system of unknown etiology, there is degeneration of motor neurons in the spinal cord and the lower brainstem, with the clinical manifestation of disturbance in motility. It is a disease of later life, with a

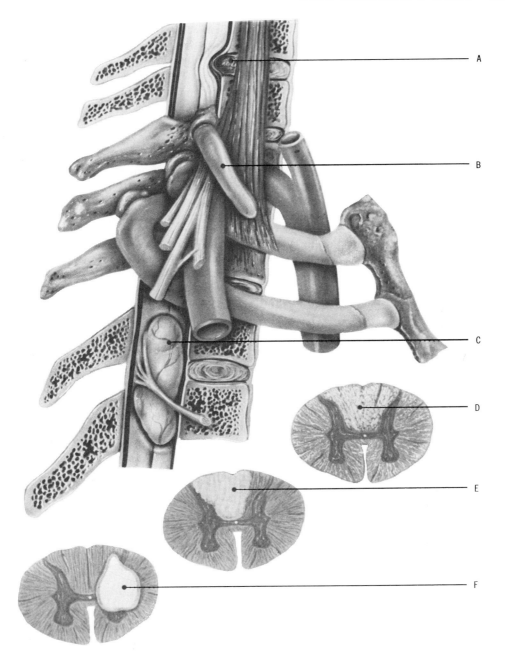

A. INTERVERTEBRAL DISC Lesions of sensory nerves and of posterior roots give rise to paresthesias within the area they supply. The location of paresthesia is of great value in determining the level of a herniated intervertebral disc.

B. SCALENUS ANTICUS SYNDROME Paresthesias are common symptoms in cervicodorsal outlet syndromes. The paresthesias may involve the whole hand but more frequently are confined to the ulnar half and the corresponding portion of the forearm.

C. MENINGIOMA Pressure on the spinal cord, by lesions such as meningiomas, may produce paresthesias in the form of feelings of intense cold, deadness, or numbness.

D. TABES DORSALIS Paresthesias occur in approximately 25 per cent of cases of tabetic neurosyphilis. The feeling of constriction or girdle sensation of tabes dorsalis is a classic example of paresthesia.

E. MULTIPLE SCLEROSIS Presenting symptoms in the spinal form of multiple sclerosis are usually paresthesias in the extremities accompanied by weakness or awkwardness. Their intensity may vary from day to day or shift from one extremity to another.

F. SYRINGOMYELIA Intramedullary lesions, including syringomyelia, disseminated sclerosis, and tumors, may give rise to paresthesias.

Fig. 18-30. Paresthesia. (From Therap. Notes **71**:193, July-Aug., 1964, Parke, Davis & Co.)

peak incidence in the fifth and sixth decades. Twitchings (fasciculations) are widely distributed in muscles. The distal muscles of the upper limb are most often affected, and they have the appearance of wasting. As the disease progresses, proximal and trunk muscles become involved. Less commonly, progressive bulbar palsy occurs, with muscles of the palate, pharynx, and tongue most often affected. In this disease two signs are the "simian hand" (thumb falling into the plane of the palm of the hand from involvement of lateral and medial thenar groups leading to the thumb) and the footdrop caused by involvement of motor units in the leg. Death usually occurs within 3 to 4 years after onset of the symptoms. The terminal event is usually bronchopneumonia, caused by inability to handle secretions because of weakness of respiratory muscles.

When peripheral nerves are stretched or subjected to pressure, transient paresthesias occur. Ischemia of the peripheral nerves produces paresthesia over the affected limb in vascular lesions, such as Raynaud's syndrome, Buerger's disease, atheroma with thrombosis, and costoclavicular compression of the subclavian artery. Paresthesia is an early symptom of peripheral neuropathy caused by diabetes or alcoholism.

SEIZURES[7, 10, 30, 49, 100, 121]

Seizures are symptom complexes encompassing the epilepsies. Seizures may be convulsive with loss of consciousness or nonconvulsive with only slight changes in consciousness.

The term "epilepsy" comes from a Greek word meaning a condition of seizure.[47] In ancient times people afflicted with epilepsy were believed to be under the influence of evil spirits or "possessed." It was not until about the mid-nineteenth century that epilepsy received medical and humanistic consideration. However, many misguided and uninformed people still persist in thinking of epilepsy as a social stigma. According to one authority, epilepsy is the only common disorder "where the sufferer is more handicapped by the attitude of society than by his disability."[116] Persons who become seizure free under the new medications and those having only infrequent seizures are capable of physical and mental activity of a normal person, provided mental capacity is not impaired from other reasons. Many epileptics have normal or above normal intelligence. Indeed, some famous people in history have been victims of epilepsy. They include leaders, such as Julius Caesar, Alexander the Great, Napoleon, and William Pitt; writers such as Lord Byron and Dostoevski; the artist van Gogh; and the composer Handel.[121]

It is estimated that there are 1 to 2 million persons or more in the United States who have epilepsy.[121] There are many hidden cases, however, who are never brought to medical attention and hence cannot be counted.

Epilepsy is a condition in which there are aberrant electric discharges in the brain; it is characterized by disturbances of consciousness and in some types by seizures. The seizure is the sign of abnormal release of energy within the brain. The brain has millions of neurons that control or direct whatever we do. These neurons build up their supply of electricity or energy through chemical actions. When the nerve cells become overactive and discharge irregularly, the disturbance can spread from a focal area to neighboring or even to distant areas in the brain. This spread of disturbance over areas of the brain causes the epileptic seizure.[49, 121]

There are a number of disorders or conditions in the brain that can irritate the nerve cells, causing them to abnormally discharge and disturb brain wave patterns. Any damage to the brain may result in seizures. This damage may be from congenital malformations, induced chromosomally or otherwise, and include microgyria (abnormally small, malformed convolutions of the brain), porencephaly (presence of cavities in the brain), and hemangiomas. Perinatal difficulties that cause birth trauma and asphyxia resulting in cerebral damage may later be manifested as epilepsy. Multiple cerebral abnormalities may also be caused by maternal infection with rubella and toxemia of pregnancy. These structural abnormalities may later be associated with seizures.

Meningitis, encephalitis, and brain abscesses may also be the cause of seizures during the course of the infection or later when healing produces cerebral scars. Cerebral neurosyphilis is often associated with seizures. Seizures may also be associated with cysticercosis and schistosomiasis in highly endemic areas. In infants and young children, nonspecific infections that are not from direct infection of the nervous system are commonly accompanied by febrile convulsions (convulsions from high rise in temperature). Later these children may develop epilepsy in the absence of fever.

Head injury is a major cause of acquired epilepsy. The penetrating missile wounds of the head are accompanied by epilepsy in about 40% of the patients,[121] but only about 10% of the patients with blunt injuries of the head develop epilepsy. Depressed skull fracture is associated with epilepsy in about 30% of the cases, particularly if brain damage is severe. The convulsive seizures following head injuries occur within the first week after injury in almost all cases. These seizures are typically focal motor in type and may not recur. Seizures that develop after the first week of head injury are prone to recur and may be persistent.

Between 30% and 40% of all patients with brain tumors are subject to seizures, and in many cases a seizure is the first symptom of the tumor. The brain tumors most often implicated are astrocytomas, meningiomas, and metastatic lesions.

Cerebral vascular disease is a rather common cause of seizures, especially in the older age groups. They result from localized vascular ischemia and secondary ischemic hypoxia, or they may be the result of residual scars following embolism, thrombosis, or hemorrhage of cerebral vessels. Loss of consciousness caused by diminished cerebral blood flow may progress to seizures. The small vascular lesions involving the brain in some collagen disorders, such as systemic lupus erythematosus and periarteritis nodosa, are other causes of seizures.

A significant number of seizures occur in several generalized cerebral degenerative and demyelinating diseases, such as multiple sclerosis, Alzheimer-Pick dementia, tuberous sclerosis, and Tay-Sachs disease. The seizures may be generalized or myoclonic (spasms of muscles).

Toxic and metabolic disorders are important causes of seizures. These include withdrawal from drugs such as barbiturates, sedatives, tranquilizers (chronic drug intoxication), and alcohol. Seizures from alcohol withdrawal may precede delirium tremens. Some of the metabolic disorders that may be associated with seizures are pyridoxine deficiency, phenylketonuria, hypocalcemia, porphyria, and hypoglycemia. Seizures are common in acute and chronic renal insufficiency. Convulsions in terminal renal failure may be precipitated by water intoxication, but the most important precipitating factor in renal failure is severe hypertension. The seizures in terminal renal failure may occur without any obvious precipitant and are usually the grand mal type, but may occasionally be jacksonian (see p. 356).

Grand mal epilepsy

Grand mal epilepsy is characterized by generalized convulsions and is the most common manifestation of epilepsy in both adults and children. The term "grand mal" comes from French, meaning great sickness or major attack.[121] The convulsions may range from a brief, mild muscular rigidity and jerking to one of demoniacal violence. An attack is usually preceded by a preliminary aura, during which the patient may cry out. Next follows a tonic spasm of the voluntary muscles of the entire body, causing the patient to lose his upright position and fall to the floor or ground. Consciousness is ordinarily lost before the tonic spasm begins, but occasionally the patient is aware of muscular contraction, or he may hear himself phonate. Rarely, consciousness is retained through a short, generalized convulsion. During the seizure there is hypersalivation (Fig. 18-21) and incontinence, and the patient may bite his tongue and thrash around. When he regains consciousness, he is groggy but has no recollection of what has occurred.

Petit mal

Petit mal is French, meaning little sickness or minor attack.[121] It occurs most commonly in children. A transient loss of consciousness lasting for about 5 to 30 seconds may occur anywhere from 5 to 40 or more times a day.[49] Although the convulsions may not be obvious, some muscular movement occurs in most of the patients. These may vary from barely perceptible to extreme. There may be rolling or blinking of the eyes and rhythmic swaying of the head and neck or upper part of the body, which may be forward, lateral, or backward. Posture is usually maintained, but on the basis of brain wave patterns, some neurologists consider petit mal to be of two types when muscles are involved: in one type the muscles suddenly go limp, and the patient falls to the ground but usually gets up by himself and continues with whatever he was doing. In the other type the arms and legs may move jerkily. Some authorities call these minor motor seizures. In petit mal the brain wave records indicate that the disordered release of energy covers the entire brain, as it does in grand mal.[47] In petit mal there is no drooling or hypersalivation, and incontinence occurs infrequently. The petit mal attacks are often referred to as blackouts, fainting, trances, dazes, dreaming, and dizziness. This type of epilepsy intereferes with work because, although brief, it occurs dozens of times during a day in many patients.

Other specific epileptic types

Some types of epilepsy are called focal seizures because abnormal electric discharges are traced to one small area of the brain or to a number of such areas. One of these is called jacksonian seizure, in which overactive neurons are located in the part of the brain governing movements of muscles. Patients with a superficial cortical lesion retain consciousness during a jacksonian seizure. The focal seizures generally start in the toes of one foot, fingers or a hand, or the corner of the mouth. The affected parts start to tremble violently, or it may just feel numb. As more and more neurons are affected, trembling moves up a limb or numbness increases. It may stop suddenly, or it may cross to the other side of the body in a few seconds or minutes. The person then loses consciousness, and the attack is similar to that of a grand mal. The exception to loss of consciousness is noted above.

The most common type of focal seizure is generally known as psychomotor epilepsy.[49] In this type both the muscles and mental processes are affected during an attack. These seizures are temporal lobe seizures. About one half of the patients have serious psychologic or mental disorders. Most of the epileptics admitted to mental institutions are suffering with psychomotor epilepsy. There are three recognized types —automatic, subjective, and tonic. In the automatic type, there is amnesia for events; in the subjective type, awareness is retained; and in the tonic type, there are focal features of arrest of motion or mentation and loss of awareness and memory. The classic features of temporal lobe epilepsy are auditory, olfactory, or visual hallucinations and illusionary phenomena such as micropsia, macropsia, and deja vu phenomenon[10] (an illusion in which a new situation is incorrectly identified as a repetition of a previous situation). There is mental confusion, with automatic movements or semipurposeful activity. In children there is frequent abnormal motor movement, such as the extension of an arm, turning to the side, or falling to the floor. This may be followed by 3 to 5 minutes of unconsciousness.[10] People driving a car may experience a psychomotor seizure and continue to drive following traffic regulations.[30] Consciousness may not be regained until they have driven several miles. These drivers are accident prone. During the seizure children do not exhibit the bizarre behavior seen in adults. A period of aura is almost always present in young children, in which they cry out, reach for support, or run to a parent. Enuresis is a symptom of psychomotor epilepsy; a family history of enuresis is observed more frequently in epileptics than in nonepileptics.

Diagnosis

The electroencephalogram (EEG) provides the most valuable findings in the evaluation of a convulsive disorder. An EEG is a record of the tiny electric currents given off by the brain, and approximately one third of the brain's electrical activity can be assessed from the outside by this means.[121] The recording of the brain waves is a painless process and is done through electrodes placed on the scalp, each picking up an electric current from a different area of the brain. These electrodes are attached by wires to a receiver where the amplified current by moving a pen records the activity of the brain in a series of long, wavy lines for each section of the brain. The higher the wavy lines and the faster they are recorded, the greater the electrical activity of the brain's nerve cells. An EEG of an infant 3 months old shows three to six waves per second; the adult pattern is about ten waves per second, at least until the age of 60, after which waves become slower. Brain waves give no clue to the intelligence of the person or his thoughts or mental health. But they do provide information as to whether or not a person has epilepsy.[121] The EEG of most persons with epilepsy will show some irregularity of wave patterns even between seizures.

There should also be a thorough diagnostic evaluation to determine causative and precipitating factors. The selected laboratory investigations should include blood chemistry tests and cerebrospinal fluid analysis, in addition to electroencephalography. Special roentgenologic studies may also be helpful. A family history should be obtained to determine if there is a susceptibility to seizures and to ascertain if the patient experienced febrile seizures in infancy or childhood. A family history may reveal neurologic abnormalities and genetically determined cerebral disorders that are associated with seizures.

SPLENOMEGALY[54, 109]

Enlargement of the spleen or splenomegaly (Fig. 18-31) is present in adults if the spleen can be palpated. In children the normal spleen is palpable.

Hypersplenism is a spleen malfunction in which destruction of normal blood cells is increased. It causes splenomegaly as well as hemolytic anemia, neutropenia, thrombocytopenia, and rarely pancytopenia. Hypersplenism may be primary or secondary to another disease. Antibodies autoimmune to erythrocytes may or may not be demonstrated. They are present in the following diseases associated with hypersplenism: carcinoma, myeloma, dermoid cysts, ovarian cysts, ulcerative colitis, rheumatoid arthritis, systemic lupus erythematosus, and periarteritis. They are not found in hypersplenism associated with subacute or chronic leukemia (discussed on p. 359), myeloid metaplasia, portal hypertension, Gaucher's disease (Chapter 7), and Niemann-Pick disease (discussed on p. 359). Chronic lymphocytic leukemia, lymphomas, and sarcoidosis may or may not have antibodies present. The antibodies are passively transferred in hemolytic disease of the newborn and erythroblastosis fetalis (Chapter 9).

There are a number of congenital or acquired erythrocytic and hemoglobin abnormalities that produce splenomegaly and hemolytic disease. The congenital forms are hereditary nonspherocytic anemia and hemoglobinopathies such as thalassemia. Ac-

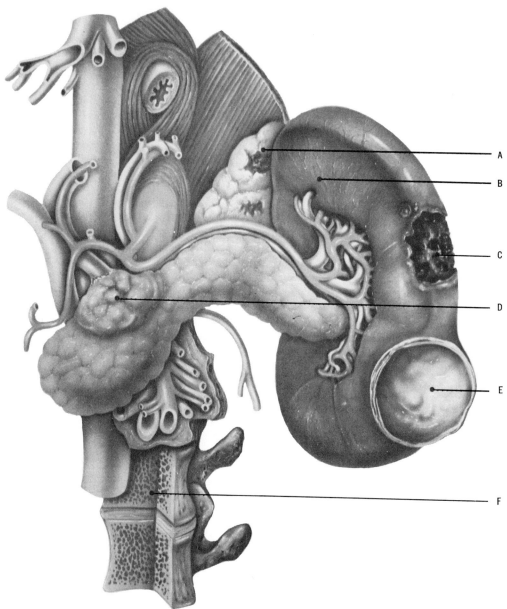

A. TUMORS Lymphosarcoma, reticulum cell sarcoma, Hodgkin's disease, and follicular lymphoma frequently cause splenomegaly. Uncommon tumors causing splenomegaly are hemangioma, lymphangioma, and endothelial sarcoma. Leiomyosarcoma, fibrosarcoma, and myoma are rare causes. Direct extension from tumors of other abdominal organs and hematogenous spread from tumors of the breast, lung, or a malignant melanoma may cause splenomegaly.

B. HYPERSPLENISM A malfunctioning spleen which excessively destroys normal blood cells becomes enlarged; the syndrome may be associated with a wide variety of diseases. Autoimmune antibodies may or may not be demonstrated.

C. INFECTIONS Direct involvement of the spleen by chronic granulomatous processes, such as tuberculosis, histoplasmosis, or brucellosis, and by parasitic infections, such as kala-azar or malaria, may cause splenomegaly. Abscesses of the spleen are uncommon and are usually secondary to pyemia.

D. PORTAL HYPERTENSION A chronically congested spleen may result from portal hypertension secondary to cirrhosis, thrombosis or compression of the portal vein caused by fibrosis or tumor of the pancreas, or splenic artery aneurysm.

E. CYSTS Splenic cysts are uncommon. They may be classified as true, such as dermoid or mesenchymal inclusion cysts; false, which are probably secondary to intrasplenic hemorrhage; or parasitic cysts, as in Echinococcus infestation.

F. ERYTHROCYTIC ABNORMALITIES The various abnormalities of erythrocytes and hemoglobin which result in hemolysis are important causes of splenomegaly.

Fig. 18-31. Splenomegaly. (From Therap. Notes **72:**115, July-Aug., 1965, Parke, Davis & Co.)

quired forms are pernicious anemia, paroxysmal nocturnal hemoglobinuria, myeloid metaplasia, and chronic myelocytic leukemia.

Numerous infections (Fig. 18-31) are associated with hemolysis and splenomegaly, such as bacterial endocarditis, miliary tuberculosis, infectious hepatitis, infectious mononucleosis, malaria, psittacosis, septicemia caused by beta hemolytic streptococci, and *Clostridium welchii* and *Bartonella bacilliformis* infections. Some of the chemicals that can cause hemolysis are lead, arsenic, toluene, and nitrobenzene. Splenomegaly without hemolysis may occur in infections with salmonellae, rickettsiae, spirochetes and viruses. Splenomegaly is often present in polycythemia vera, acute infectious polyneuritis, rheumatoid arthritis, and chronic constrictive pericarditis.

Niemann-Pick disease[11, 54]

Niemann-Pick disease is a disorder in lipid metabolism. The lipid material is sphingomyelin, which accumulates in the bone marrow and may lead to osteoporosis (porous condition of bones). It is a rare and usually rapidly fatal affliction in infancy. There is splenomegaly, but hepatomegaly is more striking.

Leukemia[22, 54]

Leukemia is a fatal disease characterized by a greatly increased production of white cells, failure of their precursors to reach maturity, and the accumulation of white cells not only at normal sites of their formation but also in the tissue spaces or organs in which they are not ordinarily present. In most cases they will appear in large numbers in the circulating blood, but immature forms are also found in increased numbers in the bone marrow.

In unusual forms of leukemia the bone marrow cannot mobilize cells, and the white count is decreased. The marrow is hypertrophic, but for some reason there is no release of cells to the peripheral blood. These states are spoken of as aleukemic, subleukemic, or leukopenic leukemia. The blood picture varies from case to case and many change both qualitatively and quantitatively during the disease. Only the most common types of leukemia will be discussed.

The etiology of leukemia is unknown. Investigations indicate that it is a neoplasm, differing from other types of neoplasms mainly in the type of cell involved and in the easy dissemination through the bloodstream. Recently there has been evidence to support the theory that a viral agent is involved, but this theory has also been applied to other neoplasms. Leukemia has been transmitted experimentally by a particular virus in mice, but the implication of the virus as the cause is still a matter of investigation in human beings. There have been local outbreaks of leukemia suggesting a viral transmission. At the present time leukemia is considered as a neoplasm.

Leukemia may be acute or chronic. The disease is usually classified clinically on the basis of the type of leukocyte involved. The following classification according to cell types is commonly recognized: (1) myelocytic leukemia, in which granulocytes or their precursors are involved; (2) lymphocytic or lymphatic leukemia, in which the lymphocytes or their precursors are involved; and (3) monocytic leukemia, in which monocytes and their precursors are involved. A rare form is mast cell leukemia. The clinical course is acute.

Leukemia begins insidiously in most cases. It may have been present for weeks, months, or even years, before the patient and his physician become aware of its existence.[72] Its presence may have been discovered when an asymptomatic patient had a routine blood count made for an insurance or other type of physical examination, or for pending surgery, or during observation for some infection.[72] This seemingly innocuous type of leukemia will eventually become fulminant and cause the death of the patient. In these patients with a smoldering type of leukemia, on the average the fulminant type of leukemia developed in a year or so. In smoldering acute leukemia the bone marrow is diagnostic of acute leukemia when first examined. Preleukemia has been variously defined, but most agree that it represents bone marrow dysfunction that preceded the onset of diagnostic acute leukemia.[50]

The clinical manifestations differ with the type of leukemia. In almost all cases however, the anemia is progressive and internal hemorrhage may occur. In nearly all forms the spleen and lymph nodes are infiltrated and enlarged. Inflamed and bleeding gums are often manifestations of the lymphocytic and monocytic leukemias. The acute forms usually begin with symptoms of acute infection and may be associated with acute inflammatory and sometimes gangrenous lesions of the oral mucosa. The duration may be as short as a few days or several weeks or months. The latter is more typical. The onset of chronic leukemia is insidious, with the first symptoms usually being enlarged lymph nodes and spleen. Chronic myelocytic leukemia is probably the most common type. It begins with uncontrolled proliferation of leukocytes of the myeloid series. There is widespread infiltration of organs, toxemia, and often hemorrhage. The spleen is markedly enlarged. This type is seen predominantly in middle life. The chronic lymphocytic leukemia is seen most often in middle or older age groups. Acute lymphocytic leukemia is more predominant in the first three decades in life, usually occurring in young children. The acute myelocytic leukemia occurs at any age, as well as the acute monocytic type. A common characteristic of acute monocytic leukemia is the hypertrophy of the gums with ulceration and bleeding. The bone marrow, spleen, and lymph nodes are usually involved, and other organs may be infiltrated.

Both sexes are affected in leukemia, but it is more common in males. Although it may occur at any age, most of the acute cases occur in children and young adults, and the chronic cases occur in middle or older age groups. These, of course, are not hardbound rules.

The blood pictures in the types of leukemia are generally as follows: In chronic myelocytic leukemia the white cell count in the majority of cases is somewhere between 100,000 and 500,000, but higher counts have been recorded. Immature cell types appear in large numbers. All stages in the development of granulocytes usually are present, including neutrophilic, eosinophilic, and basophilic forms. Myelocytes in the middle and late stages of development are as a rule more numerous, but myeloblasts are also found. In acute myelocytic leukemia the total white count is between 15,000 and 50,000, usually with a low count at first. There is a preponderance of early developmental forms, the myeloblasts, constituting more than 90% in many cases.

In chronic lymphocytic leukemia the white count is between 40,000 and 200,000, with the majority being lymphocytes. The blast forms are uncommon and appear only in terminal cases. Blood platelets are reduced in number. In acute lymphocytic leukemias the blood changes are similar to those of acute myelocytic leukemia, with increased white cells and a high proportion of primitive cells. Anemia is severe, and reduction of platelets is a frequent concomitant, with bleeding as in the myelocytic form.

In monocytic leukemia two varieties are recognized, myelomonocytic and histiocytic which is rare.

SYNCOPE[15, 29, 37]

Syncope is transient loss of consciousness resulting from a decrease in cerebral blood flow, usually accompanied by a fall in blood pressure. It is commonly referred to as "fainting." Syncope differs from shock in that the onset is sudden and usually brief. The best known example of syncope is the common faint or vasovagal syncope, also termed vasodepressor faint. It is caused by a sudden and precipitous fall in peripheral resistance. The loss of consciousness may not be complete, but there will be varying degrees of sensorium impairment, such as blurring of vision, weakness, and loss of posture. The subject refers to these symptoms as dizziness, faintness, or light-headedness. The subject is pale, in a cold sweat, usually has a slow pulse rate, and he may be nauseated. Recovery usually occurs when the subject is placed in a recumbent position or when he falls down. The postsyncopal symptoms or manifestations are confusion, weakness, and headache.

Syncope may occur in hot surroundings, referred to as the heat syncope. This type of attack ranges in severity from a feeling of faintness to severe fatigue and loss of consciousness. There is hypotension, marked pallor, flaccid muscles, and visible sweating. Recovery occurs shortly after the subject is removed from the heat and placed in a recumbent position.

Hysterical fainting is usually seen in young women with emotional illness. They are usually free of anxiety, and the attack generally occurs in the presence of others when the subject will drop gracefully and dramatically and appear motionless. It has been compared to the mid-Victorian drawing-room swoon. It now occurs in young women during periods of mass excitement, such as the appearance of a favorite movie idol, TV personality, or singer or musician. Pulse, blood pressure, and skin color are normal. The attack may last only a few minutes or it may extend for an hour or more. The EEG indicates no actual loss of consciousness.

Syncope may result from changes in the chemical composition of the blood as in hyperventilation or hypoglycemia. Syncope is also a manifestation of chronic orthostatic hypotension, a condition that sometimes occurs in diabetic neuropathy and tabes dorsalis. Chronic orthostatic hypotension is a disorder of the autonomic nervous system. The attack occurs when the subject attempts to assume an upright position. There is no pallor, sweating, or nausea, but the subjects may exhibit other aspects of autonomic dysfunction such as impotence, bladder disturbances, and anhidrosis in the lower extremities.

Syncope may occur with myocardial infarction or valvular lesions, angina pectoris, and generalized atherosclerosis with coronary or cerebrovascular involvement. It is one of the three cardinal symptoms of aortic stenosis, the others being exertional dyspnea and angina pectoris. In these patients the syncopal episode may be prolonged and accompanied by convulsions and loss of sphincter control.

The brief loss of consciousness that occurs in syncope must be differentiated from other diseases such as epilepsy, vertigo, cataplexy, and stroke. These conditions also produce disturbances of consciousness and generalized weakness or inability to stand erect. The diagnosis of syncope depends upon careful history of attacks (time, duration, setting, and any precipitating factors), postsyncopal manifestations, and evaluation of the electroencephalographic findings.

TREMOR[18, 110]

Tremor or involuntary quivering of one or more parts of the body is produced by alternate contractions of opposing muscle groups. The severity and distribution of the tremor depends on the underlying disease process (Fig. 18-32).

Tremors are described as coarse, fine, rapid, or slow. Some tremors occur when the affected part is at rest and decrease during activity. Intention tremors (action) occur during voluntary movement, or they may be increased by such action. As a rule, tremors do not occur during sleep. Tremors termed physiologic occur with fatigue, hunger, excitement, physical exertion, during convalescence from exhausting illnesses, or exposure to cold. A congenital or familial tremor involving especially the hands, lips, tongue, or head occurs without any evidence of disease being the initiating factor.

Some of the most prominent central nervous system disorders associated with tremor are illustrated in Fig. 18-32.

In addition to these, tremor is also a feature in Friedreich's ataxia (Chapter 16), cerebral palsy (discussed on p. 363), Wilson's disease (hepatolenticular degeneration),

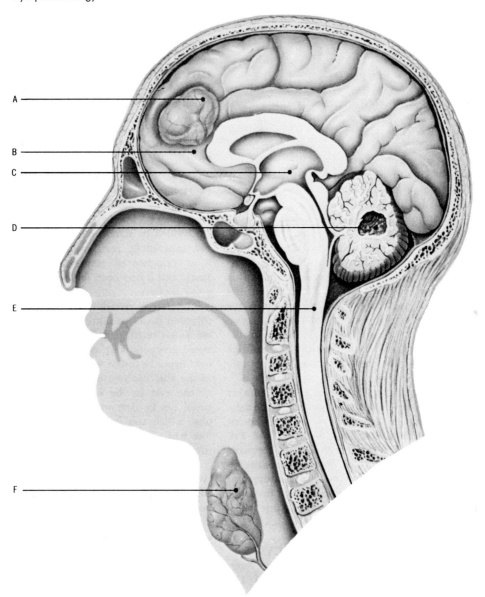

A. FRONTAL LOBE TUMOR A rapid, fine tremor of the contralateral arm and leg may be elicited by tumor, focal injury, or abscess of the frontal lobe. Diagnosis is commonly based on associated signs and symptoms.

B. HYSTERICAL TREMOR Characterized by irregularity, hysterical tremor decreases when the patient's attention is distracted and increases when attention is directed to the affected part.

C. PARKINSON'S DISEASE A coarse, resting tremor is often the first of the symptoms and signs of this disease, which include rigidity, slowness and weakness of movements, and masklike facies. Tremor is usually present in the fingers, forearm, tongue, and head. It is increased by excitement and usually disappears during sleep.

D. CEREBELLAR ABSCESS Focal signs of cerebellar abscess include ataxia, intention tremor, nystagmus, and other cerebellar and vestibular symptoms. Unless the infection is active, symptoms are usually those of increased intracranial pressure.

E. MULTIPLE SCLEROSIS In this disease, the tremor is the intention type, which occurs only during voluntary movement and disappears at rest. Occasionally there is a static tremor of the head.

F. HYPERTHYROIDISM A regular, rapid, fine tremor of the outstretched hands and fingers is characteristic. The tremor is aggravated by emotion and exertion; in severe cases, tremor may involve the legs also.

Fig. 18-32. Tremor. (From Therap. Notes **72**:171, Nov.-Dec., 1965, Parke, Davis & Co.)

generalized cerebral arteriosclerosis, and Parkinson's disease (discussed below).

Endocrine disorders associated with tremor are hyperthyroidism (Chapter 17) and hypoglycemia (below normal concentrations of glucose in the blood).

The most common toxic tremor occurs in alcoholism, the severest form of which is called delirium tremens. Toxic tremor also occurs with drug addiction (barbiturates, cocaine, opiates) and in poisoning with heavy metals (mercury, lead, manganese, antimony, gold, bismuth).

A coarse tremor occurs in uremia. A characteristic flapping tremor of the outstretched hands occurs in hepatic coma,[79] which is usually associated with Laennec's cirrhosis or acute viral hepatitis.

Parkinson's disease[18, 45, 123, 188]

Parkinson's disease, also known at times as parkinsonism, paralysis agitans, and shaking palsy, is a progressive neurological disorder that affects the brain centers responsible for control and regulation of movements. It is characterized by a symptom complex consisting of rigidity, akinesia, tremor, and a loss of postural reflexes. The intellect is ordinarily unimpaired. The stooped, shuffling, festinating gait, and the pill-rolling resting tremor are almost always correctly diagnosed by the physician. Although there is disturbance of equilibrium and motion, paralysis does not result, but the disease can be extremely crippling over a period of years. While the disease is rarely the primary cause of death, it often weakens the victim so that he falls prey to other diseases. It can occur in either sex at any age from childhood to advanced years but is more common in the sixth and seventh decades of life. The disorder has been known since Biblical times. Galen, a Greek physician and medical writer in the second century A.D., described it as shaking palsy. In an "Essay on Shaking Palsy," Dr. James Parkinson, an English physician, gave an apt and still-used description of this disease

in 1817 and distinguished the ailment from other diseases characterized by tremor. As a memorial to him, the disease has been called Parkinson's disease or parkinsonism.

Loss of postural reflexes resulting in sudden episodes of falling can be the initial symptom or complaint of the disease.[45] The signs and symptoms of Parkinson's disease or parkinsonism are generally believed to be related to decreased levels of dopamine within the striatum. It is believed that there is a balance between acetylcholine and dopamine that is important to the regulation of the activity of the striatal neurons and that parkinsonism represents an absolute loss of dopamine effect with a relative increase of acetylcholine effect.[123] One theory on the cause is that coordinated muscle control depends upon a balance of two neurochemical systems, cholinergic and dopaminergic, and that the symptoms of parkinsonism are caused by overactivity or underactivity of one or the other of these symptoms.[123] Recent research has shown that depletion of dopamine, one of the biogenic amine substances in the brain necessary for nerve transmissions, is found in parkinsonism. To date, however, except for one form (postencephalitic) that appears to be the direct result of encephalitis, the cause or causes of Parkinson's disease are not known. There also seems to be a hereditary tendency.

Cerebral palsy[118]

Cerebral palsy is not a single disease but refers to a group of ailments having a variety of symptoms and all being brain centered and affecting muscular control. Names for the disease are "Little's disease," a nineteenth century name; "spastic palsy," meaning abnormally tight, stiff muscles; "spastic paraplegia" when both legs are spastic; "spastic hemiplegia" when an arm and a leg on one side are affected; "spastic quadriplegia" when all four limbs are affected; and "infantile cerebral palsy or infantile paralysis," which is the popular picture of cerebral palsy.

Cerebral palsy is now described according to type. Spastic comprises the largest group, and these patients have tense, contracted muscles. Patients with the athetoid type show constant uncontrolled motion. In the rigid type the children have rigid muscles that resist moving and they are slow-moving. The ataxic patients have a poor sense of balance and are prone to fall. Patients with the tremor type have shaking of the hands and feet, making their use difficult. Some group the patients with excessive motion under the term "hyperkinetic." Athetoid, tremor, and less common types of unnatural motion would be classified in this category.

In addition to the symptoms of the types of cerebral palsy, as described above, mental deficiency may occur in many cases, as well as convulsive disorders caused by central neuronal degenerations. A number of patients, however, have normal intelligence. The muscles and tendons may be shortened by tension, and the bones may be twisted by the tense muscles. Facial grimaces may occur from afflicted head muscles, and involvement of the tongue causes speech defects. Some will be able to utter only guttural sounds. Deafness and partial blindness may be complications. The symptoms vary from patient to patient, and there are many mixed types, all dependent upon the extent of brain damage.

The etiology can be traced to brain injuries in a number of cases, but sometimes no cause can be found. Cerebral palsy can result from malformation of the brain caused by a variety of influences operating in the early stages of fetal development. Poor nutrition and poor health of the mother both before and during pregnancy can affect brain development of the baby. Infections in the mother, such as German measles (rubella), toxoplasmosis, or cytomegalovirus, and such maternal ailments as anemia and toxemia, can affect the brain of the unborn child. A conflict between the mother and unborn child in their Rh blood factor may also be responsible for cerebral palsy in the neonate. All Rh-negative blood type mothers should receive Rh immune globulin within 72 hours after each birth of an Rh-positive baby or an Rh-positive or unknown type in miscarriage of an unsensitized mother.[118] This protects future children from possible Rh-conflict cerebral palsy. Some babies have suffered birth difficulties without damage, but complications during delivery and injury or infection after birth sometimes cause cerebral palsy.

A rather uncommon type of cerebral palsy, Lesch-Nyhan cerebral palsy,[118] is caused by an enzyme defect, inherited through the mother. In families known to carry the enzyme defect of purine metabolism, affected children can be identified while still in the uterus at an early stage of pregnancy.

Accurate figures of the number of cerebral palsy victims are not available, since it is not a disease that has to be reported to state health departments. The United Cerebral Palsy Association has suggested that there are about 750,000 persons with cerebral palsy and that about 15,000 babies are born with cerebral palsy each year, or one newborn in every 200 live births.[118]

URINARY FREQUENCY[111, 115]

Urinary frequency is associated with a number of inflammatory or obstructive lesions of the bladder and adjacent structures, as illustrated in Fig. 18-33. Some of these are described in more detail below. Dysuria (difficult urination), tenesmus (ineffectual and painful straining to urinate), urgency, burning, and strangury (slow and painful urination) occur in conjunction with urinary frequency. Urinary frequency often results from increased intracystic pressure on the bladder and from irritative lesions of the upper urinary tract through reflex stimulation of the bladder.

Acute or chronic inflammation of any part of the urinary tract may produce urinary frequency, even when no infection is present. Cystitis, prostatitis, and posterior

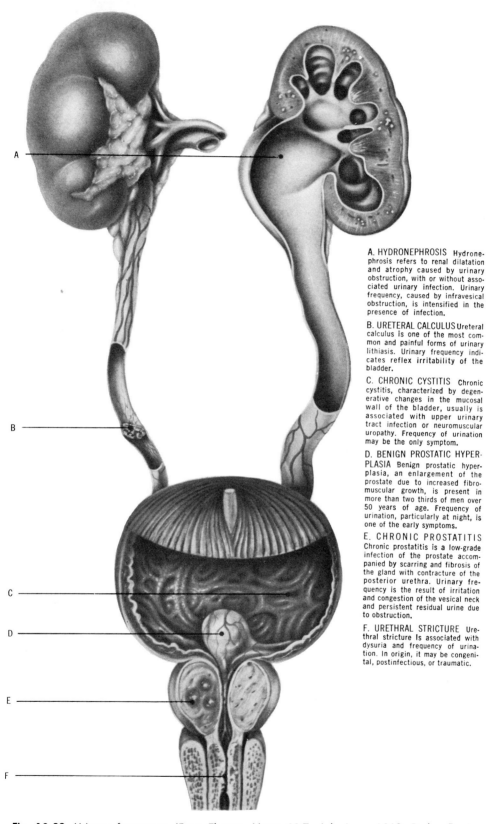

A. HYDRONEPHROSIS Hydronephrosis refers to renal dilatation
and atrophy caused by urinary
obstruction, with or without associated urinary infection. Urinary
frequency, caused by infravesical
obstruction, is intensified in the
presence of infection.

B. URETERAL CALCULUS Ureteral
calculus is one of the most common and painful forms of urinary
lithiasis. Urinary frequency indicates reflex irritability of the
bladder.

C. CHRONIC CYSTITIS Chronic
cystitis, characterized by degenerative changes in the mucosal
wall of the bladder, usually is
associated with upper urinary
tract infection or neuromuscular
uropathy. Frequency of urination
may be the only symptom.

**D. BENIGN PROSTATIC HYPER-
PLASIA** Benign prostatic hyperplasia, an enlargement of the
prostate due to increased fibromuscular growth, is present in
more than two thirds of men over
50 years of age. Frequency of
urination, particularly at night, is
one of the early symptoms.

E. CHRONIC PROSTATITIS
Chronic prostatitis is a low-grade
infection of the prostate accompanied by scarring and fibrosis of
the gland with contracture of the
posterior urethra. Urinary frequency is the result of irritation
and congestion of the vesical neck
and persistent residual urine due
to obstruction.

F. URETHRAL STRICTURE Urethral stricture is associated with
dysuria and frequency of urination. In origin, it may be congenital, postinfectious, or traumatic.

Fig. 18-33. Urinary frequency. (From Therap. Notes **69**:7, July-Aug., 1962, Parke, Davis
& Co.)

urethritis are almost invariably accompanied by urinary frequency.

Urinary frequency may occur with excessively acid or alkaline urine, pronounced crystalluria, Reiter's syndrome (nongonorrheal arthritis, conjunctivitis, and urethritis), periurethritis, and periurethral abscess. Phimosis, balanitis, or helminthiasis may cause urinary frequency in children.

The conditions associated with polyuria (Chapter 8) usually cause urinary frequency because of more rapid filling of the bladder. Nervous polyuria, polydipsia (excessive fluid intake), diabetes, and nephritis often are accompanied by urinary frequency.

Vesical spasm caused by infection or calculi and neurogenic spasm of bladder muscles reduce the capacity of the bladder and induce urinary frequency. Pelvic masses, such as ovarian cysts or uterine tumors and pregnancy, create external pressure on the bladder or ureters and cause urinary frequency. Severe urinary frequency may accompany chronic infections that produce contracture of the bladder. This is particularly true of tuberculous infection.

Hydronephrosis[4, 115]

In hydronephrosis there is dilatation of the renal pelvis, with associated atrophy of renal tissue caused by obstruction to the outflow of urine. This is a common disease of the kidneys. Urinary calculi are a frequent cause. The congenital etiology includes atresia of the urethra, congenital valve formations either of ureters or the urethra, aberrant renal arteries, and torsion or kinking of the ureter caused by displacement of the kidney. The acquired causes are prostatic hypertrophy, carcinoma of the prostate, uterine procidentia producing angulation of the urethra, and pregnancy. Spinal cord damage and neurogenic paralysis of the bladder are other causes. Obstruction may also be caused by neoplastic invasion of the ureter or bladder, or the ureters or bladder can be compressed by

tumors from the ovaries, uterus, or other pelvic structures. When obstruction of a ureter is unilateral, the unaffected kidney may exhibit a compensatory hypertrophy. This represents the most extreme degree of hydronephrosis. Obstruction of the ureter caused by prostatic enlargement produces bilateral hydronephrosis and dilated ureters.

Urinary calculi[13, 68, 135]

Urinary calculi are one of the major disorders of the urinary system and can lead to irreversible damage in the kidney. The stones may form in the kidney, pass into the ureter and become lodged or impacted, or they may form in the bladder. Most of the vesical and ureteral calculi are of renal origin. The stones that form in the kidney are composed of one or several chemical constituents—calcium, phosphate, oxalate, magnesium, ammonium, cystine, and uric acid. They may be single or bilateral.

The two important metabolic factors that appear related to the formation of renal stones are an increased urinary output of one or more of the chemical constituents and persistent and significant acidity or alkalinity of the urine. A high concentration of crystalline salts in the urine favors precipitation. Colloids in the urine hold the crystalloids in solution in a supersaturated state. This delicate balance may be upset by hyperexcretion of crystalloids, as often occurs in primary hyperparathyroidism, which is a common cause of calcium stone formation. The balance may also be disturbed by a decrease of colloids caused by infection. Solid material may become encrusted with urinary salts. A nidus for such precipitation may be bacteria, necrotic or degenerated tissue, shed epithelium, a tiny blood clot, or foreign bodies. Urinary reaction is important in maintaining the urinary salts in solution and largely determines the composition of the stones. Cystine calculi form only in acid urine and are dissolved by alkalinizing the urine. Phosphatic stones form in alkaline or neutral urine. Oxalate stones may also form in acid urine. Xanthine calculi will form only in acid urine. The calcium oxalate stones may be formed in urine at any pH. Urinary reaction alone, however, is probably never the cause of stone formation. When there is obstruction anywhere in the urinary tract, the stasis or stagnation favors crystallization and also promotes infection. Stagnation, however, is rarely the sole factor in stone formation. Stones containing calcium are often associated with an elevated excretion of this chemical in the urine. The resultant hypercalciuria can be caused by renal tubular acidosis, primary hyperparathyroidism, or prolonged recumbency as required in treatment of fracture of the spine or hip in the elderly. Other causes include milk-alkali syndrome, hypervitaminosis D, and renal sarcoidosis.

Urinary calculi produce a variety of symptoms related to obstruction, infection, and local irritation. Stones in the kidney, however, may be asymptomatic, or they may be manifested by back pain, hematuria, nausea, and vomiting. The complications are hydronephrosis from partial or intermittent obstruction and pyelonephritis caused by stasis or obstruction. The renal stones may pass from the kidney into the ureter, obstructing the passageway.

Ureteral stones almost always cause obstruction and usually produce clinical manifestations of ureteral colic. The pain is episodic and excruciating, occurring in the back and side and radiating into the lower part of the abdomen and to the testes in the male. There may be associated hematuria, urinary frequency, nausea, and vomiting. Fever may occur with a stone in the kidney or ureter if infection is present. If the obstruction is acute, a tender, enlarged kidney may be palpated. The majority of ureteral calculi occur in males between the ages of 20 and 50 years. The site of impaction of ureteral stones is most commonly at the ureteropelvic junction, where the ureter crosses the iliac vessels, at the base

of the broad ligaments in females and the ductus deferens in males, or at the entrance of the ureter at the external muscle layer of the bladder and ureteral orifice. In addition to hydronephrosis and pyelonephritis other complications are periureteritis and periureteral abscess.

Vesical calculi are usually of renal origin and are associated with pyelonephritis. Stones that develop in the urinary bladder may be of inflammatory or noninflammatory origin. The most common causes are imperfect emptying of the bladder caused by obstruction or paralysis, infection, foreign bodies, inadequate vitamin A, and faulty metabolism of calcium, uric acid, cystine, or xanthine. The incidence of vesical calculi is low in the United States compared to other parts of the world, especially southern China and India. The vesical stones may be no larger than sand particles but may range up to several centimeters. In addition to hydronephrosis or pyelonephritis there may be bladder hypertrophy.

Roentgenologic examination will demonstrate calculi in most cases. The radiopacity of stones is usually caused by the presence of calcium or magnesium salts in the crystalline shells. In cystine stones, however, the crystals are packed tightly or are dense enough to impede passage of x rays.[13] With the rare exception of xanthene stones, radiolucent stones are most often made of uric acid. Stone analysis may be made by sophisticated techniques, which include x-ray diffraction and infrared spectral analysis.[13]

Chronic prostatitis[19, 58, 65]

Chronic prostatitis is one of the most common chronic infections in men of the middle and later years. It usually occurs in a younger age group than does the carcinoma of the prostate. On examination the prostate feels somewhat enlarged, soft, and boggy. The surface outline is often irregular, with areas of induration and periprostatic adhesions that may fix it to the pelvis. Generally the seminal vesicles are palpable and are involved in the inflammatory and infectious process. They may be irregular, nodular, indurated, and not compressible.

Chronic prostatitis frequently produces no symptoms and is discovered during a routine physical examination. Chronic inflammation of the prostate gland has been considered to harbor the foci of infection responsible for arthritis, myositis, neuritis, and iritis. Allergic manifestations have also been attributed to chronic prostatitis.

Acute prostatitis is a triad of symptoms of malaise, fever, and chills. In addition, there may be sexual and urinary symptoms. It is usually an extension from pyelonephritis, epididymitis, cystitis, or posterior urethritis. It may also follow manipulation of the urethra by catheterization, urethral dilatation, transurethral examination of the bladder, or partial transurethral resection of the prostate. The common bacterial agents are staphylococci, streptococci, gonococci, and the coliform group of bacilli. On examination the prostate is swollen and exquisitely tender. There may be multiple abscesses and foci of necrosis, and the suppurative inflammation is diffuse.

Calculi may be present in both acute and chronic prostatitis. Corpora amylacea may obstruct the acini, causing them to become closed cavities where prostatic secretions stagnate and become infected. The corpora amylacea form the nucleus of an endogenous calculus. Exogenous or false calculi are of urinary origin.

Benign prostatic hypertrophy[19, 58, 65]

Benign prostatic hypertrophy is primarily a disease of senescence. It occurs in approximately one third of all males over 60 years of age. The prostate becomes from two to four times larger than normal. The prostate is one of the most important of the accessory sex glands. Because of its strategic location surrounding the posterior urethra and the vesical orifice, disease of this gland whether from infection, enlargement, or malignancy can produce obstructive symptoms that vary from insidious to severe and life threatening. Prolonged obstruction may result in profound changes in the bladder, ureters, and kidney and thus jeopardize the integrity of the urinary system.

The etiology of prostatic hypertrophy is unknown, but it has been variously attributed to inflammation, arteriosclerosis, sexual indulgence, or perversion. The benign nodules that are the cause of the hypertrophy are akin to the benign tumors of adenoma and leiomyoma.

The size and contour of the hypertrophied prostate bear no relation to the severity of the symptoms. The prostate gland is normally about the size of a chestnut, but with benign prostatic hypertrophy it can reach the size of an orange. A very small nodule at the vesical orifice may produce complete retention, although hypertrophy of the gland to the size of an orange may produce relatively few symptoms. Hypertrophy affects certain areas within the prostate and is not a diffuse hyperplasia of the entire gland. The area adjacent to the urethra is the portion that becomes hypertrophied most frequently. On rectal examination an enlargement may be detected that on occasion may be so extensive that it almost obliterates the rectal cavity.

One of the most common complications of benign prostatic hypertrophy is cystitis.

VAGINAL DISCHARGE[112]

Any discharge from the vagina other than blood is called leukorrhea. It is one of the complaints most frequently encountered by gynecologists. The discharges vary in viscosity and color and are accompanied by symptoms of burning, itching, and soreness of the vulva.

A large percentage of vaginal discharges are the result of infections. *Trichomonas vaginitis* is a parasitic protozoan sometimes found in the vagina. It produces a profuse, yellowish discharge. It is also found in the bladder, prostate, and urethra of males, and it is considered by some to be a form

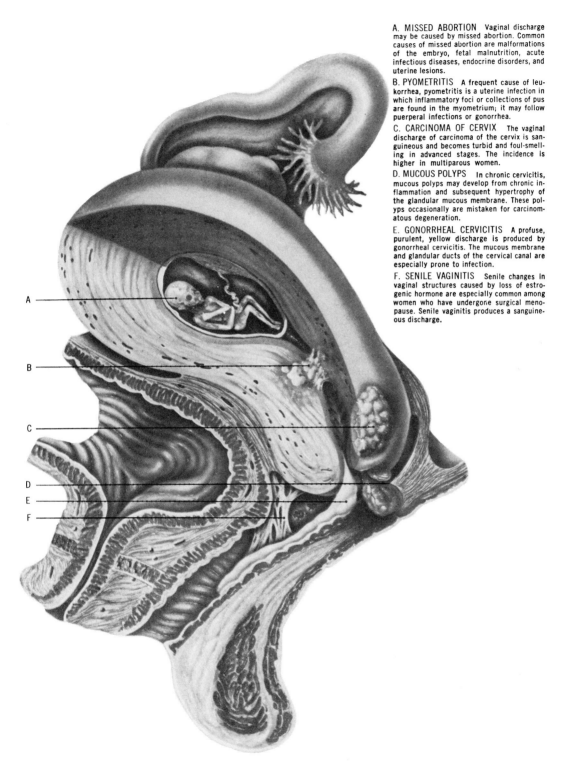

A. MISSED ABORTION   Vaginal discharge may be caused by missed abortion. Common causes of missed abortion are malformations of the embryo, fetal malnutrition, acute infectious diseases, endocrine disorders, and uterine lesions.

B. PYOMETRITIS   A frequent cause of leukorrhea, pyometritis is a uterine infection in which inflammatory foci or collections of pus are found in the myometrium; it may follow puerperal infections or gonorrhea.

C. CARCINOMA OF CERVIX   The vaginal discharge of carcinoma of the cervix is sanguineous and becomes turbid and foul-smelling in advanced stages. The incidence is higher in multiparous women.

D. MUCOUS POLYPS   In chronic cervicitis, mucous polyps may develop from chronic inflammation and subsequent hypertrophy of the glandular mucous membrane. These polyps occasionally are mistaken for carcinomatous degeneration.

E. GONORRHEAL CERVICITIS   A profuse, purulent, yellow discharge is produced by gonorrheal cervicitis. The mucous membrane and glandular ducts of the cervical canal are especially prone to infection.

F. SENILE VAGINITIS   Senile changes in vaginal structures caused by loss of estrogenic hormone are especially common among women who have undergone surgical menopause. Senile vaginitis produces a sanguineous discharge.

A
B
C
D
E
F

Fig. 18-34. Vaginal discharge. (From Therap. Notes **69**:5, Jan.-Feb., 1962, Parke, Davis & Co.)

of venereal disease in that the infection is transmitted through sexual intercourse.

Candidiasis or moniliasis, a fungal infection caused by *Candida albicans,* may involve the vagina (vulvovaginitis) and produce a whitish discharge. Gonorrheal infections also produce vaginal discharges. Gonorrhea is discussed in Chapter 14. Infection with gonorrhea produces a profuse yellow discharge. A thick tenacious leukorrhea is a common symptom of chronic cervicitis that occurs as a result of puerperal trauma or attempted abortion. The causative organisms are streptococcus, staphylococcus, and *Escherichia coli.* Infections of the vulva, such as urethritis, skenitis (Skene's glands), and batholinitis (Bartholin's glands), may also contribute to leukorrhea. Chronic pelvic inflammatory disease is nearly always associated with leukorrhea, but the discharge is caused by concurrent cervicitis.

Anemia, tuberculosis, and debilitating diseases of the heart, kidney, and liver may give rise to vaginal discharge.

Endocrine disorders of certain types may produce scanty discharge, often occurring on a cyclic basis. Premenstrual mucoid discharge may occur in normal women, and a small amount of mucoid discharge may occur in patients with functional uterine bleeding. Leukorrhea frequently occurs in pregnant women. It is partly from endocrine factors and partly from gestational hyperemia.

Some of the major causes of vaginal discharge are illustrated in Fig. 18-34.

REFERENCES

1. Almy, T. P.: In Beeson, P. B., and McDermott, W., editors: Cecil-Loeb textbook of medicine, ed. 13, Philadelphia, 1971, W. B. Saunders Co. (disorders of motility).
2. American Heart Association: Heart disease in children, New York, 1963, The Association (rheumatic fever).
3. Aman, R. W., and Bockus, H. L.: Arch. Intern. Med. 107:504, 1961 (regional enteritis).
4. Anderson, W. A. D., and Jones, D. B.: In Anderson, W. A. D., editor: Pathology, ed. 6, St. Louis, 1971, The C. V. Mosby Co.
5. Angrist, A. A.: J.A.M.A. 183:249, 1963 (pathogenesis of bacterial endocarditis).
6. Azar, R. F.: J. La. State Med. Soc. 115:317, 1963 (glaucoma).
7. Baird, H. W. III: Pediatr. Clin. North Am. 10:705, 1963 (epilepsy).
8. Becklake, M. R.: In Beeson, P. B., and McDermott, W., editors: Cecil-Loeb textbook of medicine, ed. 13, Philadelphia, 1971, W. B. Saunders Co. (pneumoconioses; emphysema).
9. Beeson, P. B.: In Beeson, P. B., and McDermott, W., editors: Cecil-Loeb textbook of medicine, ed. 13, Philadelphia, 1971, W. B. Saunders Co. (epidemic diarrhea; bacterial endocarditis).
10. Bennett, A. E.: Calif. Med. 97:346, 1962 (epilepsy).
11. Bennett, G. A.: In Anderson, W. A. D., editor: Pathology, ed. 6, St. Louis, 1971, The C. V. Mosby Co. (Paget's disease of bone; Niemann-Pick disease).
12. Bennett, G. A.: In Anderson, W. A. D., editor: Pathology, ed. 6, St. Louis, 1971, The C. V. Mosby Co. (joints—rheumatoid arthritis; osteoarthritis).
13. Berman, L. B.: J.A.M.A. 231:865-866, 1975 (renal geology).
14. Black, W. P.: Practitioner 187:337, 1961 (abnormal uterine bleeding).
15. Braunwald, E.: In Beeson, P. B., and McDermott, W., editors: Cecil-Loeb textbook of medicine, ed. 13, Philadelphia, 1971, W. B. Saunders Co. (syncope).
16. Bricker, N. S.: In Beeson, P. B., and McDermott, W., editors: Cecil-Loeb textbook of medicine, ed. 13, Philadelphia, 1971, W. B. Saunders Co. (acute renal failure).
17. Bodian, D., and Horstmann, D. M.: In Horsfall, F. L., Jr., and Tamm, I., editors: Viral and rickettsial diseases of man, ed. 4, Philadelphia, 1965, J. B. Lippincott Co. (poliomyelitis).
18. Chason, J. L.: In Anderson, W. A. D., editor: Pathology, ed. 6, St. Louis, 1971, The C. V. Mosby Co. (multiple sclerosis; hemiplegia; Parkinson's disease).
19. Colby, F. H.: Essential urology, ed. 2, Baltimore, 1953, The Williams & Wilkins Co. (prostatic lesions).
20. Couch, R. B.: In Beeson, P. B., and McDermott, W., editors: Cecil-Loeb textbook of medicine, ed. 13, Philadelphia, 1971, W. B. Saunders Co. (mycoplasmal pneumonia).
21. Dagradi, A. B., and Rappaport, I.: Geriatrics 18:642, 1963 (esophageal hiatal hernia).

22. Dameshek, W., and Gunz, F.: Leukemia, ed. 2, New York, 1963, Grune & Stratton, Inc.

23. Des Prez, I.: In Beeson, P. B., and McDermott, W.: editors: Cecil-Loeb textbook of medicine, ed. 13, Philadelphia, 1971, W. B. Saunders Co. (tuberculosis).

24. Dodds, J. J.: J. Tenn. Med. Assoc. **57**:53, 1964 (acute pancreatitis).

25. Drew, W. L., and others: J.A.M.A. **230**:713-715, 1974 (diagnosis of *Pneumocystis carinii* pneumonia by bronchopulmonary lavage).

26. Ebert, R. V.: In Beeson, P. R., and McDermott, W., editors: Cecil-Loeb textbook of medicine, ed. 13, Philadelphia, 1971, W. B. Saunders Co. (interstitial lung disease; emphysema; lipid pneumonia).

27. Edmondson, H. A., and Peters, R. L.: In Anderson, W. A. D., editor: Pathology, ed. 6, St. Louis, 1971, The C. V. Mosby Co. (cirrhosis; portal hypertension).

28. Feinstein, A. R.: In Beeson, P. B., and McDermott, W., editors: Cecil-Loeb textbook of medicine, ed. 13, Philadelphia, 1971, W. B. Saunders Co. (cough in cancer of lung).

29. Fishman, A. P.: In Beeson, P. B., and McDermott, W., editors: Cecil-Loeb textbook of medicine, ed. 13, Philadelphia, 1971, W. B. Saunders Co. (cough in heart failure; syncope).

30. Forster, F. M., and Liske, E.: Neurology **13**:301, 1963 (epilepsy).

31. Goodwin, R.: In Beeson, P. B., and McDermott, W., editors: Cecil-Loeb textbook of medicine, ed. 13, Philadelphia, 1971, W. B. Saunders Co. (cough in pulmonary tuberculosis).

32. Gordon, D. M.: Clinical symposia, Summit, N. J., Oct.-Dec., 1962, Ciba Pharmaceutical Co. (diseases of the eye).

33. Gore, I.: In Anderson, W. A. D., editor: Pathology, ed. 6, St. Louis, 1971, The C. V. Mosby Co. (Kaposi's sarcoma).

34. Gutre, T.: In Beeson, P. B., and McDermott, W., editors: Cecil-Loeb textbook of medicine, ed. 13, Philadelphia, 1971, W. B. Saunders Co. (relapsing fever).

35. Halpert, B.: In Anderson, W. A. D., editor: Pathology, ed. 6, St. Louis, 1971, The C. V. Mosby Co. (cholecystitis).

36. Hertig, A., and Gore, H.: In Anderson, W. A. D., editor: Pathology, ed. 6, St. Louis, 1971, The C. V. Mosby Co. (endometriosis; abruptio placentae; placenta previa; abortion).

37. Heyman, A.: In Beeson, P. B., and McDermott, W.: editors: Cecil-Loeb textbook of medicine, ed. 13, Philadelphia, 1971, W. B. Saunders Co. (syncope).

38. Horn, R. C., Jr.: In Anderson, W. A. D., editor: Pathology, ed. 6, St. Louis, 1971, The C. V. Mosby Co. (ascites; regional enteritis; hernias; ulcerative colitis; peptic ulcer).

39. Howell, J. B. L.: In Beeson, P. B., and McDermott, W., editors: Cecil-Loeb textbook of medicine, ed. 13, Philadelphia, 1971, W. B. Saunders Co. (bronchiectasis; emphysema).

40. Hurst, J. W.: In Beeson, P. B., and McDermott, W., editors: Cecil-Loeb textbook of medicine, ed. 13, Philadelphia, 1971, W. B. Saunders Co. (arterial insufficiency; Leriche syndrome; pulseless disease).

41. Jaffee, B. F.: Arch. Otolaryngol. **86**:81, 1967 (sudden deafness).

42. Jawetz, E.: In Beeson, P. B., and McDermott, W., editors: Cecil-Loeb textbook of medicine, ed. 13, Philadelphia, 1971, W. B. Saunders Co. (trachoma and inclusion conjunctivitis).

43. Jeffries, G. H.: In Beeson, P. B., and McDermott, W., editors: Cecil-Loeb textbook of medicine, ed. 13, Philadelphia, 1971, W. B. Saunders Co. (cirrhosis).

44. Kim, H., and Hughes, W. T.: Am. J. Clin. Pathol. **60**:462-466, 1973 (*P. carinii* pneumonia methods for identification).

45. Klawans, H. L., and Tepel. J. L.: J.A.M.A. **230**:1555-1557, 1974 (parkinsonism as a falling sickness).

46. Kincaid-Smith, P.: In Beeson, P. B., and McDermott, W., editors: Cecil-Loeb textbook of medicine, ed. 13, Philadelphia, 1971, W. B. Saunders Co. (dialysis).

47. Koller, A. E., and Hetherington, J., Jr.: Becker-Schaffer's diagnosis and therapy of the glaucomas, ed. 4, St. Louis, 1976, The C. V. Mosby Co.

48. Lacy, P. E., and Kissane, J. M.: In Anderson, W. A. D., editor: Pathology, ed. 6, St. Louis, 1971, The C. V. Mosby Co. (pancreatitis).

49. Lennox, W. G., and Lennox, M. A.: Epilepsy and related disorders, vol. 2, Boston, 1960, Little, Brown and Co.

50. Linman, J. W., and Sarni, M. I.: Semin. Hematol. **11**:92-100, 1974 (the preleukemia syndrome).

51. Lumb, G.: Gastroenterology **40**:290, 1961 (ulcerative colitis and regional enteritis).

52. McDowell, F. H.: In Beeson, P. B., and McDermott, W., editors: Cecil-Loeb textbook of medicine, ed. 13, Philadelphia, 1971, W. B. Saunders Co. (Horner's syndrome).

53. Maher, J. E.: Ohio State Med. J. **20**:235, 1964 (dialysis).

54. Miale, J. B.: In Anderson, W. A. D., editor:

Pathology, ed. 6, St. Louis, 1971, The C. V. Mosby Co. (splenomegaly, anemia; leukemia; Niemann-Pick's disease).

55. Marciel-Rojas, R. A.: In Anderson, W. A. D., editor: Pathology, ed. 6, St. Louis, 1971, The C. V. Mosby Co. (malaria).

56. Millard, M.: In Anderson, W. A. D., editor: Pathology, ed. 6, St. Louis, 1971, The C. V. Mosby Co. (bronchiectasis; emphysema; tuberculosis; pneumonia).

57. Morton, W.: Proceedings of Workshop, University of Colorado Medical Center, 1962, Washington, D. C., 1963, U.S. Department of Health, Education, and Welfare, Division of Chronic Diseases, Heart Disease Control program (rheumatic heart disease in children).

58. Mostofi, F. K., and Leestma, J. E.: In Anderson, W. A. D., editor: Pathology, ed. 6, St. Louis, 1971, The C. V. Mosby Co. (acute prostatitis; benign prostatic hypertrophy).

59. Myers, D., Schlosser, W. D., and Winchester, R. A.: Clinical symposia, Summit, N.J., April-June, 1962, Ciba Pharmaceutical Co. (otologic diagnosis and treatment of deafness).

60. Nelson, J. R.: In Beeson, P. B., and McDermott, W., editors: Cecil-Loeb textbook of medicine, ed. 13, Philadelphia, 1971, W. B. Saunders Co. (hearing loss; Meniere's disease).

61. Nursing Education Service Bulletin No. 12, Columbus, Ohio, 1963, Ross Laboratories (abnormalities of the placenta).

62. Obley, F. A.: You and your emphysema, Philadelphia, 1968, J. B. Lippincott Co.

63. Parks, J., and Barker, H.: Ariz. Med. 20:155, 1963 (placenta previa).

64. Payne, F. L., Wright, R. C., and Fetterman, M. D.: Am. J. Obstet. Gynecol. 77:1216, 1959 (abnormal uterine bleeding).

65. Pessin, S. B., and Anderson, W. A. D.: In Anderson, W. A. D., editor: Pathology, ed. 5, St. Louis, 1966, The C. V. Mosby Co. (chronic prostatitis; benign prostatic hypertrophy).

66. Phibbs, B.: The human heart, the layman's guide to heart disease, ed. 3, St. Louis, 1975, The C. V. Mosby Co. (rheumatic fever; endocarditis).

67. Pinkerton, H.: In Anderson, W. A. D., editor: Pathology, ed. 6, St. Louis, 1971, The C. V. Mosby Co. (poliomyelitis; rabies).

68. Prince, C. L., and Scardino, P. L.: J. Urol. 83:561, 1960 (urinary calculi).

69. Radman, H. M.: Am. J. Obstet. Gynecol. 59:1, 1960 (abnormal uterine bleeding).

70. Redman, Jack C.: J.A.M.A. 230:1561-1563, 1974 (*Pneumocystis carinii* pneumonia in an adopted Vietnamese infant).

71. Reis, D. J.: In Beeson, P. B., and McDermott, W., editors: Cecil-Loeb textbook of medicine, ed. 13, Philadelphia, 1971, W. B. Saunders Co. (neurofibromatosis in kyphosis; amyotrophic lateral sclerosis).

72. Rheingold, J. J.: J.A.M.A. 230:985-986, 1974 (acute leukemia—its smoldering phase).

73. Robbins, S. L.: Pathology, ed. 3, Philadelphia, 1967, W. B. Saunders Co. (cholecystitis; cirrhosis; multiple sclerosis; bronchiectasis; arthritis; kidney diseases).

74. Rogers, D. E.: In Beeson, P. B., and McDermott, W., editors: Cecil-Loeb textbook of medicine, ed. 13, Philadelphia, 1971, W. B. Saunders Co. (psittacosis).

75. Sanford, J. P.: In Beeson, P. B., and McDermott, W., editors: Cecil-Loeb textbook of medicine, ed. 13, Philadelphia, 1971, W. B. Saunders Co. (Friedländer's pneumonia).

76. Schiffer, M. A.: Am. J. Obstet. Gynecol. 86:264, 1963 (ectopic pregnancy).

77. Schuster, B.: Ohio State Med. J. 59:993, 1963 (emphysema).

78. Scotti, T. M.: In Anderson, W. A. D., editor: Pathology, ed. 6, St. Louis, 1971, The C. V. Mosby Co. (bacterial endocarditis; rheumatic fever).

79. Sherlock, S.: In Schiff, L., editor: Diseases of the liver, ed. 2, Philadelphia, 1963, J. B. Lippincott Co. (hepatic coma; liver diseases).

80. Siltzbach, L. E.: In Beeson, P. B., and McDermott, W., editors: Cecil-Loeb textbook of medicine, ed. 13, Philadelphia, W. B. Saunders Co. (cough in sarcoidosis).

81. Sleisenger, M. H.: In Beeson, P. B., and McDermott, W., editors: Cecil-Loeb textbook of medicine, ed. 13, Philadelphia, 1971, W. B. Saunders Co. (diseases of bile duct and gallbladder; celiac disease).

82. Strohl, E. L., Diffenbaugh, W. G., and Anderson, R. E.: Ill. Med. J. 124:29, 1963 (cholecystitis).

83. Therapeutic Notes: Feb., 1963, Parke-Davis & Co. (abdominal distention).

84. Therapeutic Notes: Sept.-Oct., 1963, Parke-Davis & Co. (abdominal rigidity).

85. Therapeutic Notes: March-April, 1965, Parke-Davis & Co. (abnormal uterine bleeding).

86. Therapeutic Notes: Jan., 1964, Parke-Davis & Co. (acute renal failure).

87. Therapeutic Notes: Sept. 1964, Parke-Davis & Co. (anhidrosis).

88. Therapeutic Notes: April, 1964, Parke-Davis & Co. (anuria).

89. Therapeutic Notes: July-Aug., 1962, Parke-Davis & Co. (arterial insufficiency).
90. Therapeutic Notes: March, 1964, Parke-Davis & Co. (ataxia).
91. Therapeutic Notes: Nov.-Dec., 1963, Parke-Davis & Co. (chills).
92. Therapeutic Notes: May, 1962, Parke-Davis & Co. (earache).
93. Therapeutic Notes: July-Aug., 1962, Parke-Davis & Co. (epiphora).
94. Therapeutic Notes: May-June, 1965, Parke-Davis & Co. (fatigue).
95. Therapeutic Notes: Feb., 1964, Parke-Davis & Co. (fever).
96. Therapeutic Notes: Jan., 1963, Parke-Davis & Co. (hearing loss).
97. Therapeutic Notes: Nov.-Dec., 1962, Parke-Davis & Co. (heartburn).
98. Therapeutic Notes: March, 1962, Parke-Davis & Co. (hemiplegia).
99. Therapeutic Notes: Sept., 1963, Parke-Davis & Co., (hyperhidrosis).
100. Therapeutic Notes: Oct., 1964, Parke-Davis & Co. (hypersalivation).
101. Therapeutic Notes: Nov.-Dec., 1964, Parke-Davis & Co. (insomnia).
102. Therapeutic Notes: Jan.-Feb., 1965, Parke-Davis & Co. (joint enlargement).
103. Therapeutic Notes: Jan., 1964, Parke-Davis & Co. (kyphosis).
104. Therapeutic Notes: March, 1964, Parke-Davis & Co. (leg ulcers).
105. Therapeutic Notes: Sept.-Oct., 1962, Parke-Davis & Co. (muscular weakness).
106. Therapeutic Notes: Oct., 1963, Parke-Davis & Co. (nuchal rigidity).
107. Therapeutic Notes: May-June, 1964, Parke-Davis & Co. (pallor).
108. Therapeutic Notes: July-Aug., 1964, Parke-Davis & Co. (paresthesia).
109. Therapeutic Notes: July-Aug., 1965, Parke-Davis & Co. (splenomegaly).
110. Therapeutic Notes: Nov.-Dec., 1965, Parke-Davis & Co. (tremor).
111. Therapeutic Notes: July, 1962, Parke-Davis & Co. (urinary frequency).
112. Therapeutic Notes: Jan., 1962, Parke-Davis & Co. (vaginal discharge).
113. U.S. Department of Health, Education, and Welfare, Division of Chronic Diseases, Diabetes and Arthritis Program, Public Health Service Publication No. 29, Health Information Series 9, revised 1965 (arthritis, osteoarthritis, gout).
114. U.S. Department of Health, Education, and Welfare, Division of Chronic Diseases, Neurological and Sensory Disease Service Program, Public Health Service Publication No. 1030, 1965 (glaucoma).
115. U.S. Department of Health, Education, and Welfare, Division of Chronic Diseases, Public Health Service Publication, No. 1307, Health Information Series 123, revised Aug., 1966 (kidney diseases).
116. U.S. Department of Health, Education, and Welfare, National Institute of Arthritis and Metabolic Diseases, Public Health Service Publication No. 280, Health Information Series 71, revised 1965 (peptic ulcer).
117. U.S. Department of Health, Education, and Welfare, National Institute of Neurological Diseases and Stroke, DHEW Publication No. (NIH) 74-103, 1974 (myasthenia gravis).
118. U.S. Department of Health, Education, and Welfare, National Institute of Neurological Diseases and Stroke, DHEW Publication No. (NIH) 75-159, revised 1975 (cerebral palsy).
119. U.S. Department of Health, Education, and Welfare, National Eye Institute, DHEW Publication No. (NIH) 73-410, 1973 (corneal disease).
120. U.S. Department of Health, Education, and Welfare, Public Health Service Publication Series No. 30, 1970 (tuberculosis).
121. U.S. Department of Health, Education, and Welfare, National Institute of Neurological Diseases and Stroke, DHEW Publication No. (NIH) 73-1956, 1973 (epilepsy).
122. U.S. Department of Health, Education, and Welfare, Public Health Service, DHEW Publication No. (NIH) 74-614, 1974, (chronic obstructive lung disease, emphysema, and chronic bronchitis).
123. U.S. Department of Health, Education, and Welfare, Public Health Service, DHEW Publication No. (NIH) 74-629, 1974 (the NINDS Parkinson's disease research program).
124. U.S. Department of Health, Education, and Welfare, National Institute of Neurological Diseases and Stroke, DHEW Publication No. (NIH) 72-75, 1975 (multiple sclerosis).
125. U.S. Department of Health, Education, and Welfare, Public Health Service, DHEW Publication No. (NIH) 74-332, 1974 (the NINDS multiple sclerosis research program).
126. U.S. Department of Health, Education, and Welfare, Public Health Service Publication No. 116, Health Information Series 41, revised May, 1967 (malaria).
127. U.S. Department of Health, Education, and Welfare, Public Health Service Publication No. 97, Health Information Series 30, revised Aug., 1963 (rabies).
128. Weinstein, L.: In Beeson, P. B., and McDermott, W., editors: Cecil-Loeb textbook of

medicine, ed. 13, Philadelphia, 1971, W. B. Saunders Co. (poliomyelitis).

129. Whalen, G. E., Soergel, K. H., and Geenen, J. E.: Gastroenterology **56**:1021, 1969 (diabetic diarrhea).

130. Wheeler, E., Jr.: In Beeson, P. B., and McDermott, W., editors: Cecil-Loeb textbook of medicine, ed. 13, Philadelphia, 1971, W. B. Saunders Co. (inherited ectodermal defect).

131. Wilkes, J. D.: In Anderson, W. A. D., editor: Pathology, ed. 6, St. Louis, 1971, The C. V. Mosby Co. (otosclerosis).

132. Wood, B. S., Jr.: In Beeson, P. B., and McDermott, W., editors: Cecil-Loeb textbook of medicine, ed. 13, Philadelphia, 1971, W. B. Saunders Co. (cough in pneumonia; pneumococcal pneumonia).

133. Yahr, M. D.: In Beeson, P. B., and McDermott, W., editors: Cecil-Loeb textbook of medicine, ed. 13, Philadelphia, 1971, W. B. Saunders Co. (Parkinson's disease).

134. Zimmerman, L. E.: In Anderson, W. A. D., editor: Pathology, ed. 6, St. Louis, 1971, The C. V. Mosby Co. (ophthalmic lesions).

135. Zinsser, H. H.: J.A.M.A. **174**:2062, 1960 (urinary calculi).

INDEX

375